Health Psychology

Health Psychology
A Discipline and a Profession

Edited by
George C. Stone
Stephen M. Weiss
Joseph D. Matarazzo
Neal E. Miller
Judith Rodin
Cynthia D. Belar
Michael J. Follick
Jerome E. Singer

The University of Chicago Press
Chicago and London

The University of Chicago Press, Chicago 60637
The University of Chicago Press, Ltd., London

96 95 94 93 92 91 90 89 88 87   5 4 3 2 1

The University of Chicago Press gratefully acknowledges a subvention from the John D. and Catherine T. MacArthur Foundation in partial support of the costs of production of this volume.

Library of Congress Cataloging-in-Publication Data

Health psychology.

   Based on a conference held in 1983 at the Arden House in Harriman, N.Y. and sponsored by the MacArthur Foundation.
   Includes bibliographies and index.
   1. Medicine and psychology—Congresses.   2. Medicine and psychology—Study and teaching—Congresses.   I. Stone, George Chester.   II. John D. and Catherine T. MacArthur Foundation. [DNLM: 1. Delivery of Health Care—congresses.   2. Psychology, Medical—congresses. W 84.1 H4375 1983]
R726.5.H4335   1987   610'.1'9   86–27254
ISBN 0–226–77557–7

Contents

Preface   ix

PART ONE   **The Emergence of the Field**   1
Stephen M. Weiss, editor

1   Education for a Lifetime of Learning   3
Neal E. Miller

2   Historical Highlights in the Emergence of the Field   15
Judith Rodin and George C. Stone

3   The Scope of Health Psychology   27
George C. Stone

4   Relationships of Health Psychology to Other
Segments of Psychology   41
Joseph D. Matarazzo

5   Health Psychology and Other Health Professions   61
Stephen M. Weiss

PART TWO   **The Knowledge Base**   75
Neal E. Miller, editor

6   Basic Laboratory Research in Health Psychology   77
Neil Schneiderman

7   Basic Field Research in Health Psychology   91
Nancy E. Adler, Shelley E. Taylor, and Camille B. Wortman

8   Training for Applied Research in Health Psychology   107
Jerome E. Singer

PART THREE   **Applications of Health Psychology**   119
Michael J. Follick, editor

9   Health Care Services   121
Steven R. Tulkin

10   Health Psychology at the Worksite   137
*Michael J. Follick, David B. Abrams,
Rodger P. Pinto, and Joanne L. Fowler*

11   Community Interventions and Health Psychology:
An Ecologically Oriented Perspective   151
Edison J. Trickett

12   Health Psychology and Public Health   165
Ruth R. Faden

13   Health Psychology and Health Policy   175
Patrick H. DeLeon and Gary R. VandenBos

PART FOUR   **Professional Issues in Health Psychology**   189
Cynthia D. Belar, editor

14   Credentials for Health Psychologists   191
Nelson F. Jones

15   Ethical Concerns in Health Psychology   203
Charles Swencionis and Judy E. Hall

16   An Overview of Health Psychology and the Law   217
Robinsue Frohboese and Thomas D. Overcast

17   Employment Options for Health Psychologists   231
David G. Altman and Jerry Cahn

PART FIVE   **Health Psychology and Segments of the Population**   245
Judith Rodin, editor

18   Women's Health Issues: An Emerging Priority for
Health Psychology   249
Mary A. Jansen

19   Race, Ethnicity, and Health Psychology: The
Example of Essential Hypertension   265
Norman B. Anderson and James S. Jackson

20   Child Health Psychology   285
Ronald B. Kurz

21   Older Persons and Health Psychology   303
Margaret Gatz, Cynthia Pearson, and Wendy Weicker

PART SIX **Challenges and Opportunities in Training Health Psychologists** 321
Joseph D. Matarazzo, editor

22 The Current Status of Predoctoral and Postdoctoral Training in Health Psychology 325
Cynthia D. Belar

23 Predoctoral Education and Training in Health Psychology 335
Thomas J. Boll

24 Apprenticeships in Health Psychology 351
Bonnie R. Strickland

25 Postdoctoral Training for Research 361
Howard S. Friedman

26 Postdoctoral Education and Training of Service Providers in Health Psychology 371
Joseph D. Matarazzo

27 Postdoctoral Training in Health Policy 389
Lee Sechrest

28 Respecialization and Continuing Education for Health Psychology 403
Wilbur E. Fordyce and Manfred J. Meier

29 Accreditation of Training Programs 413
Paul D. Nelson

30 Curricula of Graduate Training Programs in Health Psychology 425
Joseph Istvan and Daniel C. Hatton

PART SEVEN **Sites for Training Health Psychologists** 449
Jerome E. Singer, editor

31 Health Psychology Training in University Departments 453
Judith Rodin and Johanna Freedman

32 Training Health Psychologists in the Academic Medical Center 467
Gilbert Levin and Charles Swencionis

33 Schools of the Allied Health Professions 473
Nathan Perry

34 Training Health Psychologists in Schools of
Public Health   481
Karen A. Matthews and Judith M. Siegel
35 Educating Health Psychologists: Lessons to Be
Learned at School   493
Jean R. Eagleston and Carl E. Thoresen
36 Schools of Professional Psychology as Sites for
Training Health Psychologists   505
Nelson F. Jones
37 Health Psychology in the Twenty-first Century   513
The Editors

List of Contributors   525
Index   529

Preface

The original idea of preparing a book as a consequence of the Arden House Conference was conceived during the planning of the conference. It was agreed that the conference proceedings should appear quickly and report as accurately as possible what transpired there. In order to appear quickly and report accurately, we felt that the proceedings had to stay very close to the formally reviewed materials and the addresses given. But we also believed that more would take place at Arden House than could be represented by these semiofficial documents. The conference brought together over fifty of the leaders in the new field of health psychology for an intensive consideration of what the next generation of health psychologists ought to be taught. To answer this question, we had to take stock of where we are and where we are going. Furthermore, we began to identify what we need to do, by way of research, practice, and training, to accomplish what we presently see as our objectives.

Thus, in those intensive days, we brought forth in our minds a picture of the field near the end of its first decade as a defined area in psychology. Why not, we thought, take advantage of this crystallization of ideas to create a book that would serve others in their efforts to comprehend the emerging field and would also stand as a historical document that revealed the context of the Arden House proceedings?

In setting out, we did not explicitly identify a target audience. Many different groups would be interested, we thought, in a comprehensive picture of the state of the field. For people who had been involved in its development, such a book could help to clarify and give substance to issues with which they had struggled and could provide a basis for moving ahead with greater clarity. For faculties teaching health psychology, it could provide an authoritative compilation of a range of scientific and professional issues that are not readily available in journals or are widely scattered. It could serve as a resource in their efforts to socialize students into the field. For students in the field, it might not be used as a text for any one course but more as a guidebook to this complex field they are seeking to enter. For outsiders trying to understand what was causing all this ferment of activity among a group calling themselves health psychologists, it could be a book *about* health psychologists, written by health psychologists. Such a book could help other psychologists decide whether they might be interested in moving toward the field. Undergraduate students who were considering what sort of graduate training to undertake could use it to get a much richer picture of the field than could be gained by a chapter in some later edition of "Careers in Psychology." Those who form health policy might find it valuable in gaining an overview of the field.

The book retains the focus on the education of health psychologists that characterized the Arden House Conference. To set the stage for a consideration of educational issues, the first five of its seven parts present a broad overview of the field. Part 1 discusses origins, defines the field, and sets it off from related areas of psychology and other health professions. The sources of our data in laboratory and field research are considered in part 2, along with the particular issues of basic and applied research that are so intimately related in health psychology. The application of our knowledge in a variety of settings are the subject matter of part 3. Part 4 is a consideration of professional issues that must be faced in our work as health psychologists and attempts to highlight how the special circumstances of the health settings in which we work call for modifications of the traditional working styles and approaches that psychologists have developed over the decades to deal with similar problems in other settings. Part 5 explores how the general considerations that have been developed in the first four sections need to be modified to meet the needs of certain subgroups of our population—needs that may not be fully met unless special attention is given to them.

The first five sections outline the educational task that we face in setting out to educate students who will be the next generation of health psychologists. Parts 6 and 7 present various aspects of the answer to the question, "How can we possibly impart all of the knowledge and skills that are necessary within any reasonable amount of time?" Part 6 focuses on components of the educational sequence and part 7 on the venues in which it can take place.

A final chapter, in a sense, looks back by looking ahead. We can gain a different perspective on what we are now doing by attempting to anticipate what health psychologists will be called upon to accomplish in the next quarter of a century—what new challenges they will face and what new tools they may have with which to face them. In this chapter we take the risk of going beyond the prediction that what is beginning to happen now will happen increasingly. We draw on forecasts of changes in the social context in which health psychology does its work to anticipate changes not yet attracting the attention of many health psychologists.

In putting together a book such as this, with chapters written by over thirty authors and groups of authors, all focusing on some aspect of the field of health psychology, it is inevitable that there will be some repetition. If we look at an object from many different angles, we gain multiple views of the same features. Furthermore, as we try to provide a graceful context for the assertions we set forth, we call upon a limited pool of rhetoric. The editors have tried to reduce unwarranted repetition where it was possible to do so without creating structural damage to a particular viewpoint. Some repetition inevitably remains. We invite readers to view this repetition as a kind of validation by replication and to consider it a strength rather than a weakness of the book.

We are indebted to the John D. and Catherine MacArthur Foundation for an editorial grant that greatly facilitated the preparation of the book. We acknowledge with appreciations the support and encouragement of William Bevan and Idy Gittelson at the MacArthur Foundation.

This book is presented just a decade after the publication of the report of the APA's Task Force on Health Research, which pointed to the need for a field of health psychology. We believe we can take pride in our progress to date and that we can proceed with confidence on the basis of the foundations that are described here.

George C. Stone

Part One

The Emergence of the Field

Editor: Stephen M. Weiss

Fittingly, this book begins with a statement from the most distinguished elder statesman of health psychology. From the earliest days of his career, Neal Miller has been committed to the enterprise of bringing to bear on the task of healing human beings basic laboratory research with animals and the theories built upon such research. For many years, his work and that of his students has provided the basis for the clinical applications of biofeedback, applications that have provided one of the mainstays in the development of health psychology. Professor Miller was asked to give the opening address at the Arden House Conference to provide a context for beginning our work. There he spoke about the need for the conference and the challenging task of educating students for effective participation in a world where the research literature would have doubled three times before they reached the end of their careers. He has adapted and expanded those introductory remarks to set the stage for this volume and to establish the link between the book and the Arden House Conference.

In the second chapter, Judith Rodin and George Stone draw upon earlier accounts and their own experience to trace the history of psychology's engagement with health issues from the earliest beginnings to the burst of activity in the 1970s that gave rise to a new named area of concentration in psychology. The main focus of this chapter is on the recent period and on the organizational developments that led to the formal recognition of the field and the identification of many psychologists with it. The primary psychological organization that resulted from this activity was the Division of Health Psychology in the American Psychological Association, but a number of interdisciplinary organizations also took form at about the same time.

Chapter 3 presents a broad overview of the potential areas of research and application that fall within the purview of health psychology given the comprehensive definition of the field adopted by the Division of Health Psychology at an early meeting. The chapter's author, George Stone, has consistently stressed the importance of locating one's individual work within a framework that defines the field of health psychology as the intersection of the competence of psychology with the problems of the health system. In this chapter he gives the most complete expression of this point of view and identifies portions of the domain of work thus defined in which there is as yet little being done.

In chapters 4 and 5 attention is turned to the relationships between health psychology and other segments of psychology and also related disciplines and fields. These relationships are not only conceptual. There are political and collegial interrelationships that both facilitate and constrain the development of health psychology within the social context. Joseph Matarazzo addresses relationships within psychology from the viewpoint of organizational pressures toward standardization of graduate curricula and resistance to such pressures. Taking a strong stand for the existence of a common, generic core of psychology that should be taught to all students, he argues that health psychology cannot yet claim the status of a specialty—indeed, in his view, there is no field of psychology that can make such a claim. Matarazzo outlines the steps that he believes must be surmounted before full-fledged specialty status can be achieved, and he develops the somewhat controversial position that health psychology is generic psychology applied in a variety of health venues.

In the final chapter of the section, Stephen Weiss considers the many ways in which psychologists are brought into contact with researchers, health care providers, administrators, and policymakers from many disciplines and professions as they move out into increasing numbers of niches in the health system. Weiss emphasizes not only the opportunities offered by these interdisciplinary contacts, but the demands they place on psychologists for preparation that will facilitate collaboration. His overview of these issues anticipates many topics treated at greater length in the following sections on research, applications, and training.

1

Education for a Lifetime of Learning

Neal E. Miller

Origins of This Book
EXPANDING ROLE OF PSYCHOLOGY IN HEALTH

In the past, psychology's chief contact with medicine had been largely via a single specialty, psychiatry, with a few secondary contacts with pediatrics and neurology. In these contacts, psychology's main role was assessment, with a gradually increasing role in psychotherapy. More recently, a number of developments have come together to foster the use of psychologists for a greater variety of purposes in a wider range of areas of medicine.

One of these developments was the change in the burden of illness produced by the conquest of the major infectious diseases. As the Surgeon General's report on Health Promotion and Disease Prevention (1979) points out, "At the beginning of this century, the leading causes of death were influenza, pneumonia, diphtheria, tuberculosis, and gastrointestinal infections. Since then, the yearly death rate from these diseases per 100,000 people has been reduced from 580 to 30!" Thus, the burden of illness has changed to deaths and disabilities caused by chronic diseases and by conditions such as injuries from accidents, poisonings, or violence. A number of studies have shown that a major role in current causes of mortality and morbidity is played by behavioral factors, especially by long-standing habits such as smoking, overeating of high-fat diets, and abuse of alcohol. For example, the Center for Disease Control (1980) of the U.S. Public Health Service estimated that fifty percent of mortalities from the ten leading causes of death in the United States can be traced to life styles. Other authors (Lalonde 1974; Knowles 1977) have reinforced this conclusion and believe that the major opportunities for further improvements in health will come from changing unhealthy behaviors. For example, a recent Surgeon General's report (1982) estimates that one-third of all cancers are caused by smoking, which also contributes to cardiovascular and other diseases. In 1977, the direct and indirect costs of alcohol abuse were estimated at $43 billion (Berry et al. 1977).

Another major factor responsible for the increased interest in the behavioral aspects of medicine has been increasing evidence of the effects on the health of the body of psychological factors such as stress, social isolation, hostile, impatient Type A behavior, and of the availability of suitable coping responses or of social support. Such evidence has come from an increasing number of clinical and epidemiological studies supported by rigorously controlled experiments on animals. In addition, an increasing number of physiological mechanisms have been discovered by means of which the brain can affect the health of the body.

Physicians are becoming increasingly aware of the fact that many of their patients do not take the drugs that are prescribed or do not comply with other medical regimens and that certain illnesses can produce severe emotional problems. Furthermore, certain behavioral techniques, such as relaxation training, behavior therapy, and biofeedback have been found to be therapeutically useful in treating certain physical illnesses, in managing pain, and in rehabilitation. Other psychological techniques have been found useful in preventing the acquisition of unhealthy habits, such as smoking, and in dealing with a considerable range of other problems. As increasing numbers of psychologists have been employed in medical institutions for longer periods of time, a larger number of medical departments have found them useful in a greater variety of ways. But there is much room for further improvement.

THE TRAINING CONFERENCE

As a result of these and other factors, there has been, at first, a slow and, more recently, a rapid development in the area of health psychology. The largest single area of placements of psychologists over the past ten years has been in medical centers (Matarazzo 1980). In 1978, the Division of Health Psychology of the American Psychological Association was founded with 600 charter members. Within three years, 2,000 additional psychologists had joined the Division and a new scientific journal, *Health Psychology,* had been started.

The psychologists who are now working in a wide range of medical environments have come from virtually all of the different areas of psychology; they have been trained in clinical, social, experimental, physiological, developmental, and other areas of psychology. But, as they are being used in settings that are new to them in their rapidly developing cooperation with physical medicine, dentistry, public health, and biomedical research, it is becoming increasingly evident that health psychologists need new types of training. And new training programs have been initiated. At least ten academic institutions have or are developing training programs for psychologists that focus on health-related issues. Therefore, the Division of Health Psychology felt that this was a critical time in the development of the field when it would be particularly worthwhile to hold a training conference to bring together approximately fifty leaders representing the different facets of the field of psychology concerned with different aspects of health.

Intensive preparations were made by a series of committees headed by Dr. Stephen Weiss. These included an open forum at the 1982 meeting of the American Psychological Association, preparation by Dr. Cynthia Belar of a large briefing book composed of volunteered and solicited papers, and a four-day, intensive working conference held at Arden House, 23–27 May, 1983.

The conclusions of this training conference were published in the fall of 1983 as a supplement to volume 2 (issue no. 5) of *Health Psychology* (National Working Conference 1983). It was felt, however, that the thoughts about training for health psychology stimulated by the conference, and continuing after it, merited a more thorough publication. That was the reason for deciding to write this book.

The remainder of this chapter will summarize briefly some of the author's conclusions about the main themes and highlights of the conference and his ideas about the principal problems that they pose for the training of health psychologists.

Highlights of the Conference
SCIENTIST-PRACTITIONER MODEL

Both aspects of the scientist-practitioner model ("Boulder" Conference 1949; see Raimy 1950) are especially important, particularly in the early stages of the rapidly developing field of health psychology. Elsewhere I have emphasized the symbiotic value of two-way interactions between the laboratory and the clinic (Miller 1983). The clinic suggests significant new problems for laboratory investigation, and the laboratory produces new knowledge that provides the foundation for innovative clinical applications. Practitioners need a sound understanding of research techniques and processes in order to be able to critically evaluate the results of studies reported in the literature so they can take advantage of those that are good but not be misled by those that are inadequate. Clinicians have found research training to be valuable also in gaining entry into new medical settings by being useful research consultants to their medical colleagues. This training also is useful in developing and evaluating new procedures. The systematic collection of clinical data by the individual clinician can help him evaluate his own techniques and refine his skill. On a larger scale, cooperative cost-effectiveness studies can convince administrators who are being increasingly hard-pressed to hold down rapidly escalating medical expenses that it is in their interest to pay for the services of clinicians with behavioral training. The research training of psychologists has been, and will continue to be, one of the greatest strengths in opening up significant new areas of applications. But, in addition to securing new ideas about significant problems from contact with clinical phenomena, the psychologist whose primary interest is in research often needs some of the skills and sensitivity of the clinician in order to deal effectively with human subjects in a medical setting.

ETHICAL AND LEGAL PROBLEMS

The fact that health psychologists, whether primarily involved in research or in applications, are likely to be dealing with injured or ill people who are more vulnerable to, and a higher risk for, medical catastrophes than are healthy people means that they must be especially sensitive to a new range of ethical and legal problems. Health psychologists need special education concerning such problems; they must know how to handle them, how to stay within the limits of their professional competence and legal license. Ethical issues will be discussed in more detail in later chapters.

THE BREADTH OF HEALTH PSYCHOLOGY

All aspects of psychology—ranging from physiological through social—can be relevant to medical problems; therefore, a solid and broad foundation in psychology is valuable for the health psychologist. But one cannot apply the principles and techniques of any science without an adequate understanding of the conditions to which they are to be applied. Thus, it is essential for the health psychologist to acquire understanding of the organization, functioning, folkways, *mores,* and vocabulary of the health care system. Health psychologists also need to know the somewhat different types of statistical procedures that are used by medical people and by epidemiologists.

Health psychologists may potentially make contributions in connection with virtually all aspects of the broad spectrum of health activities. But, in order to contribute, they must know something about the special problems with which their medical colleagues are dealing—for example, the type of pathophysiology or clinical symptoms of the particular disorder. Such knowledge is the only way to discover the problems that the medical specialist considers to be important and to which the psychologist can make a contribution. In the potentially cost-effective area of prevention, health psychologists need to know something about public health. For applications in industry, they need to know something about industry. There also is a need for at least some health psychologists to know enough about the world of health economics and legislative affairs to be able to contribute to the extremely important task of formulating health policy. Different chapters of this book will give further illustrations of the breadth of the potential activities of health psychologists.

THE IMPORTANCE OF QUALITY

The best way to advance health psychology is to turn out graduates of the highest quality who will be better able than those of any other profession to solve behavioral aspects of the most difficult problems confronting the health care system. If health psychologists are more narrowly trained as technicians, their field is likely to be limited to inferior contributions and a lower status. Starting out with students who are selected and trained to be highly qualified and creative professionals will open up possibilities at a later date for the employment of a larger number of more narrowly trained technicians.

Education for a Lifetime of Learning

From the foregoing brief summary, it can be seen that the problem of adequately training the type of people that are needed in health psychology is a formidable one. It demands a coherent, organized program with adequate time, staff, and facilities. This fact will become still clearer in the subsequent chapters of this book.

With the multitudinous useful things that are desirable to know, there is considerable danger of designing a curriculum that is so broad that it must inevitably be too shallow. There is danger that too much forced feeding will spoil the appetite for the intellectual feast.

Graduate students educated in health psychology now may be expected to have a career of thirty to forty years in length. Judging from the past, we may expect radical changes during those years. A number of the things that we now consider important may be outmoded before then, and we may not even be able to imagine now some of the things that will be important for our students later on in their careers. Therefore, our students will have to be prepared to continue to learn from their own and related disciplines through their early, middle, and even later careers. Twenty years ago, how important was the behavior therapy of sickness behavior or the biofeedback treatment of neuromuscular disorders, and who had thought of endorphins and other neuropeptides, or silicon chips, microprocessors, and home computers? In a world of increasingly rapid changes, which hopefully will be especially rapid in the new field of health psychology, the only solution is to educate our students for a lifetime of continued learning.

How can we best prepare our students to continue to learn on their own after they have completed their formal education? The most important thing is to pose this crucial question. But I have a few tentative answers based on some success in teaching graduate students to learn things that I never knew.

CONFIDENCE FROM EXPERIENCE WITH LEARNING WITHOUT A TEACHER

One of the important goals is to teach students confidence in their ability to learn new things by themselves—not to be cowed by superficially formidable new terminology or techniques. The way to teach students to teach themselves is to give them practice in doing it, to confront them with the need and the opportunity to learn unfamiliar things on their own initiative to a functional level of understanding and skill. For example, they might be required to teach themselves two quite different, unfamiliar but not too extensive areas of subject material and one or two different unfamiliar techniques. To facilitate interdisciplinary learning, one such unit of self-instruction should be in a relevant social science and another in a relevant biomedical science.

Students should discover that, where necessary, they can start with an elementary textbook. Then, by sampling the original literature, they should be exposed to situations in which they can discover that statements in an elementary textbook sometimes may be only partially true or even completely false or out of date. One may not learn as many facts this way as one would if consistently force-fed, but what is learned about autonomous learning will be far more valuable than most facts.

BASIC ELEMENTS OF EFFICIENT TEACHING

Of course, there are certain basic types of knowledge that will provide a foundation for further education. Ideally, students should come already having a high level of ability to read and write the English language. They should have a background in mathematics, in biology, and at least some social science. They should learn basic facts and techniques of areas of psychology relevant to their special interest and something about enough areas to be able to choose their special interests wisely. One way to make the curriculum more efficient will be to teach as many basic elements and psychological principles as possible in the context of their application to problems of health psychology. Principles of statistics, experimental design, how to be alert to and control for artifacts can also be taught by using examples of their application to health psychology, thus simultaneously exposing the student to both types of material.

UNDERSTANDING SCIENCE

One of the most basic things for students to learn, with the widest applicability, is a general understanding of how science develops and progresses, sometimes by having the wit to exploit an accidental observation, sometimes by building a cathedral-like structure systematically, one small building block at a time, and occasionally by a revolutionary change to an opposite point of view. Students need to understand how increases in pure knowledge may sometimes quite unpredictably lead to practical applications and how such applications may in turn contribute to basic research. They need to understand the role of new techniques in enabling rapid advances in new directions. Some of this understanding can be acquired by exposure to materials like Conant's book "On Understanding Science" (1947), which presents case histories of the foregoing type in physical science. We need books of this type that are more directly relevant to biomedical issues and to health psychology; Swazey's book on chlorpromazine (1974) is nearer our field. I have made short steps in this direction in one brief chapter (Miller 1985a) and in a few parts of another one (Miller 1983).

LEARNING TO JUDGE QUALITY OF RESEARCH

Another of the basic units fundamental to preparation for a lifetime of continuous, autonomous learning is the ability to judge the quality of research. This obviously is important for a career of research; it also is important for the practitioner who wants to be able to take advantage of the results of the best new research and theory and not be misled by faulty interpretations or an inadequately evaluated therapeutic technique. One of the strengths of the well-trained psychologist is his ability to design and evaluate research involving complex individual and group behavior. Students should be repeatedly exposed in widely different complex contexts to common sources of artifacts, such as selection errors, regression to the mean, halo and placebo effects, and others. Teachers should occasionally, without warning, assign plausible articles in which, ideally, a prestigious individual has used an inappropriate statistical approach, failed to control for an important artifact, or made some other error. Through a journal club or in classroom reports on original articles, students should secure practice in spotting artifacts, misinterpretations, or inadequately supported conclusions. They should be exposed to examples in which a firmly established dogma, such as only one neurotransmitter used by a given neuron, is proved to be false.

CASE HISTORIES OF SCIENTIFIC DEVELOPMENTS

Teachers should assign series of original papers in the literature illustrating how a commonly accepted explanation can be turned upside-down. For example, early experiments on rearing puppies in isolation in an environment of extreme sensory deprivation produced dramatic, long-lasting deficits in social and other behavior. The obvious explanation seemed to be that, if such behaviors were not learned during an early critical period of development, they could not be learned later. But Fuller and Clark (1966) found that, if such dogs were given chlorpromazine when first tested in the normal complex environment, they showed sophisticated, normal, social behavior. Obviously, these were innate behavior patterns that had been maturing in spite of the deprived environment. The cause of the pathology turned out to not be the deprivation but the trauma of being suddenly plunged into the new, complex, confusing test situation. If a small hole was cut between the deprived and normal environments, dogs exposed themselves very gradually and exhibited virtually no deficits.

Students should be exposed to long-lasting, misleading conclusions and to the development and resolution of certain controversies. For example, Mott and Sherrington (1895) found that if the sensory nerves from a monkey's limb were cut, the animal failed to use the deafferented limb. They and others following them had theoretical reasons for expecting this. For fifty years, virtually no one thought to ask whether a monkey could be motivated to relearn the use of such a limb. Then, Knapp, Taub, and Berman (1963) found that such animals could be trained to make a conditioned avoidance response with a deafferented limb. Further extensive work by a number of investigators uncovered other abilities to use deafferented limbs; these conclusions and a hypothesis of learned disuse (Taub 1980) have led directly to useful clinical applications (Miller 1985b).

Another possible example is Brady and Mason's (Brady 1958) original experiments in which the "executive" monkey who had to control the situation was the one to get the stomach ulcers. Then Jay Weiss got exactly opposite results: the rat that had a coping response to control the situation got far fewer stomach lesions. Later, it was found that while an easy coping response reduced the number of lesions, a conflict-inducing or a too difficult one increased them (Tsuda and Hirai 1975; Weiss 1971a, 1971b). In other words, there was a strong interaction so that, under different circumstances, the same type of manipulation could produce opposite results. But I have considerably oversimplified this development.

The development of biofeedback could be made into another instructive example. There were early wildly inflated claims for alpha rhythm and a subsequent controversy about the nature of the learned modification of that rhythm. There were experiments with normal animals on the modification of visceral responses by instrumental learning that have been repeated, and experiments from a number of laboratories on animals paralyzed by curare appeared to be extremely convincing. These experiments on paralyzed rats had a strong impact but at present do not appear to be repeatable—a puzzling phenomenon! But, via acquiescence by Brucker and Ince (1977) to a patient's pleas, an attempt to get similar results on paralyzed people led to experiments that have provided quite convincing proof of the conclusion, reached in the original work on paralyzed rats, about the instrumental learning of visceral responses (Miller and Brucker 1979). After an initial period of discrediting disillusionment from the failure to realize the impossible claims made by a few injudicious individuals, clinical experience indicates that biofeedback is a valuable component of a broader therapeutic package in the treatment of a number of afflictions. The alert teacher can no doubt find additional, and perhaps more instructive, examples within the brief history of health psychology.

Exposure to Case Histories of Successful and Unsuccessful Examples of Application

Students also should be exposed to case histories which enable them to understand the problems involved in successful applications of psychological knowledge and techniques to practical situations. While not directly involving health psychology, the history of the Army Air Force Program in World War II could provide some material. Essentially, the success of this program resulted from three factors: (*a*) finding something that the Air Force needed (which initially was selection of personnel), (*b*) that psychologists could deliver, and (*c*) providing data proving that it had been delivered. An example of a difficulty was a program in which the executive officer of the Command Headquarters had been deceived when he was the head of a large business into purchasing a worthless system for the selection of junior executives. This strategically placed senior officer was instrumental in keeping the psychology unit assigned to his command from gaining any access to most of the activities of the entire organization.

DIFFERENT PATTERNS OF TRAINING FITTED TO THE INDIVIDUAL STUDENT

There is not time enough for training of the foregoing kind to be completely comprehensive. The best that can be done is to sample strategically selected portions of knowledge, going into each of these deeply enough to develop standards of what is high quality work at the frontier of knowledge.

Since no one person can have all the knowledge and skills that are desirable for health psychology, it will be important to educate a variety of students in tailor made programs that fit their particular strengths and interests. Each of them should have enough experience in learning a number of new things on their own as a basis for continued learning. All of them should have a good knowledge of some area of psychology and of the area of health in which they plan to work. Some may be rather narrow specialists and some broad generalists, with the primary criterion being that their program makes sense and that it is of high quality.

It will require considerable ingenuity to adapt the foregoing strategy to the relatively rigid standardization of training that is easiest to administer for the purposes of accreditation and providing credentials. But I believe that at this stage of the development of health psychology special efforts to combine flexibility with quality control will be beneficial for both the profession and the public.

REFERENCES

Berry, R. E., J. P. Boland, C. N. Smart, and J. R. Kanak. 1977. *The economic cost of alcohol abuse, 1975. Final Report.* Contract No. ADM 281−76−0016. Bethesda: National Institute for Alcohol Abuse and Alcoholism.

Brady, J. V. 1958. Ulcers in "executive" monkeys. *Scientific American* 199:95−100.

Brucker, B. S., and L. P. Ince. 1977. Biofeedback as an experimental treatment for postural hypotension in a patient with a spinal cord lesion. *Archives of Physical Medicine and Rehabilitation* 58:49−53.

Center for Disease Control. 1980. *Ten leading causes of death in the United States, 1977.* Washington, D.C.: Government Publishing Office.

Conant, J. B. 1947. *On understanding science.* New Haven: Yale University Press.

Fuller, J. L., and L. D. Clark. 1966. Genetic and treatment factors modifying the postisolation syndrome in dogs. *Journal of Comparative and Physiological Psychology* 61:251−257.

Knapp, H. D., E. Taub, and A. J. Berman. 1963. Movements in monkeys with de-afferented forelimbs. *Experimental Neurology* 7:305–16.

Knowles, J. H., ed. 1977. *Doing better and feeling worse.* New York: Norton.

Lalonde, M. 1974. *A new perspective on the health of Canadians: A working document.* Ottawa: Government of Canada.

Matarazzo, J. D. 1980. Behavioral health and behavioral medicine: Frontiers for a new health psychology. *American Psychologist* 35:807–17.

Miller, N. E. 1983. Behavioral medicine: Symbiosis between laboratory and clinic. *Annual Review of Psychology* 34:1–31.

———. 1985a. Prologue to *Psychology and life,* edited by P. Zimbardo. Glenview, IL: Scott, Foresman, i–vii.

———. 1985b. The value of behavioral research on animals. *American Psychologist* 40:423–40.

Miller, N. E., and B. S. Brucker. 1979. A learned visceral response apparently independent of skeletal ones in patients paralyzed by spinal lesions. In *Biofeedback and self-regulation,* edited by N. Birbaumer and H. D. Kimmel, 287–304. Hillsdale, NJ: Lawrence Erlbaum Associates.

Mott, F. W., and C. S. Sherrington. 1895. Experiments upon the influence of sensory nerves upon movement and nutrition of the limbs. *Proceedings of the Royal Society* 57:481–88.

National Working Conference on Education and Training in Health Psychology. 1983. Health Psychology 2(5): 1–153, supplement section.

Raimy, V. C. 1950. *Training in clinical psychology.* New York: Prentice-Hall.

Surgeon General. 1979. *Healthy people.* Washington, D.C.: Government Printing Office.

Surgeon General. 1982. *Report.* Washington, D.C.: Government Printing Office.

Swazey, J. P. 1974. *Chlorpromazine in psychiatry: A study of therapeutic innovation.* Cambridge, Mass.: MIT Press.

Taub, E. 1980. Somatosensory deafferentation research with monkeys: Implications for rehabilitation medicine. In *Behavioral psychology in rehabilitation medicine: Clinical applications* edited by L. P. Ince, 371–401. Baltimore: Williams & Wilkins.

Tsuda, A., and H. Hirai. 1975. Effects of the amount of required coping response tasks in gastrointestinal lesions in rats. *Japanese Psychological Research* 17:119–32.

Weiss, J. M. 1971a. Effects of coping behavior in different warning signal conditions on stress pathology in rats. *Journal of Comparative and Physiological Psychology* 77:1–13.

———. 1971b. Effects of punishing the coping response (conflict) on stress pathology in rats. *Journal of Comparative and Physiological Psychology* 77:14–21.

2

Historical Highlights in the Emergence of the Field

Judith Rodin and George Stone

In the preceding chapter, Neal Miller has outlined some of the factors that gave rise to a discovery of the potential contributions of psychology to the prevention of illness and the provision of effective health care. Other chapters in later sections elaborate on some of these issues. In this chapter we will look at the response of the discipline and the profession of psychology to the opportunities that were presented. In doing so, we have to recognize that many of the techniques and much of the knowledge that psychologists now consider to be within their province were known and used long before they were embodied in psychological theory and practice. Also, psychologists were participating actively in the health system long before a field of health psychology had been identified and labeled. In our view, however, the self-conscious recognition that began to appear less than twenty years ago has played a significant part in the rapid growth of the field in recent years. Reflection on and analysis of opportunities cannot take place except in the most specific form until the field is cognized as a field and made the subject of study. This chapter is intended as a contribution to the reflexive analysis of health psychology.

Defining the Field

How do we set the boundaries that mark out the domain of health psychology and distinguish it from other disciplines and professions that deal with related problems and issues? This question is addressed at length in the remaining chapters of this first part, so at this point we offer only a bare definition that will serve to bound this historical survey. By psychology we mean the scientific study of the nature and determinants of human experience and behavior and the application of the knowledge thus gained in professional practice. Health psychology, in our definition, is any aspect of psychology that bears upon the experience of health and illness and the behavior that affects health status. It includes basic research into the psychophysiological mechanisms that link environmental events with health outcomes, including laboratory research on human and animal subjects. It includes as well applied research on the structure and content of communications designed to alter health behaviors and on the responses to such communications. This definition covers approximately the same domain as the official definition adopted by the Division of Health Psychology in 1979 (see chapter 3).

Contemporary psychology also incorporates professional practice. Definitions of the boundaries of such practice are the subject of much discussion and legal and quasi-legal activity. Without elaborating on the details of practice, we can define professional health psychology as the conduct of interventions, derived from psychological science, aimed at altering health-related experience or behavior of individuals, either directly or through action upon the experience or behaviors of persons whose activities affect the health of others. Since psychological science has studied such matters as the design of educational materials, the impact of contingencies of reinforcement, and the role of cognitive appraisal in regulating bodily response to stress, health psychologists often use interventions that make use of educational materials, contingency management, or redirection of stress appraisals. Clearly, many psychologists other than those practicing health psychology use these interventions and so also do health educators, parents, and pastors, the latter groups having done so long before the word "psychology" was invented. Psychology does not claim to have invented these techniques but merely to have systematized their application and developed the theoretical structures on which they are based. Professional health psychologists have contributed to both of these activities.

The Beginnings of Health Psychology

It is conventional to date the beginnings of psychology as a separate discipline from the opening of psychological laboratories and the publication of textbooks bearing the word "psychology" in their titles during the closing years of the nineteenth century by the German, Wilhelm Wundt, and the American, William James. Neither of these founders of the discipline gave significant attention to the subject of health in their textbooks. The closest Wundt came to treatment of health issues was in his material on pain as one of the basic senses. James, perhaps because of his lifelong struggle with poor health, dealt with matters relevant to health in many places, although not in his *Principles*. He published a book, *On Vital Reserves: The Energies of Men; The Gospel of Relaxation* in 1922, based in considerable part on portions of an earlier book (James 1899) and a lecture delivered to the American Philosophical Society in 1906. In this book he discussed the "hyperesthetic condition of chronic invalidism," the spiritual exercises of Ignatius Loyola, Yoga systems, and "the unlocking of energies in the persons of those converts to 'New Thought', 'Christian Science', 'Metaphysical Healing' or other forms of spiritual philosophy, who are so numerous among us today." He foreshadowed the discovery of the Type A personality in the following quotation:

> We say that so many of our fellow-countrymen collapse, and have to be sent abroad to rest their nerves, because they work so hard. I suspect that this is an immense mistake. I suspect that neither the nature nor the amount of work is accountable . . . but that their cause lies rather in those absurd feelings of hurry and having no time, in that breathlessness and tension, that anxiety of feature and that solicitude for results . . .
>
> (James 1922, 214)

Another leading figure in the beginnings of American psychology, G. Stanley Hall, was literally preoccupied with health as a central value in life. In his massive work on adolescence (Hall 1904), he included a chapter on "Diseases of the Body and Mind." He bemoaned the fact that "until now, there has been little time and less motive to consider preventive medicine or the more general problems of regimen and hygiene" (p. 238). He speculated that the disinterest and distaste for such matters "perhaps could be overcome only by some such philosophic device as having physicians insure the health of their patients . . ." (p. 238). In an address before a meeting of the Young Men's Christian Association delivered in 1901 (published in Hall 1904), Hall said, "Health means holiness or wholeness. The words healthy, holy, hale, heal, and whole all come from the same Anglo-Saxon root. Physiological psychology is now restoring this deep philosophy embedded in the words."

Early issues of the *Psychological Index* listed articles such as these: "The Power of the Mind in the Cure of Disease"; "On Certain Psychological Phenomena Accompanying the Administration of Anesthesia"; "Mental Symptoms Occurring in Bodily Diseases"; "Neural and Psychic Manifestations Subsequent to Fractures or Dislocations"; and "The Nervous System in Disease; A Plea for Greater Recognition of the All-pervading Influence of the Nervous System upon Diseases in General." In the first few volumes, such subjects were represented in one to two percent of the titles, but a decade or two later they had virtually disappeared as psychologists increasingly focused their attention on abnormalities of attitude, mentation, and behavior.

The first semiofficial action of organized psychology, in the form of the American Psychological Association, regarding the health system was the outcome of a panel discussion at the annual meeting of that organization held in December 1911 to consider how psychology could contribute to medical education and practice. (See Stone [1979] for a fuller account of this symposium and subsequent developments.) The APA appointed a committee to survey the current beliefs and practices regarding the teaching of psychology in medical schools. Widespread agreement was found with the idea that medical students should receive some instruction in psychology, either as a part of their premedical training or in the medical schools themselves. However, less than a third of the medical schools were providing any such training, and less than ten percent indicated that they had psychologists teaching medical students. The committee commented on serious deficiencies in the comprehension of the nature and potential of psychology shown in the replies and recommended that courses should be established and taught by persons trained in both psychology and in medicine.

Implementation of the recommendations of the committee was slow. A review of teaching in medical schools published sixteen years later (Bott 1928) spoke of a wide and growing recognition of the importance of psychological factors crucial to health but cited no studies. In 1950, the University of Pittsburgh sponsored eight lectures on "The Relation of Psychology to Medicine" (Dennis 1950). Contributors optimistically spoke of ending a period of neglect and an emerging collaboration with health professions and medical educators. A series of surveys documented a sustained growth in the numbers of psychologists on faculties of medical schools and in responsibilities assigned to them, beginning in the early 1950s (Buck 1961; Lubin, Nathan, and Matarazzo 1978; Matarazzo 1955; Matarazzo, Carmody, and Gentry 1981; Matarazzo and Daniel 1957; Mensch 1953; Webster 1971).

Although the incorporation of psychological competence into medical practice via the instruction of health professional students was the early focus of interest on the part of organized psychology, entry of professional psychologists into the health care system probably developed more rapidly. Two factors make it hard to be more precise in this assertion: first, professional activities are not as well documented as are those of teachers, and second, the traditional distinction between mental health problems and physical health problems has clouded the writings of the histories. Since the early days of psychology, lip service has generally been given to the idea that there should be no sharp distinction made between physical and mental health. In practice, however, psychologists and psychiatrists have, until very recently, generally restricted their practice and their consultations to problems of psychopathology and serious behavioral disturbances, while health psychology, in its emergent state, focused primarily on physical health and disease, perhaps to position and distance itself from the subdiscipline of clinical psychology. A more appropriate logical structure, now apparent, is that health psychology—as the subdivision of psychology concerned with health—could be further divided into clinical and nonclinical branches. Within the branch of clinical health psychology, one subdivision would be concerned with those situations in which the psychological state or behavior of the individual is the presenting problem. While we are not proposing a revolutionary reorganization of professional allegiances, it is important to note that, conceptually, treating the mental state of individuals would be seen as a subcomponent of attending to their overall health.

Research in clinical psychology has also focused at times on physical rather than psychological symptoms. The most extensive early work dealt with applying psychotherapy to problems presenting physical as well as psychological symptoms (Olbrisch 1977). A couple of articles concerning "over-utilizers" appeared in the 1930s. Efforts to ameliorate conditions believed to be affected by life stress (the "psychosomatic" conditions) were studied during the 1940s and 1950s, and the first studies of the impact of preparing patients psychologically for surgical procedures were published in the late 1950s. Much of this work was done by persons other than psychologists. From the mid-1950s through 1970, Olbrisch found about three studies per year. After that the rate increased sharply, probably in relation to an event to be described shortly.

In addition to the clinical research just described, research on topics now considered to be a part of health psychology began to appear some time before the field was cognized. We scanned *Psychological Abstracts* for the years 1950–60 to gain some feeling for the number of published studies in areas we now consider to be within the purview of health psychology, for example: the effects of personality or mental states on physical health; studies of pain that examined psychosocial variables; compliance with medical regimens, health attitudes, and decision making; and reproductive health behavior. In 1950, 136 articles covering such health psychology topics were abstracted. The largest numbers of them dealt with pain, the effects of stress, and the psychological and behavioral determinants of reproductive health. The total number had increased to 257 by 1960, with far fewer entries on pain, more on health attitudes and behavior, and a reemergence of work on the effects of psychological processes on physical health. While this work provided a starting point from which the research of the 1970s and 1980s proceeded, it was sparse and involved very few psychologists until certain organizational changes transpired.

The Emergence of an Organized Health Psychology

In June 1969 William Schofield published an article in the *American Psychologist* that precipitated a period of rapid development in health psychology (Schofield 1969). He categorized articles listed under twenty-two headings in the *Psychological Abstracts* for 1966 and 1967. Only nineteen percent of the approximately 4700 articles dealt with topics not traditionally included within the field of mental health. Several psychologists published articles or letters directly responsive to Schofield's call which addressed both the need for more research and for a wider scope for psychological services (Crary and Steger 1972; McMillan 1970; Psychology and National Health Care 1971; Weisenberg 1970).

The most significant consequence of Schofield's article was the APA appointment in 1973 of a Task Force on Health Research. Schofield was named chair of this group, which was charged to "collect, organize, and disseminate information on the status of health behavior research" (APA 1976, 270). The Task Force carried out a comprehensive search of the *Psychological Abstracts*, covering the years 1966–73. The search was intended to retrieve only the articles that would have fallen in the nineteen percent found by Schofield that were not concerned with mental health topics. The first return consisted of 3500 articles, or about 440 per year, a return entirely consistent with the approximately 450 per year in Schofield's study. This set was closely examined to eliminate those that actually dealt with mental health (in spite of their classification heading) and those that were not direct reports of research. This screening reduced the total number of articles to 350, of which about two-thirds addressed psychobiological aspects of health and about fifty dealt with all aspects of health care delivery and with the measurement and modification of health attitudes.

On the basis of their review, the Task Force concluded, "Up to the present time, American psychologists have not been attracted in large numbers to the problems of health and illness as fruitful areas for both basic and applied research activity; nor have these psychologists perceived the potentials for their work in effecting improvements in health maintenance, illness prevention, and health care delivery" (APA Task Force 1976, 271). Their report also recommended, "We need to blueprint programs for graduate education of researchers that will provide an early awareness of the needs and opportunities to apply psychological principles and methods to the understanding and improvement of health behaviors."

Attainment of these goals was substantially aided by another activity of the Task Force, the development of a roster of psychologists interested in health research. The final mailing list had just under 500 names, and it was used for distribution of a fifth newsletter, in August 1975, which announced plans for an organizational meeting to be held at the meetings of the American Psychological Association in Chicago later that month.

Section on Health Research, Division of Psychologists in Public Service

At those meetings, some of the psychologists interested in this emerging area came together to discuss a proposal presented by Schofield to organize as a section under the auspices of the Division of Psychologists in Public Service (Division 18). At that meeting there was considerable discussion of the question of a name, specifically whether it should include the words "health research" and thus indicate that the section was not to be construed as a venture by clinicians seeking to open new territories for practice. The other side of the discussion favored the term "health psychology" in order to be more inclusive and to make a fresh start in the effort to keep practitioners and researchers in one camp. The name chosen was Section on Health Research, and William Schofield was elected first president. Charter members of the section numbered about one hundred and fifty.

Those involved in the Section on Health Research were grateful to the Division of Psychologists in Public Service for their hospitality in providing an interim home for the fostering of a new area of specialization in psychology. As they viewed the rapid growth of interest, however, they realized that the section would soon outnumber the rest of the division and believed that their growth and development would be enhanced by gaining separate division status in the APA. During the life span of the Section on Health Research, another proto-organization also appeared to bring together the rapidly increasing number of clinical psychologists working in medical settings. David Clayman was the focus of this activity, using a newsletter to build communication among the members of the Medical Psychologist's Network. In the summer of 1978, therefore, members of the section, the network, and others recruited by them circulated a petition seeking divisional status, and by the time of the 1978 APA meetings in Toronto, they had collected well over 400 signatures, enough to ensure acceptance of their petition. The formation of the Division of Health Psychology (Division 38) was approved. At its organizational meeting, Joseph Matarazzo was elected president in recognition of his exceptional contributions in bringing the division into being, and David Clayman was elected Secretary/Treasurer. In the seven years since its formation, the Division of Health Psychology has grown to 2500 members. Its presidents, following Matarazzo, include Stephen Weiss, Neal Miller, Jerome E. Singer, Judith Rodin, Gary Schwartz, Edward Blanchard, and George Stone, with Richard Evans scheduled to follow.

A year after its formation, the Division of Health Psychology decided to establish a divisional journal. At the next annual meeting, in August 1980, George Stone was named editor, and the first issue of *Health Psychology* appeared in January 1982. The journal increased its frequency from quarterly to bimonthly in 1984 in response to a clear increase in outstanding manuscripts, and the editorship passed to Neil Schneiderman in 1985.

Developments in Other Organizations

Other psychological organizations have been active in the area of health psychology. The Division of Rehabilitation Psychology (Division 22) was formed in APA in 1958 and continues to support research and practice on the rehabilitative aspect of health psychology. The Society for Pediatric Psychology also antedates the formation of the Division of Health Psychology by several years. Although many of its members now have dual memberships in the Division of Health Psychology, the society continues to function as a subspecialization within clinical health psychology on the basis of the ages of patients served or research subjects described.

Health psychology functions in a highly interdisciplinary context. As described more fully in chapter 4, some of the early leaders in the division were also instrumental in bringing into existence the interdisciplinary field of behavioral medicine. The critical event in that development was the Yale Conference, 4–6 February 1977, which resulted in the formation of the Society for Behavioral Medicine in April 1978 and the establishment of the *Journal of Behavioral Medicine*, which began publication in 1978 under the editorship of W. Doyle Gentry. The Academy of Behavioral Medicine Research was also founded in 1978 to "foster the integration of research in biomedical and behavioral science" and to engage in various activities to guide and promote such research. About a hundred invitations were initially extended to those who had been most active in establishing the field. Membership has since grown to about 200, as other productive researchers have been asked to join. In these groups, psychologists constitute a third to a half of the membership, as an interdisciplinary membership is actively promoted.

Health psychology also has a significant interface with the field of public health. From a historical point of view, psychologists working in the U.S. Public Health Service studying the acceptance of measures aimed at prevention of illness (Hochbaum 1958; Rosenstock 1966; Rosenstock, Derryberry, and Carriger 1959) originated the "Health Belief Model," which has been a major theoretical influence in health psychology. Following this early beginning, however, there was a period of mutual disenchantment between the public health approach and that of psychologists, which is only now being overcome (see chapter 34; Runyan et al. 1982; Williams 1982).

Other Developments

Recognizing the explosion of work in the area of health and behavior and its enormous theoretical and practical significance to medicine, the Institute of Medicine (IOM) of the National Academy of Sciences formed a committee in 1979 to evaluate the field and set a research agenda for this area. Psychologists constituted over half the membership of the committee, which was chaired by David Hamburg, then President of the IOM. Judith Rodin was vice-chair. The committee held six major conferences at the IOM: Smoking and Behavior; Combining Psychosocial and Drug Therapy for Hypertension; Depression and Diabetes; Biobehavioral Factors in Sudden Cardiac Death; Infants at Risk for Developmental Dysfunction; Health, Behavior and Aging; and Behavior Health Risks and Social Disadvantage. A report, subsequently published by the IOM, examined the extent of behavior-related disease and disability and evaluated scientific approaches to understanding, treating, and preventing such illness. The book was significant because of its influence on stimulating Congressional interest in the area, leading to increased funding initiatives for behavioral factors in disease prevention and health promotion proposed by Congressional mandate to the National Institutes of Health budget. In 1983, the influential John D. and Catherine MacArthur Foundation also added a network on "The Determinants and Consequences of Health Damaging and Health Promoting Behavior" to the three others it had organized to facilitate research in mental health.

A developing field of scholarship and practice is shaped to a significant degree by publications in which it is represented and presented. Commentaries on the field and textbooks play an important part in defining just what comes to be included as a part of the field and guide developing training programs and curricula. Research summaries shape decisions about what kinds of research will be proposed and funded. Evaluative reviews of interventions influence practitioners and clinical researchers. It would be impossible to present here a comprehensive bibliography of the burgeoning literature in health psychology, but we list a few of the formative works of the first decade of health psychology.

Health psychology: A handbook (Stone, Cohen, and Adler 1979)
Behavioral approaches to medicine (McNamara 1979)
Handbook of clinical health psychology (Millon, Green and Meagher 1982)
Handbook of psychology and health, volumes 1–5 (1982–83)
Behavioral health: A handbook of health promotion and disease prevention (Matarazzo et al. 1984)
Handbook of behavioral medicine (Gentry 1984)

Finally, the Arden House Conference, held in May 1983, examined complex issues related to training health psychologists and made numerous important recommendations. While it is too soon to determine the extent of dissemination or impact of these recommendations, the meeting certainly was successful in focusing attention on the existing theoretical and empirical bases of health psychology; on the nature, strengths, and limitations of settings where health psychologists are trained; on the academic and professional disciplines within the field; and on the potential breadth and impact of this now well-cognized field. We leave prognostication about the future of the discipline to the final chapter; suffice it to say here that its roots seem firmly established.

References

American Psychological Association Task Force on Health Research. 1976. Contributions of psychology to health research. *American Psychologist* 31:263–74.

Bott, E. A. 1928. Teaching of psychology in the medical course. *Bulletin of the Association of American Medical Colleges* 3:289–304.

Buck, R. L. 1961. Behavioral scientists in schools of medicine. *Journal of Health and Human Behavior* 2:59–64.

Crary, W. G., and H. G. Steger. 1972. Prescriptive and consultative approaches to psychological evaluation. *Professional Psychology* 3:105–9.

Dennis, W. 1950. *Current trends in the relation of psychology to medicine.* Pittsburgh: University of Pittsburgh Press.

Gentry, W. D., ed. 1984. *Handbook of behavioral medicine.* New York: Guilford.

Hall, C. S. 1904. *Health, growth, and heredity.* Edited with an introduction and notes by C. E. Strickland and C. Burgess. Classics in Education no. 23. New York: Teachers' College Press.

Handbook of psychology and health. 1982–83. Volumes 1–5, edited in various combinations by A. Baum, R. Gatchel, D. Krantz, J. E. Singer, and S. Taylor. Hillsdale, NJ: Lawrence Erlbaum and Associates.

Hochbaum, G. M. 1958. *Public participation in medical screening programs: A sociopsychological study.* Public Health Service Publication no. 572. Washington, D.C.: Superintendent of Public Documents.

James, W. 1899. *Talks to teachers on psychology; and to students on some of life's ideals.* New York: Henry Holt.

———. 1922. *On vital reserves: The energies of men; the gospel of relaxation.* New York: Henry Holt.

Lubin, B., R. G. Nathan, and J. D. Matarazzo. 1978. Psychologists in medical education. *American Psychologist* 33:339–43.

Matarazzo, J. D. 1955. The role of the psychologist in medical education and practice. *Human Organization* 14:9–14.

Matarazzo, J. D., T. P. Carmody, and W. D. Gentry. 1981. Psychologists on the faculties of medical schools: Past, present, and possible future. *Clinical Psychology Review* 1:293–317.

Matarazzo, J. D., and R. S. Daniel. 1957. The teaching of psychology by psychologists in medical schools. *Journal of Medical Education* 32:410–15.

Matarazzo, J. D., S. M. Weiss, J. A. Herd, N. E. Miller, and S. M. Weiss, eds. 1984. *Behavioral health: A handbook of health enhancement and disease prevention.* New York: Wiley.

Mensch, I. N. 1953. Psychology in medical education. *American Psychologist* 8: 83–85.

McMillan, J. J. 1970. Agenda for the 1970s in professional affairs: Some first thoughts. *Professional Psychology* 1:181–84.

McNamara, J. R. 1979. *Behavioral approaches to medicine.* New York: Plenum.

Millon, T., C. Green, and R. Meagher, eds. 1982. *Handbook of clinical health psychology.* New York: Plenum.

Olbrisch, M. E. 1977. Psychotherapeutic interventions in physical health: Effectiveness and economic efficiency. *American Psychologist* 32:761–77.

Psychology and national health care. 1971. *American Psychologist* 26:1025–26. Adopted as a position statement of The American Psychological Association by its Board of Directors, 8 July.

Rosenstock, I. M. 1966. Why people use health services. *Millbank Memorial Fund Quarterly* 44:94–124.

Rosenstock, I. M., M. Derryberry, and B. Carriger. 1959: Why people fail to seek poliomyelitis vaccination. *Public Health Reports* 74:98–103.

Runyan, C. W., R. F. DeVellis, B. M. DeVellis, and G. M. Hochbaum. 1982. Health psychology and the public health perspective: In search of the pump handle. *Health Psychology* 1:169–80.

Schofield, W. 1969. The role of psychology in the delivery of health services. *American Psychologist* 24:568–84.

Stone, G. C. 1979. Psychology and the health system. In *Health psychology: A handbook,* edited by G. C. Stone, F. Cohen, and N. E. Adler. San Francisco: Jossey-Bass.

Stone, G. C., F. Cohen, and N. E. Adler. 1979. *Health psychology: A handbook.* San Francisco: Jossey-Bass.

Webster, T. G. 1971. The behavioral sciences in medical education and practice. In *Psychosocial aspects of medical training,* edited by R. H. Coombs and E. V. Clark. Springfield, IL: Thomas.

Weisenberg, M. 1970. The role of psychology in the delivery of health services. *American Psychologist* 25 : 472.

Williams, A. F. 1982. Passive and active measures for controlling disease and injury: The role of health psychologists. *Health Psychology* 1 : 399–409.

3

The Scope of Health Psychology

George C. Stone

At its annual meeting in 1980, the Division of Health Psychology adopted an "official" working definition of the field of health psychology: "Health Psychology is the aggregate of the specific educational, scientific, and professional contributions of the discipline of psychology to the promotion and maintenance of health, the prevention and treatment of illness, the identification of etiologic and diagnostic correlates of health, illness and related dysfunction, and the analysis and improvement of the health care system and health policy formation." This definition, based on modest revisions of a proposal offered by Matarazzo from an article of his then in press (Matarazzo 1982), was recognized as a starting point from which the field would grow and was not in any sense intended to limit the application of psychological competence to those aspects of the health system specified in it. The definition lists a broad array of activities, ranging from prevention of illness to the formation of health policy to which health psychology can make contributions.

In the chapters that follow, many specific examples are provided of the ways in which psychologists are currently fulfilling this definition. As described in the previous chapter, in fifteen years this field has grown from virtually nothing to a highly visible, highly productive enterprise involving thousands of psychologists. Rather than define the scope of the field by what these workers have chosen to do to date, it is my intention to approach the matter more abstractly. I hope in this way to provide a basis for locating the large amount of work now being done within an even larger domain of opportunity.

At the outset it is important to clarify one aspect of the definition given above. In attending to health psychology's bringing "contributions of the discipline of psychology to . . ." problems of the health system, we must not lose sight of the other function of specialized fields in psychology—their contributions to the growth of the discipline itself. Some fields contribute especially (and indeed may be defined) in terms of the substantive and methodological problems that they pose. Personality, social, and clinical psychology are examples of "major" fields (American Psychological Association 1981, xlviii) that bring problems to our discipline—problems solutions to which may lead to the discovery of new knowledge and the development of new theory. Other fields are defined by their special approaches to the solutions of problems—experimental psychology by its methodology, comparative psychology by its study of animals to address questions that cannot be answered by research using only human subjects, and physiological psychology that seeks answers at a particular level of explanation.

Health psychology can contribute both new problems and new approaches to old problems. Humankind has had some concept resembling that of "health" for more than 4,000 years, but we have not yet been able to formulate a clear definition of the concept that fully embodies our view that it is more than the simple absence of disease (Stone 1979a). Psychology may be able to contribute to such a formulation, and in so doing, it will have to gain a clearer understanding of the nature of human values as psychological constructs. Whatever else it may be, health is a value standard used to compare that which is with that which might be. I will return to this issue in the section on the definition of the health system.

Health psychology also poses challenging questions to many segments of the parent discipline to explain the relationships between beliefs and the operation of bodily systems, such as the immune system. The old mind-body problem now emerges in a sufficiently concrete form so that we may be able to gain new perspectives on this traditionally nettlesome problem. In the third section of this chapter I propose to identify some of the psychological problems that are of special importance in the health system.

As a setting for research, the health system offers some special advantages that promise to open the way to testing existing theories in ways that have been heretofore impossible and to clarifying theoretical problems that we have as yet been unable to test. Some explication of these opportunities will constitute the fourth section of this chapter.

In pursuing both of these issues—psychological problems that present themselves in the health system and special opportunities for psychological research in the health system—we need to have agreed upon definitions of the discipline and profession of psychology and a psychologically meaningful description of the health system. In the next two sections, I will attempt to provide brief outlines of the required characterizations.

The Scope of Psychology

Since its emergence as a self-identified science about a hundred years ago, psychology has concerned itself with intraorganismic and extraorganismic influences on three domains of phenomena—experience, cognitions, and behavior. Different groups of psychologists, working in the same or different time periods, have placed more or less emphasis on one or another of these domains, and some have even sought to rule out one or more of them as uninteresting, inaccessible to study, or nonexistent. After many decades of wrestling with problems of definition and measurement, most psychologists today are ready to grant the existence of feelings and mental representations of information while recognizing that our only access to these phenomena is through the behavior of the organism to which we attribute them.

Psychology is the science that seeks laws and functions that relate antecedent states of almost any kind to consequent states of experience, cognition, or behavior of individual organisms. Psychology is distinguished from other behavioral sciences by the fact that its laws and functions are intended to predict the behavior of conscious *individuals*. Since our predictions are far from perfect, we typically look to group averages or percentages to verify that we are actually succeeding with our predictions, but our focus is on the individual. Anthropology, sociology, economics, political science, and the like seek theories that predict behavior of groups or group members.

When we look at macrobehavior, at feelings, or at cognitions as *dependent* variables, then no restriction need be placed on the antecedent states we study. When we measure the behavior of an organ or some reflex-controlled behavior, then we must require that the antecedent states include previous psychological states—states measured or inferred from conditions imposed on the organism. Without these restrictions we would fail to distinguish psychological and physiological investigations. If a kidney secretes more sodium or a heart contracts more frequently in part because of stimulation from the nervous system, understanding the phenomenon may be equally the concern of psychologist and physiologist, but their interests will be different. The physiologist will probably be interested in the interaction of these influences with others that do not involve the central nervous system, while the psychologist will probably want to know how these CNS effects arose and how they can be modified through the experience or cognitions of the organism.

It may be noted that this definition leads to the inclusion of some other scientists, notably ethologists and some anthropologists, within the field of psychology. And, of course, Pavlov did his studies of the modification of salivation behavior in his laboratory of physiology. These scientists are distinguished from psychologists by their traditions, their methods, their explanatory theories, but not by the phenomena that they study.

How are these considerations applicable to our definition of health psychology? Essentially, they tell us what it is that is to be mapped. By this definition, we can consider as problems of health psychology those in which prior experience of health, illness, and interactions with the health system are salient; those in which the immediate circumstances are in the health system; and those in which the psychological consequences—the experience, cognitions, and behavior of the individual—are likely to affect future interactions with the health system. We must turn to our consideration of the health system to see just how large a domain of psychology is thereby defined.

The Health System
DEFINITION OF THE HEALTH SYSTEM

Webster's New World Dictionary (1974) gives as its first definition of the term "system" the following: a system is "a set of things so related or connected as to form a unity or organic whole." The focus is on the *relationships* among a set of elements.

In the present day, many of us have come to think of the universe as a total system within which we more or less arbitrarily carve out subsystems for analysis. We recognize the nested or hierarchical nature of these subsystems, and we "focus down" through levels of hierarchy until we locate a subsystem that serves our purpose. One of the useful ways of isolating a subsystem is to specify that all of the relationships among its elements exist in relation to some defining principle or concept. Thus, we can define the health system as that set of elements related to each other through a mediating relation to the defining concept, "health." For example, the relation between a physician and a patient or a health insurance company and a hospital depends on the relation of each of these elements to the general concept of "health." We must turn to a definition of health to define the system.

Definitions of "health" tend to fall into one of two categories (Stone 1979a). First, there are those that consider health as an *ideal state* of an organism from which disease and injury are deviations. We seek to restore an organism to the healthy state by removing disease and disability. The principal difficulty with this kind of definition is its inability to describe the ideal. Specifying that in the ideal state the organism is able to "survive," "adapt," "express its potential fully," or "enjoy life" falls short on two counts: It fails to deal with the unattainability of the ideal, and it has difficulty in handling those situations in which individuals with obvious shortcomings of bodily function are nevertheless producing work that is deemed more socially valuable than that accomplished by others with bodies free from defect. Should a dying poet or a deafened musician who continues to produce work of great beauty and power be considered healthy?

Definitions of the second kind avoid the difficulty of judging a particular state as healthy or unhealthy by considering the term "health" to represent a positively valued *direction* in the world. It is always good to move in the direction of greater health, although in choosing behavior one must weigh the gain in health against the costs (or losses) in other value dimensions such as money, time, and personal appearances. Reflecting upon this concept, we see that there are innumerable aspects of a particular organism that can be changed in a direction of greater or lesser health and that the health status of the organism must represent the (vector) sum of the individual statuses in all of these aspects. Without specifying all of the individual values and their relative weights, it is not possible to make an analytic comparison of the relative health of two organisms, but it may be possible to compare two states of the same organism, so long as the change from one to the other does not result in opposite impacts upon the health of different aspects.

In recognizing health as a fundamental direction of value, similar to beauty, wealth, justice, and the like, we have not yet specified the principle by which we can determine that a change is in the direction of greater or lesser health. (Of course, we might have some difficulty in specifying the principles for the other great values, also.) In a discussion at a recent meeting of the John D. and Catherine MacArthur Foundation Network for the Study of the Determinants and Consequences of Health Promoting and Health Damaging Behavior, at least five distinct subdivisions of health value were identified (Irwin and Stone 1985). They included:

1. The subjective feeling of well-being
2. Capacity for a high level of social productivity
3. Superior values in measures of bodily function such as blood pressure, cardiac output, respiratory volume, etc.
4. Low drain upon the health care system
5. Ability to withstand stress, infectious challenges, and physical insults with minimum loss to criteria 1−4

These different aspects are by no means independent, but neither are they perfectly correlated. No one has yet devised a way to establish units of equal exchange among them. As in all matters of value we have no agreed means for adjudicating differences in preference, but as is commonly done, we can form policy on the basis of consensual preferences.

It should also be clear that some, if not all, of the criteria of health listed above are influenced to a greater or lesser extent by psychological states that can be affected by educational, religious, familial, and other sociocultural factors that we do not usually think of as being part of the health system. We can take refuge in the view that these factors become a part of the health system only when we are considering their impact upon health outcomes.

Thus we come to a somewhat unsatisfying definition of the health system as those elements of our human environment that have impact on the multiple aspects of the health of individuals. Even though we might wish for a firmer, more explicit basis for proceeding, we can still set forth some major categories of the system (Stone, 1979a, 1981, 1983, 1984, 1986).

ELEMENTS OF THE HEALTH SYSTEM

A basis for describing the elements of the health system can be established around the *person whose health is at issue*. I will use the acronym PHAI in referring to this element of the system. The PHAI exists in an environment that contains many *hazards* that are capable of affecting the health of the PHAI adversely and many *resources* (including human resources) that can be used to enhance it. The PHAI interacts with the resources in two ways: directly, as in feeding behavior and certain kinds of exercise to promote the healthy growth of the body and indirectly, using them to mitigate the impact of the hazards on health. The PHAI, interacting with hazards and resources, encounters *barriers* (protective and obstructive) and uses *tools* (including skills). These hazards, resources, barriers, and tools can be called the primary elements of the health system. In addition to these there are many secondary elements that act not upon the PHAI but upon the primary elements of the system or the PHAI's relationship to those primary elements. And, there are tertiary elements that act on secondary elements, and so forth. The degree of remoteness from the PHAI that we are willing to permit, while still recognizing an entity as an element of the health system, no doubt depends upon the impact that it can create upon the health of the PHAI.

Human society creates experts, agencies, and institutions that act with intent upon the primary elements of the health system to alter their relationship to the PHAI. These can be called the intentional elements of the health system. A subsystem of the intentional elements, called the health care system, is defined by its intent to intervene directly in the relationship between the PHAI and health hazards and health resources. Another subsystem, the public health system, has traditionally addressed itself to the elimination of hazards from the environment. Of late, public health professionals have also begun to add resources, mostly informational, to the environment. Other elements of the system include insurance companies and government agencies whose intent is to support the secondary intentional entities, and so on.

The point of this elaboration of relationships among the elements of the health system is to emphasize the defining role of the PHAI interacting with the primary elements. We can profitably look more closely at this central relationship. The PHAI may or may not be aware of the existence or potential impact of the hazards and resources in the environment. In more behavioral terms, the PHAI may or may not discriminate them as entities to be approached or avoided. Whether or not they are recognized, the hazards or resources may or may not actually exert their harmful or beneficial impact upon the PHAI. (The PHAI may have been lucky or immune.) If they do have impact, they may or may not give rise to discernible changes in the state of the PHAI. Up to this point in the developing transaction, health-oriented interventions directed toward hazards and resources will be similar or symmetrical. Health agents will strive to make the PHAI aware of the existence of both hazards and resources, to reduce or increase contact with them, and to make their impact more apparent. Beyond this point, the two patterns diverge, at least in traditional health care. The PHAI who has a discernible decrease in health may elect to enter the role of patient in the health care system. The variations by which diagnosis, treatment plan, compliance, and evaluation are carried out have been the subject of much discussion in recent years (Stone 1979b; DiMatteo and DiNicola 1982). Until recently, PHAI who were defined as sick were managed by health care providers while those who were well looked after themselves. Increasing emphasis on outpatient care for chronic illness has led to increasing recognition of the necessity for active participation by the PHAI in the health care process. At the same time, we note the emergence of "wellness" programs, in which plans for systematic interaction with health resources are formulated, implemented, and evaluated with professional assistance.

The final phase of the PHAI's interaction with hazards, namely rehabilitation—the effort to restore lost potential—does not appear to have a counterpart in the case of health resources.

PSYCHOLOGICAL COMPETENCE IN THE HEALTH SYSTEM

This classification of the elements of the health system provides a framework within which we can systematically consider the potential contributions of health psychologists. Such a task calls for far more space than is available here. In papers written for other purposes I have given examples of the potential for indirect contributions to direct health care (Stone 1986), and contributions in hospital settings (Stone 1983). These are but two of many regions of the health system in which psychologists can work. They can study or intervene in the impact of hazards on the PHAI, investigate the impact of alternate forms of payment for service on the curative health care transactions, or examine the relationships between health beliefs of legislators and health policy legislation.

In confronting such diverse opportunities, we have to ask whether we could train a health psychologist who could do all of these things. The answer is, obviously, we could not. Then we may ask, is a health psychologist who studies the impact of job stress on blood pressure more like another health psychologist that studies copayment and utilization of health care services or more like an academic psychophysiologist? I would answer that the common focus on psychophysiology creates more resemblance than that of shared interest in quite distant aspects of health. What is the purpose, then, of defining a field of health psychology that is so broad that resemblance across its boundaries may be much greater than those within them? This is a question that is explored implicitly or explicitly by many of the authors in this volume. My response to it is that we are studying components of a system, and it behooves us to have some conception of the entire system, even though each of us can focus on only a small portion of it. Such a broad conception will help to protect us from becoming confused or misled by perturbations that loop through remote parts of the system. So, the PHAI's response to job stress may be affected by the company's medical plan while that of the laboratory subject is probably not. And the psychologist who studies the impact of copayment had better have some notion of the contribution of stress-induced psychophysiological states on individual economic decisions. It is the fact that health psychologists work within a context of the health system and have it represented to a greater or lesser extent always in their problem analyses—that gives them their identity as psychologists.

Some Salient Psychological Problems of the Health System

Having now sketched out an enormous domain within which health psychologists could function, I propose to consider briefly where they are working and where they might profitably devote more effort at this time. In chapter 2, reference was made to William Schofield's article (1969) which gave a major impetus to the emergence of the field by his analysis of the research then being done by psychologists in the health area. His major point was that a very large proportion of the work was focused on only that part of the system that was concerned with mental health.

Prompted by Schofield's study, the American Psychological Association established a task force under his direction to do a more extensive review which came to essentially the same conclusion. In eight years of the *Psychological Abstracts*, 1966–73, this group found only about sixty articles addressed to health care delivery and to health attitudes and behavior. Although there have been no further large-scale reviews of the literature addressing this issue, there do appear to have been substantial increases in the number of articles about general health and in the proportion that focus on some aspect of the health care process, such as provider-patient interactions, patient adherence or compliance, utilization of care, and so on.

Not long ago I reviewed the *Psychological Abstracts* for 1979–84 under the headings of "Health Care" and "Health Care Services" (Stone 1986). Excluding all articles that were descriptions of the direct delivery of psychological services, which I would judge to have been something over half of the total, I found 770 articles representing psychological studies of health care processes. This number reflects a rate of almost 130 such articles a year, nearly twenty times the rate of seven per year found on such topics by the APA task force. Notably missing in this review were reports of the use of psychological assessment techniques for the guidance of health care service providers.

I also reviewed the *Abstracts* for the period from January 1982 through June 1983, looking for articles about the activities of psychologists in hospitals. Again excluding those about direct delivery of psychological services, I found thirty-eight abstracts, of which twenty-six concerned the PHAI and their relations to others, mostly (eleven cases) providers. Only three articles were about providers individually; only eight were concerned at all with the hospital organization, again in most cases with interactions; and only two of the thirty-eight articles were concerned with psychological aspects of the larger health system and the role of hospitals in it.

A breakdown of the subjects of 191 manuscripts submitted to the journal, *Health Psychology*, between January 1981 and April 1983 indicated that less than twenty percent involved physiological measures as either independent or dependent variables. A very large proportion involved psychological states or behavior of the PHAI as dependent variables (about 65%) and patients' characteristics (40%) and interventions (25%) as the independent variables. Less than ten percent of these submissions addressed organizational or system level issues.

What is apparent from these surveys, biased and incomplete as they may be, is that the research of health psychologists has been concentrated to a very large degree on professional health care processes and on the PHAI in relation to those processes. We can create one dimension of an area of research opportunity by recognizing a temporal/causal progression from concerns with prevention of illness through removing hazards from the environment and avoiding contact with them, to recognition of symptoms, seeking of treatment, participating in treatment, and undergoing the processes of rehabilitation. Psychological studies of hazard removal and resource promotion—an area that has been referred to as "managerial prevention"—are almost nonexistent. By contrast, there is a great deal of research on avoidance of risk and a lesser but still appreciable amount on personal use of health promoting resources (see Kirscht 1982 for a recent review). Most of this work is oriented toward developing, implementing, and evaluating professional interventions that will enhance such "personal prevention." The area of recognizing symptoms and deciding what to do about them, Suchman's "illness behavior," has been left to sociologists and anthropologists for the most part. In the past year or two some excellent work by psychologists regarding symptom appraisal has begun to appear (e.g., Lau and Hartman 1983; Leventhal, Nerenz, and Steele 1984; Pennebaker 1984). Once the PHAI have entered the health care system as patients, a good deal of psychological research has focused on their interactions with the health care providers in terms of the stress of illness and its treatment (Cohen and Lazarus 1979), participation in and adherence to treatment regimens (DiMatteo and DiNicola 1982), and making the consequential decisions that are called for (Janis and Mann 1977). Psychologists have also participated in studies of medical decision-making (Elstein and Bordage 1979), staff interactions, and the stresses of the health professions (Cartwright 1979), although such work is relatively rare. There is a long tradition of psychological research on the rehabilitation process, reflected in the field of rehabilitation psychology. Until recently, this branch of health psychology directed its efforts mostly toward a few conditions, such as schizophrenia and spinal cord injury, in which the disabilities often occurred early in life and profoundly impaired the capacity of the disabled to participate in the activities of everyday life. Increasing attention is now being directed to speeding recovery and enhancing the capacity of the chronically ill to engage as fully as possible in life following a variety of major illnesses.

A second dimension for the location of research opportunities can be conceptualized in relation to the distance of the psychological processes to be studied from the PHAI. At one extreme of this dimension are the individual psychological processes of the PHAI themselves. Next would come their health-relevant interactions with health care providers, health educators, family and community members, and the like, and then the psychological processes of these collaterals who are in direct contact with the PHAI. There are substantial quantities of research regarding these elements of the health system.

Beyond this region lie the psychological processes of support personnel that influence health care environments, of the people who directly influence the presence of health hazards and resources in the environment, and of the people who plan, finance, regulate, and manage the procedures, agencies, and institutions that directly or indirectly affect the environment and the health care system. These large areas have been almost totally neglected by health psychologists. When we study occupational health, we consider the participation of employees in the programs and the impact on their health and productivity, but I know of no psychological studies concerned with what causes companies to institute such programs. When we study problems of toxic waste disposal, we consider the stress on members of affected communities but not the psychology of the company managers who are responsible for the decisions about disposal, nor of the legislators who make laws to mediate between health and economic values. Obviously, there are problems of access to these remote regions of the health system. But even these problems are potentially susceptible to psychological analysis. Perhaps we need a psychology of health psychology.

Contributions from Health Psychology to the Core Discipline

One of the primary aspects of health psychology is its application of the knowledge and methods of psychology to problems of the health system. In the concluding section of this chapter I intend to address what appears to me as an equally important aspect, that of expanding and transforming that core knowledge which is to be applied. The distinction between applied and basic science is acknowledged to be difficult to draw sharply, and many of the major advances in basic science have come about as applied questions have been pursued to their roots. Thus, we could expect in principle that any area of psychological application would contribute to the development of basic knowledge and methodology in psychology.

There are several special aspects of the health system, however, that make it an especially favorable site for research. First, the values that people hold regarding health matters are unusually coherent. There are few if any other aspects of life in which we could expect such widespread, crosscultural agreement as with believing it is better to be alive than dead, free from pain than suffering pain, able to conduct one's activities than constrained by bodily incapacities from pursuing them. This coherence of values creates the opportunity to study decision-making and behavior choice in situations where relatively little variance is associated with differences in value *structures*. This is not to say that all people value health to the same degree. The widespread occurrence of health destructive behavior assures us that they do not. But regardless of how a person values health relative to other aspects of life, there is stronger consensus about what is better than what *within the sphere of health values themselves* than there is concerning what paintings or musical compositions are beautiful, what foods are delicious, what practices are just and right, and so on.

The business world also offers good opportunities in this regard, since it operates with a highly quantifiable token value system that appears to bypass concern with the intrinsic values that underly it. Many people aver, however, that the principles educed in the study of token values give a distorted view of those that actually guide human behavior. In the health system, we have an opportunity to examine most explicitly the relationships between monetary values and the intrinsic values of human life and its quality, since the health-related actions that are taken are inevitably influenced by very significant monetary costs.

A second major source of opportunity in the health system is the nearly universal acceptance of deeply invasive procedures performed in the interest of restoring health. With proper ethical and humane sensitivity, this openness can provide the basis for examining with a wide range of persons matters that could never be studied in most of their settings and circumstances, and certainly not in laboratory settings.

Coupled with this openness to study is the fact that humans in large numbers undergo extremes of stress and pain in their encounters with the health care system. Thus, there are opportunities to investigate these aspects of human life that are unparalleled elsewhere. There is no need to deceive people or to contrive simulations of real world experiences. Again, there are ethical considerations involved in further burdening suffering people with our research procedures, but many people are magnificent in their willingness—even eagerness—to give meaning to their suffering by making it the instrument of help for others.

The fourth, and last to be mentioned, merit of the health system as a site for basically important research is that the confrontation of the ancient boundary between mind and body is not only continuously possible but essential. As we study the processes of biofeedback, the interactions between stress, cognitions and the immune system, the relationships between coping styles and the reports of pain and other pain-related behaviors, and a host of other such problems, we are required to press toward explicit specification of the mechanisms by which symbols and cells interact.

For these and other reasons, it seems probable that psychologists whose interests are entirely in discovering the fundamental principles of psychology will turn in increasing numbers to the arenas of the health system for their research. As they do, it will be important that they be oriented and guided in the social and ethical norms that they will encounter, in the special vocabularies they will need to know, in the means for avoiding the organizational and methodological pitfalls that have been discovered by earlier settlers. Such orientation and guidance, whether of seasoned researchers recognizing the potential of the arena or of students striving to establish their careers in the health system, constitutes a major part of the work of health psychologists. It is the traditional work of the teacher in any art or profession, and it is the focus of many of the chapters that follow.

REFERENCES

American psychological association directory. 1981.

American Psychological Association Task Force on Health Research. 1976. Contributions of psychologists to health research: Patterns, problems, and potentials. *American Psychologist* 31:263–74.

Cartwright, L. K. 1979. Sources and effects of stresses in health careers. In *Health psychology,* edited by G. C. Stone, F. Cohen, and N. E. Adler. San Francisco: Jossey-Bass.

Cohen, F., and R. S. Lazarus. 1979. Coping with the stresses of illness. In *Health psychology,* edited by G. C. Stone, F. Cohen, and N. E. Adler. San Francisco: Jossey-Bass.

DiMatteo, M. R., and D. D. DiNicola. 1982. *Achieving patient compliance: The psychology of the medical practitioner's role.* New York: Pergamon Press.

Elstein, A. S., and G. Bordage. 1979. The psychology of clinical reasoning. In *Health psychology,* edited by G. C. Stone, F. Cohen, and N. E. Adler. San Francisco: Jossey-Bass.

Irwin, C. E., and G. C. Stone. 1985. Report on the plenary session on "Good Health." Unpublished proceedings of the Summer Meeting of the John D. and Catherine MacArthur Foundation Network for the Study of Determinants and Consequences of Health Promoting and Health Damaging Behavior. St. Petersburg, Florida.

Janis, I. L., and L. Mann. 1977. *Decision making: A psychological analysis of conflict, choice, and commitment.* New York: Free Press.

Kirscht, J. P. 1982. Preventive health behavior: A review of research and issues. *Health Psychology* 2:277–301.

Lau, R. R., and K. A. Hartman. 1983. Common sense representations of common illnesses. *Health Psychology* 2:167–86.

Leventhal, H. F., Nerenz, and D. J. Steele. 1984. Illness representations and coping with health threats. In *Social psychological aspects of health,* edited by A. Baum, J. E. Singer, and S. E. Taylor. Hillsdale, NJ: Lawrence Erlbaum and Associates.

Matarazzo, J. D. 1982. Behavioral health's challenge to academic, scientific, and professional psychology. *American Psychologist* 37:1–14.

Pennebaker, J. W. 1984. Accuracy of symptom perception. In *Social psychological aspects of health,* edited by A. Baum, J. E. Singer, and S. E. Taylor. Hillsdale, NJ: Lawrence Erlbaum and Associates.

Schofield, W. 1969. The role of psychology in the delivery of health services. *American Psychologist* 24:565–84.

Stone, G. C. 1979a. Health and the health system. In *Health psychology: A handbook,* edited by G. C. Stone, F. Cohen, and N. E. Adler. San Francisco: Jossey-Bass.

———. 1979b. Patient compliance and the role of the expert. *Journal of Social Issues* 35:34–59.

———. 1981. Training for health systems research and consultation. In *Linking health and mental health,* edited by A. Broskowski, E. Marks, and S. Budman. Beverly Hills, CA: Sage.

———. 1983. The psychologist in the hospital. Paper presented at the Invitational Conference on the Hospital: Its Psychological Effects on Patients and Staff. Northwestern University. Chicago, IL.

———. 1984. Training health professionals for health promotion. In *Behavioral health: A handbook of health enhancement and disease prevention,* edited by J. D. Matarazzo, S. M. Weiss, J. A. Herd, N. E. Miller, and S. M. Weiss. New York: Wiley.

———. 1986. Psychological aspects of health care. In *Professional psychology in transition: Meeting today's challenges,* edited by H. Dörken and G. VandenBos. San Francisco: Jossey-Bass.

4

Relationships of Health Psychology to Other Segments of Psychology

Joseph D. Matarazzo

Diversity, Commonality, and the Eye of the Beholder

An observer seeking to find *diversity* within the teachings of each of the professions of theology, law, and medicine, or within each of the scientific and cognate disciplines of mathematics, physics, and chemistry will find such diversity today, not only across widely separated countries and cultures, or within a single country but, as each reader knows from personal experience in his or her own institution of higher education, even within a *single department* of a university. Likewise, the observer seeking evidence that considerable *commonality* exists within these natural science disciplines and within theology, law, and medicine will find evidences of such commonalities and similarities not only within a single department or within a country but also across countries and cultures. In short, it is my opinion after discussions with colleagues in these other fields that whether either diversity or commonality is present within a discipline or a profession is more a function of the eye of the beholder than it is of the field itself. Depending upon predilection, an observer will perceive uniformity of ideas, subject matter, or offerings in a discipline across widely differing geographic areas or one will find diversity. I believe this also is the state of affairs in the field of psychology.

Curricular Offerings Pragmatically Define a Discipline

Specifically, it is my opinion that the graduate students and undergraduate majors in U.S. departments of psychology between 1900 and 1985 have

Preparation of this chapter was supported in part by National Heart, Lung, and Blood Institute Grants HL20910 and HL07332. The views expressed in this chapter are those of the author. Although my views as expressed here were influenced a bit from the discussions of the task group on this subject which met at the 1983 conference, they nevertheless are solely my own. Members of that task group were Nancy Adler, David Altman, Cynthia Belar, Roy Grzesiak, William Johnson, Theodore Millon, Mary Ellen Olbrisch, Bonnie Strickland, Steven Tulkin, and Gary VandenBos.

taken courses in psychology (whether required or chosen from a number of possible electives) that were almost identical in basic subject matter if not also in assigned textbooks, even though they were matriculating in universities that were geographically widely separated. Deviations from this common core of curricular offerings quite likely reflect(ed) little more than a local faculty member's idiosyncratic interest.

This is not surprising inasmuch as it is by means of such a core of knowledge that departments transmit to students what they believe is the common knowledge base of psychology. It is through assimilating this core that students of psychology (or any discipline) adopt a common frame of reference that identifies them as members of the same cultural subgroup. Furthermore, as with other fields, it is by additions to and deletions from the core that we continuously define and redefine psychology. As specialization evolves, as it clearly continues to do, that process will determine *how* and *in what directions* psychology will be applied; however, the core of knowledge determines *what* will be applied in that evolution. Study of any standard textbook in psychology will quickly reveal that there have been large increases and fundamental changes in the knowledge base of psychology during the past century. Today's best-selling introductory psychology textbook obviously contains considerably different content than did William James's *Principles of Psychology* or Boring's pre-Second World War introductory textbook. That fact notwithstanding, the major themes found in the subject matter of the introductory and graduate textbooks which define the parameters of our discipline for each succeeding generation have changed very little between 1900 and the present. Even today, such textbooks continue to be more similar than different than their predecessors in their chapter titles or core content.

Is Today's Predoctoral Education in Psychology General or Specialized?

In our country each of the *professions* of law, medicine, and dentistry decided early in this century that in order to be nationally accredited the doctoral curriculum in that field offered by each institution of higher education would have to be a relatively highly standardized, quality curriculum covering basically the same areas of knowledge in each institution. *Scientific disciplines,* such as physics, mathematics, biochemistry, sociology, and anthropology did not institute comparable formal procedures for designating the areas of content, let alone accrediting the quality of this content in the doctoral curriculum in their respective fields of knowledge.

Until 1948, psychology was also one of those cognate scientific disciplines which did not have a national accrediting body which, following *voluntary* application for accreditation, could exercise influence over each institution of higher education's own local mechanisms of peer review and quality control. However, our country's need for thousands of new mental health professionals who could provide services to the emotionally disabled among the 15,000,000 men and women being discharged immediately following the end of the Second World War markedly changed psychology from an exclusively university-based scientific discipline to a unique hybrid consisting of part scientific discipline and part service-providing profession. This change did not occur overnight but evolved in stages from 1948 to the present. One of the important concomitants of this change was that beginning in 1948, and complying with the requirements for funding programs of both the National Institute of Mental Health and the Veterans Administration, psychology established the process by which the Education and Training Board of the American Psychological Association could assess and accredit both the curricular content offered and the quality of doctoral programs offering training for the *profession* of (clinical) psychology. From 1949 until 1985 the curriculum for a student seeking a career in *academic or scientific* psychology (in contrast to clinical psychology) was *not* similarly so standardized by these outside national influences.

After 1948, psychology reaffirmed this change involving national accreditation of a part of its university programs in each of five subsequent major national conferences on graduate education and training in psychology. These were held at Boulder, Colorado, in 1949, at Stanford in 1955, at Miami Beach in 1958, at Chicago in 1965 and at Vail, Colorado, in 1973. As the major recommendations promulgated at these five national conferences have been recently reviewed (Matarazzo 1983), I will not repeat those recommendations here. What is important for the present chapter is that representatives of the national leadership in graduate education in psychology asserted and then four times reaffirmed that psychology was *both* an academic-scientific discipline and a profession. The effect of this decision in practical terms was twofold. First, participants reaffirmed their decision to continue to *not* standardize the curriculum for psychology students heading for a scientific career. Nevertheless because the content of the graduate course offerings (whether required or "elective") were highly similar across universities, from 1949 on every doctoral graduate from a *department of psychology,* whether heading for a career in the discipline or in the profession of psychology, continued to receive basically the same core of generic training in psychology. Put differently, and because of the very practical reality that the graduate students matriculating in almost every university department of psychology had to successfully complete a relatively large number of hours of studies in psychology, this first practical impact was that the "core" doctoral curriculum for *all* psychology students would, as before 1949, continue to be essentially similar. This was so even though the student's ultimate goal was a career which required an extra elective track of additional courses to facilitate his or her later work in experimental psychology, developmental psychology, industrial psychology, clinical psychology, physiological psychology or in any of psychology's other arenas of potential subsequent application. The second area of consensus was that, inasmuch as the accumulated knowledge base of psychology had persuaded leaders in government and others that psychology in 1949 also had the potential to offer services to the public as a fee-for-service profession, the predoctoral student in psychology aiming for such a professional career would specifically need to add to this common, generic core an additional track of required (or elective) advanced courses and apprenticeship experiences designed to be differentially appropriate to that particular clinical area of application.

As just suggested, despite its seeming to be, this two-part 1949 decision was not a departure from what had been the rule for *all* students in traditional doctoral education in departments of psychology. Thus, after studying essentially the same predoctoral core psychology between 1900 and 1949, the graduate student of this earlier period wishing a career in experimental psychology added to that common core a minor field or track consisting of courses in mathematics, biology, and engineering. Likewise, the graduate student wishing to do research in and be a teacher of physiological psychology added to his or her graduate psychology core courses a minor track which consisted of neurology, neuroanatomy, physiology, and the like. And, pre-Second World War graduate students aiming for a career in developmental or child psychology added as their minor track a program which included, for example, courses in embryology, the home and family, and correlation and regression analyses.

What the 1949 Boulder Conference on Training in Clinical Psychology did that was a slight departure from this earlier state of affairs was to *loosely codify* these "extras" that had to be taken by a psychology department graduate student wishing a career of professional service or research (or both) in the then societally needed arena of *clinical psychology*. Specifically, the Boulder conferees agreed informally that henceforth such a professionally oriented student would *add* to his or her required core of generic psychology graduate courses extra work in personality theory, developmental psychology, psychopathology, clinical medicine, and clinical psychiatry as well as courses and related apprenticeship experiences in assessment and psychotherapy which dealt with the applications of such extra knowledge (Raimy 1950, 68–70). Although a common *core* of subject matter already existed via use of similar textbooks in the psychology doctoral programs across different departments of psychology, the conferees at Boulder rejected the suggestion that each department offering a Ph.D. via training in clinical psychology should offer essentially the same list of standardized core (or even elective) courses in the clinical track. Interestingly, although rejecting the idea that the actual list of core courses should be mandated, the participants at Boulder did introduce a bit of standardization, even if through the back door. Specifically, the conferees agreed that, "There should be a common core curriculum for all students in graduate programs leading to the doctorate in psychology" (Raimy 1950, 61). Nevertheless, having stated this broad mandate they could not bring themselves to list, except in very general terms (Raimy 1950, 64; APA 1947, 545–51), the actual coursework or subject matter which was required by this decision to break away from the tradition of the scientific disciplines and, as was true for the professions, introduce the element of standardization of the curriculum.

Psychology as a Profession Rejected Early Codification of the Graduate Curriculum

The agenda of each of the next four major national conferences on graduate education in psychology included ample time for further discussion of *mandating* a "list" versus *recommending,* in general terms as was done at Boulder, the *common core of subject matter* which every university department of psychology offering a doctorate had to offer. Although recognizing that such standardization of predoctoral curricula was (and still is today) the rule in medicine, dentistry, and, in great part, law, between 1949 and 1973 the leadership of academic psychology rejected such an overt move to a standardized curriculum at each of these national conferences. The rejection was not total, however. In fact, the language used by the conferees at the 1958 conference in Miami Beach specifically regarding this issue quite poignantly portrays the continuing paradox the field of psychology was experiencing on this matter: "Two interesting conclusions appeared from the [Miami] conference discussions. First, there is a common core. Second, we should not specify what this is lest we in any way discourage innovation in graduate training" (Roe et al. 1959, 44). This acceptance in the first conclusion, and its concurrent rejection in the second, was in no small part a product of the fact that the attendees at Miami and at each of these conferences were almost exclusively psychologists who held full-time positions on university faculties. In retrospect one should not be surprised that the ethic (local rather than national control of curricula) which guided the recommendations of these psychologists was one that for the entire 900-year history of universities in the Western Hemisphere had been the desire of members of the academic and scientific disciplines which make up a university. The irony of this is that the curricula of these differing academic-scientific disciplines, like the curricula of the several professions, have been and are shaped in great part by the writers of what become the classic textbooks in that field. *It is the content of these text books,* in the main, which influences the aggregate product called a doctoral curriculum in a discipline more so than the pronouncements of representative educators at national conferences.

As but one example of this point, despite a full day and a half of emotionally toned review of what some suggested should be the minimum list of core courses required of the recipient of the Ph.D. degree in psychology departments at every United States university, and the overwhelming formal rejection of such a list at the Miami Beach conference (as well as the other four), informal examination at Miami Beach by some of the conferees of such curricula then being offered in departments of psychology in different universities revealed a remarkable degree of overlap. This is not surprising when one remembers that then, as now, faculties go out of their way to attempt to select the best from the textbook offerings in their discipline. Therefore, as stated above, it is not surprising that, in good part, the names of the core graduate courses offered (and required by some departments and offered as "elective" in others) and the contents of the textbooks used during the period from 1890 to the present were and are essentially indistinguishable from one psychology department to another.

Thus, from Boulder in 1949 through the 1973 Vail Conference, psychology appeared to be engaged in an interesting exercise in dissonance: loudly and formally professing that there is a core curriculum albeit adding that there should not be a standardized list of required graduate course titles and offerings, on the one hand, and using textbooks whose contents were essentially facsimiles of each other across university departments of psychology and thus practicing standardization, albeit informally, on the other. As a further example of the dissonance, in the area of the required apprenticeship experience, even the internship centers (which evolved between 1949 to the present to provide the required nationally accredited internship apprenticeship experience for students wishing a career in clinical psychology) were mandated by the APA Accreditation Committee to accept trainees from *many* universities rather than serve as a "captive" internship center for only one university's student body.

Recent Currents Fostering Codification of the Graduate Curriculum

As this dissonance continued among academic psychologists, the post-Boulder Conference generation of fee-for-service, professional psychologists faced a different set of challenges. In time these challenges would help resolve this dissonance being practiced by their university mentors. Law, medicine, dentistry, and nursing each had earlier learned that whereas a university is empowered by its state charter to grant the *academic* title of Doctor of Jurisprudence, Doctor of Medicine, Doctor of Dental Medicine, and Bachelor of Nursing, only the citizens of a state, acting through another mechanism (a state licensing board appointed by the governor and accountable to its citizens) can confer the parallel *professional* title of attorney, physician, dentist or registered nurse. I have discussed these different sets of constituencies (university, national accrediting body, and state licensing board) and their interrelationships within the field of psychology in some detail (Matarazzo 1977) and thus will not repeat the discussion here.

What is important to point out is that the post-1949 holders of a doctorate earned in a psychology department who wished to be fee-for-service providers in a clinical setting or in industry had first to join together and persuade a state licensing board that they had the *credentials* for such practice mandated in the laws in the fifty states plus the District of Columbia which were enacted beginning in 1945. One of the key passages in each of these laws was that the person wishing to become a licensed (or certified) psychologist had to have earned a doctoral degree in psychology *or its equivalent*. This latter clause was the result of a blend of humanism and a behind-the-scenes compromise the psychologist-writers of these fifty-one post-Second World War licensing laws had to make with the holders of doctorates whose studies were in such "related" fields as guidance and counseling, education, human and child development, pastoral counseling, and sociology in order that holders of the degrees from such other departments or university units would not attempt to defeat these licensing laws in each state. However, after the first groups of individuals with degrees earned in these "related" disciplines were "grandfathered" and "grandmothered" into the profession of psychology as fully licensed psychologists, and as these clauses in the statutes of each state ran out their periods of life, it became progressively obvious that it was difficult if not impossible for the psychologist members of these licensing boards to accurately judge whether or not the transcript of an applicant whose work was *not* in a bona fide department of psychology but who took some graduate courses in psychology did or did not meet the educational requirement of *a degree in psychology or its equivalent*. Help with this problem was requested by the state boards from a number of quarters, including the Education and Training Board and Board of Professional Affairs, as well as several other Committees and Divisions of the American Psychological Association (APA), the national organization of chairpersons of departments of psychology called the Council of Graduate Departments of Psychology (COGDOP), the American Association of State Psychology (Licensing) Boards (AASPB), the National Register of Health Service Providers in Psychology (National Register), the Association for the Advancement of Psychology (AAP), and related groups.

Concurrent with these pressures on psychology to define itself, which came from the psychology licensing constituencies, a new pressure from outside of psychology, per se was also coming from the arena of health insurance; it too would have a profound impact on the definition of a psychologist. Specifically, as private insurance companies, state accident insurance agencies, and other third-party payers of health care costs began to pay for mental health services provided by psychologists, these groups insisted that the profession of psychology differentiate which of its generically licensed psychologists were health service providers and which others, albeit also licensed as generic psychologists, were industrial psychologists, experimental psychologists, educational psychologists, and others whose training ipso facto did not qualify them to provide the *clinical* services to the mentally disabled which were covered by their policies.

The needs of licensing boards on the one hand and third-party payers on the other set into motion a series of ad hoc forces during the early 1970s which, over the next decade, would coalesce into a national consensus. As a result of a number of formal court challenges by applicants for licensure whose doctoral degrees were *not* earned in departments of psychology but who alleged they nevertheless met the requirement of ". . . or its equivalent," by 1975 it became clear to state psychology licensing boards that the courts (especially the ruling in *Berger vs. Board of Psychologist Examiners,* in the District of Columbia) and not the discipline of psychology would fill the vacuum left when organized psychology opted not to formally define the core curriculum which differentiated a graduate as a generic psychologist as against other graduates whose program of study was in departments or fields other than psychology. Second, as a response to the needs of third-party payers, a private corporation, the Council for the National Register of Health Service Providers in Psychology, with offices in the headquarters of the American Psychological Association, also was established in 1975. In the first ten years of its existence, and with informal input from APA committees on which standards to apply, it has examined the educational credentials of a large number of psychologists and has certified, via publication of their names in a hardcover national register available to third-party payers, some 14,600 psychologists who meet the profession's standard of education (graduation from a program designated by the *National Register* as being a doctoral program in psychology), as well as training and experience to qualify each of them as a fee-for-service health service provider. Between 1974 and 1975 these efforts of the AAASP and the National Register were coordinated with the counterpart boards and committees of the APA, notably with the Committee on Accreditation of the Education and Training Board and with the Committee on Standards for Providers of Psychological Services of the Board of Professional Affairs. And, working collectively via a National Task Force on Education and Credentialing, they launched a search for a definition which could be accepted by all of psychology's constituencies of what curricular qualifications must be met by a unit of an educational institution wishing to be publicly designated as offering a Ph.D. or Psy.D. degree following graduate study in psychology.

Psychology Accepts a Mandated Minimum Graduate Curriculum

Once psychology left the halls of academe and between 1945 and 1975 vigorously obtained licensure and the related statutory as well as quasi-legal claims to health insurance fees for its practitioners, it no longer was possible for it to define itself as both a science and a profession, as it had since 1945, but then *also* refuse to specify formally the subject matter which must be mastered by one of its doctorate-holding graduates who wishes a state license to practice that profession for a fee. By 1975 it became apparent to the APA, AASPB, the National Register, and the AAP (the latter established as an independent arm for American Psychology to lobby for needed federal and state legislation) that societal forces required psychology to define the core which differentiates it from other fields. Therefore with the advantages as well as disadvantages of some of the same persons serving on each of the parallel committees (Matarazzo 1977), after almost a decade of exchanging written communications, as well as joint meetings, at the beginning of 1985 representatives of the APA, the AASPB, COGDOP, and the National Register appeared to have reached a consensus on the minimum educational requirements ("the generic core") which must be met by a student with a doctoral degree based on study in a psychology department (or other psychology unit) in a regionally accredited institution of higher education.

That minimum core, put together from disparate drafts which have been circulating since 1975, and finally formally voted as official APA policy during the February 1985 meeting of the APA Council of Representatives, is shown in table 4.1. I feel confident that with few if any exceptions all the readers of this chapter who took their graduate work and degree in a department of psychology had courses in their doctoral program which satisfy all or most of this list of minimum core curriculum. The first two areas are not core psychology but involve tools and concepts scientists need and which have been in place in psychology for decades. The third and fourth areas are also discipline-specific and have been in place in most programs for years. The fifth area, ethics, was strongly recommended by the APA several years ago in letters to the faculties of departments of psychology not then offering such a course.

Areas 6 through 9 in table 4.1 are the core areas which involved considerable discussion before a consensus was achieved although, as a not unimportant aside, my study of the reports of the prior national conferences reveals little change in the four over the years (APA 1947, 545–51; Raimy 1950, 64). Nevertheless, even though codification was now being demanded by state boards and the insurance industry, etc., concession was made to local control by the broad wording (shown only in summary form in table 4.1) of these requisite four areas, plus the suggestion that any of a number of actual course titles or equivalent subject matter content in that area are qualifying. The examples which follow in parentheses are illustrative and, reinforcing a bit my point that there has been a consensus on the core content of psychology in every generation since 1890, have remained essentially unchanged in every Task Force draft since 1975: (*a*) *biological bases* (e.g., physiological psychology, comparative psychology, neuropsychology, psychopharmacology); (*b*) *cognitive-affective bases* (e.g., learning, memory, perception, cognition, thinking, motivation, emotion); (*c*) *social bases* (e.g., social psychology, cultural, ethnic and group processes, sex roles, organizational behavior); and (*d*) *individual differences* (e.g., personality theory, human development, individual differences, abnormal psychology, psychology of women, psychology of the handicapped, psychology of the minority experience).

TABLE 4.1 Minimum Graduate Educational Requirements Which Must Be Met by a Student Seeking Credentialing as the Holder of a Doctorate from a Psychology Department or Unit Which Has Been Nationally Designated as a Doctoral Program in Psychology

1. Research Design and Methodology
2. Statistics
3. Psychological Measurement (Psychometrics)
4. History and Systems of Psychology
5. Scientific and Professional Ethics and Standards
6. Biological Bases of Behavior
7. Cognitive-Affective Bases of Behavior
8. Social Bases of Behavior
9. Individual Differences
10. An Advanced Sequence of Studies appropriate to each graduate's later career "track" (e.g., an advanced research or professionally applied apprenticeship experience plus additional relevant courses in biology, neurosciences, chemistry, genetics, systems theory, computer sciences, mathematics, epidemiology, demography, anthropology, sociology, management science, linguistics, engineering)

In addition to the other nine required minimum offerings, listed in table 4.1, all programs must include an advanced sequence and apprenticeship experiences (area 10 of the list) appropriate to the area of psychology which represents the students' subsequent career goal (e.g., clinical, experimental, developmental, neuropsychology, health psychology, school psychology, etc.).

Formal ratification of the minimum educational requirements listed in table 4.1, by each of the four disparate constituencies, either individually, or then as a consortium, is the next step. As noted above, at its February 1985 meeting in Washington, D.C., the APA Council of Representatives, acting singly as necessary at this stage, formally adopted the criteria in table 4.1 as APA's official policy of what constitutes a doctoral program of study in psychology. This minimum program of graduate study must now be translated into practice by APA's various boards and committees. The decision was postponed to a subsequent meeting by the 1985 APA Council of Representatives as to whether APA would proceed alone (or in a consortium with AASPB, or the National Register, or COGDOP, or with others) in the next step of actually inviting applications from programs wishing to be so designated on a national roster as "doctoral programs in psychology."

My experience with each of these four constituencies suggests that ratification by the *elected* officers and members of all four national organizations may be easy for some and harder for others. Thus, APA already has ratified [1] the criteria in table 4.1, and the National Register, which has been using the criteria in table 4.1 as its official policy for some time, will very likely continue to use it as their official definition of what constitutes a doctoral program in psychology. However, given the centuries' old tradition of university faculty jealously guarding their right to decide their own curricular offerings, I would not be surprised if a majority of the members of the Council of Graduate Departments of Psychology (COGDOP) vote *not* to become official members of the proposed consortium, thereby indicating COGDOP's disapproval of a national system of designation. Additionally, after what I expect may be quick approval of the criteria by the (psychologist) members on the Executive Committee of the American Association of State Psychology Boards, themselves, I suspect the next step in AASPB (agreeing to a consortium) will take a number of years. That is, even if a consortium concept is ratified by the AASPB officers, it is well known that state legislatures move slowly. Therefore, in those states where such standards-clarification "housekeeping" actions of the nationally affiliated, member psychology Boards of AASPB are not automatically accepted by the legislature of that state but must be ratified by a specific amendment of the original authorizing legislation, such legislatures act slowly and it may be a number of years before the list in table 4.1 actually becomes mandated by *statute* in each of the fifty states and the District of Columbia. However, this quite likely will present little or no problem even in such states inasmuch as a future applicant wishing to be credentialed as a psychologist by the National Register still will have had to be educated in a department of psychology whose doctoral program is publicly designated (if not also credentialed) by APA as offering and requiring the courses listed.

This latter suggests one other point which needs to be clarified in relation to the ten criteria listed in table 4.1; namely the distinction between a doctoral program which the APA, AASP, COGDOP, and National Register, acting individually or as a consortium for the whole discipline of psychology, designate as a *psychology* doctoral program and a program to which the Accreditation Committee of APA has given its seal of accreditation. *Designa-*

1. As another index of its desire to bow to the strong feelings being expressed by some university psychology departments, at its subsequent August 1985 meeting the APA Council of Representatives reopened and thus put on temporary hold any *implementation* of its January 1985 decision which officially adopted the criteria in table 4.1. However, that same week the elected officers of the National Register and AASPB voted to proceed to develop plans for a consortium consisting of their two bodies to affect a national designation system.

tion means that a psychology program has undergone an initial evaluation of its curricular offerings by the discipline (in this case one or more members of the consortium) and has satisfied the ten criteria listed here in table 4.1 (plus several relatively less substantive criteria involving faculty and institutional administrative issues). *Accreditation* is a second-stage process and is accorded after a program designated by any member of the consortium to be a psychology doctoral program requests APA to evaluate the *quality* of the entire program, including the curricular offerings, listed in table 4.1, and is found to meet the APA's standards.

Generic Psychologist versus Specialist in Psychology

What these developments, which have led to what essentially is now the mandated generic core shown in table 4.1, have done is to codify what, as I discussed above, because of the use of similar textbooks has been the de facto requirement for graduates of psychology departments since 1890. The minimum shown in table 4.1, which, by 1985, the elected officers of APA, AASPB, and the National Register have recommended member departments should require of *all* students receiving a doctorate via psychology and not only those aiming for a professional career, *will* very nicely differentiate students with doctorates via study in psychology from their counterparts with doctorates via study in education, in the family and child, in special education, in business administration, in personnel management, etc. However, for students and faculty in psychology who increasingly are showing interest in the relationship of health psychology to other segments of psychology (the issue being addressed in this chapter), the requirements in table 4.1 which are just being promulgated will only publicly clarify what has been the fact since 1890, which is what I implied earlier in this chapter. Namely, a recipient of a doctoral degree from a university following study in a *department of psychology* in geographically widely separated institutions of higher learning throughout our country has been and today still is a *generic psychologist* upon receipt of that degree. Specifically, whether the psychology courses taken were "required" or "elective," upon graduation the transcript will show that he or she has had a core of educational experiences which had a great deal in common with recipients of doctorates from all other *departments of psychology* throughout our land.

This core of predoctoral education in psychology, despite the differing minor or advanced fields of study and the various laboratory, internship, or other apprenticeship experiences which are chosen by different graduate students in psychology, still makes each graduate of a psychology department more similar than different no matter what "extras" he or she took in their individualized minor track in psychology. Additionally, in regard to the role of these extras vis-à-vis later credentialing as a specialist, the graduate of a doctoral program which is publicly designated as one in psychology is not unlike the products of our law, medical, and dental schools, each of which permits the students a choice of electives (a "minor" track), but no one of which gives the student a *specialty* degree at the doctoral level. With few exceptions the doctoral degrees awarded in the United States in all *scientific-academic* and *professional* fields, even in 1985, are generic in that discipline. In each, as in psychology, if it exists at all "specialization" occurs in the postdoctoral and not the predoctoral period of training.

One Generic Psychology but Many Applications

Although the profession of psychology has *postdoctorally* credentialed[2] professional psychologists as "specialists" in clinical, counseling, school, industrial-organizational, neuro, and forensic psychology following the formation of the American Board of Professional Psychology in 1947, as just stated the field of psychology (operating via our APA) has continued to opt *not* to encourage university departments of psychology to offer programs of study at the *predoctoral* level which would lead to specialty credentialing at the time one received the doctorate. What this means to me is that, since 1947 what the disparate constituencies of leadership in the science and profession of psychology each have sensed is that, although there is one core body of knowledge and subject matter in psychology, a core easily ascertained from the table of contents of our best introductory psychology textbooks, after receipt of the doctorate that generic core may be *applied* by psychologists pursuing their individual interests to (or in) any of a number of widely differing areas, problems, settings, or challenges. Thus, to my mind, in 1985 physiological psychology is little more (selections from component 10, table 4.1) than generic psychology (components 6 through 9) ethically applied to individuals and problems involving the sense organs and other physiological systems; child psychology is the *same* core of knowledge applied to children (component 10); and industrial psychology is no more than the *same* core psychology applied to clients and problems in industry. Likewise, clinical, military, and consumer psychology are nothing more than the selections from a single body of knowledge (areas 6−9) which (follow-

---

2. My companion chapter on postdoctoral training in this volume asserts that, though there is *de facto* acceptance of these ABPP-designated "specialties" in psychology, not one of them, including clinical psychology, has to date achieved *de jure* recognition as a bona fide specialty.

ing selections from component 10) are applied to problems encountered, respectively, in clinical, military, or consumer settings. Although possibly
sounding by now a bit redundant, I am continuing to phrase and rephrase
this same point because, even at the May 1983 National Conference on
Graduate Education and Training in Health Psychology held at Arden House,
I found *considerable* disagreement with this thesis from colleagues whose
opinions I respect. Writing the present chapter has afforded me the needed
opportunity to better articulate my own views (and their bases) on these
issues.

Health Psychology in 1985 is Generic Psychology Applied to Health

Having arrived at this point the reader will not be surprised, therefore, that
in my mind *health* psychology is today nothing more than the application of
the accumulated knowledge from the science and profession of generic psychology to the arena of health. That is, as with each of my other examples in
the preceding paragraph, psychology is the *noun* and the term health (or
clinical, industrial, military, physiological, consumer, etc.) is the *adjective*
describing the client, setting, or problem area in which (or toward which)
psychology, including its task-specific knowledge and skills, is applied. What
I am sharing is my belief that in 1985 we still do not have *even one* bona
fide, universally acknowledged specialty in psychology. I believe this even
though, (1) I acknowledge the role of the "extras" (component 10 of the list)
we allow to be added to the core generic predoctoral curriculum which is
shown in table 4.1; (2) the credentialing process we have set in place since
1948 via accreditation by APA of each of several predoctoral specialty
"tracks" in doctoral programs; and (3) by the more mature beginning definition of a specialist since 1947 via a diploma which is conferred by the
American Board of Professional Psychology (ABPP) to successful applicants
five years after receipt of their doctorate. While individually and collectively
important, these three processes are in 1985 only the first steps toward what
in my mind (see note 2) one day will be robust, more universally acknowledged specialties in psychology.

The interested reader will find my views on the sociology of a profession
and some of the steps by which a specialty evolves, and is sanctioned,
detailed in an earlier publication (Matarazzo 1983, 92–94). In brief, in
common with "neuro" psychology, or "consumer" psychology or "child"
psychology, etc., health psychology will not become a *specialty* which is dis-
cernibly unique relative to the rest of psychology until it has gone through a
number of stages through which all fields ultimately designated as specialties

have to evolve. These stages for health psychology quite likely will need to include at a minimum (1) our own national and international associations of health psychologists (the former was accomplished in 1978 with the establishment of Division 38 within APA and the latter in 1984 with the creation of a Division of Health Psychology within the International Association of Applied Psychology), (2) a larger number of our own journals in addition to Division 38's present *Health Psychology,* and (3) acknowledgement from our peers in psychology and colleagues in sister professions, via the mechanisms of designation, accreditation and licensure, that the subject matter, methodologies, and applications of health psychology differ substantially from their own. (Despite the insistence by some Division 38 members that health psychology *is* different, it is my repeated experience that few members of other APA Divisions, intuitively recalling what was shown in table 4.1 for *all* psychologists, acknowledge that we are different in background than they, let alone practice as if we are). Furthermore, I have yet to meet a physician faculty member in any of the *many* community and university hospitals I have visited throughout our land in the past five years who differentiated a health psychologist from a clinical or medical or neuropsychologist or other health related psychologist. Once these first three hurdles are passed, there still will *not* be a bona fide *specialty* of health psychology. Other hurdles to overcome will be (4) as described in chapter 26, the development of postdoctoral training sites and a family of skills and procedures which are *specific* to health psychology as *distinct* from clinical and other areas of psychology; (5) the acknowledgement of the existence of the field of health psychology by NIH and other federal agencies which provide discipline-specific *health psychology* funds (through peer review by training committees and study sections) to support predoctoral and postdoctoral training programs, as well as research, in that field; (6) the establishment of departments of health psychology with that or a comparable name within medical schools, schools of public health, other university units, and hospitals; (7) the acceptance by our peers in and outside of psychology and by the courts that there are individuals who are experts in health psychology as differentiated from experts in clinical psychology or other areas of psychology; and (8) designation of health psychology as a bona fide, postdoctoral specialty area alongside the other specialty areas currently designated as such by the American Board of Professional Psychology, as well as still other related stages of development.

My belief that these eight steps are the minimum necessary ingredients before health psychology will be acknowledged as an emerging discipline with features distinctively different from the rest of psychology should not surprise anyone. The bases for my opinion are found in the development of our sister discipline of clinical psychology which, by 1985, has in my opinion almost surmounted all eight and may soon be acknowledged officially by APA and also de jure as well as de facto by *significant others* as a specialty area of psychology (although so designated as a specialty by the American Board during 1947–49). Specifically only today, thirty-six years after the Boulder Conference, is the APA able to reach a consensus and begin to promulgate (Sales, Bricklin, and Hall 1983) the necessary steps which one of its Divisions (or other subsets of psychologists representing special areas) must go through before its subject matter, client populations, proficiencies required, and professional services offered will be recognized as the minimum aggregate for it to be recognized as a bona fide specialty within psychology. The details of this new development are less relevant here than they are for my companion chapter (chap. 26) and therefore will be addressed there. Furthermore, only four years ago (and some thirty-two years after Boulder) was the APA, also for the first time, able to articulate the guidelines required for an agency to be officially designated as a setting (note, *not* as an individual specialist) qualified to deliver services in the area of clinical psychology (APA 1981). Anyone reading these needed ingredients to become a specialty (Sales et al. 1983) or to offer services (APA 1981) in a setting designated by our profession as offering specialty psychological services will discern from these two recent developments the many hurdles still to be surmounted by those who wish to differentiate health psychology (or neuropsychology, etc.) from generic psychology. Fortunately, the individuals representing the leadership of education and training in health psychology who were at the 1983 Arden House Conference took a few initial steps and outlined mechanisms by which to *begin* communication with the APA Accreditation Committee, ABPP, the National Register, AASPB, COGDOP, and other constituencies with which health psychology will need to interface on its way one day to being designated as a specialty.

As I reflect on the many hurdles still to be met, it is my opinion that health psychology will not be a generally recognized specialty area in psychology for at least another decade. I am not unaware that there will be some colleagues who can, will, and should muster arguments counter to mine. Clearly my opinion reflects no more than the sum of my own experiences. Nevertheless, I have not reached this opinion without considerable thought and based on some relevant experiences with a number of the different constituencies (including the two developments in APA just described) which will interface with the interested Division 38 members who wish to begin the steps needed for us to evolve through the eight processes I discussed earlier in this section. These experiences plus my thirty-five years of full-time work in a medical school as a teacher of students of medicine as well as students in our own psychology Ph.D. program, as a service provider, and as a scientist lead me to conclude that, for the moment, health psychology will continue to be defined by *significant others* as the professional and scientific *application* of the subject matter of generic psychology (items 6–9 of table 4.1) to the field of health (item 10). In sum, the noun *health psychology* is not yet a widely accepted one. Rather, it is my perception that in 1985 health is and must still be considered an adjective before the noun *psychology*.

Summary

Health psychology is a vibrant family of health-specific applications of psychology which has shown rapid growth since the establishment within the APA in 1978 of a Division of Health Psychology (Division 38). However, in my mind the term "health" is an adjective which defines the arena in which the core knowledge in the science and profession of psychology is applied, and thus, there is *not* today a health psychology which differs from psychology proper. This view may not surprise most members of Division 38 inasmuch as only in 1978–79 they accepted the following definition which I offered as the charter president of that Division: "Health psychology is the aggregate of the specific educational, scientific, and professional contributions of the discipline of psychology to the promotion and maintenance of health, the prevention and treatment of illness, the identification of etiologic and diagnostic correlates of health, illness, and related dysfunction [plus the following clause which subsequently was added by vote of the Division 38 membership], and to the analysis and improvement of the health care system and health policy formation" (Matarazzo 1980, 815; 1982, 4). In my opinion, this initial working definition, to which Division 38 members still appear to subscribe, states quite clearly that "health" psychology is the application of the common body of knowledge of psychology previously listed here in table 4.1 to any of a number of venues in the arena of health. As new information is accumulated and we add to and delete from the basic core of psychology, this continuing synthesis and resynthesis will determine *what* elements of our discipline (psychology) are applied; whereas the needs of society plus advancements in our techniques will coalesce to determine *how* and in what *directions* (including health) of potential specialization psychology will be applied by our scientists and service providers. In sum, then, it is my belief that in 1985 health psychology is best described to ourselves and others as generic psychology applied in a particular area (health) by scientists and service providers.[3] One of the necessary steps by which health psychology can begin to qualify itself as a bona fide specialty of psychology is through the establishment of nationally designated and accredited postdoctoral training programs which are publicly identified as offering preparation for work as a specialist in that field.

3. The reader will not be surprised that I hold this same view in relation to clinical, neuro-, social, child, experimental, and other areas of psychology.

REFERENCES

American Psychological Association, Committee on Training in Clinical Psychology. 1947. Recommended graduate training program in clinical psychology. *American Psychologist* 2:539–58.
American Psychological Association. 1981. Specialty guidelines for the delivery of services by clinical psychologists. *American Psychologist* 36:640–51.
Matarazzo, J. D. 1977. Higher education, professional accreditation, and licensure. *American Psychologist* 32:856–59.
———. 1980. Behavioral health and behavioral medicine: Frontiers for a new health psychology. *American Psychologist* 35:807–17.
———. 1982. Behavioral health's challenge to academic, scientific, and professional psychology. *American Psychologist* 37:1–14.
———. 1983. Education and training in health psychology: Boulder or bolder. *Health Psychology:* 2:73–113.
Raimy, V. 1950. *Training in clinical psychology.* New York: Prentice Hall.
Roe, A., J. W. Gustad, B. V. Moore, S. Ross, and M. Skodak. eds. 1959. *Graduate education in psychology.* Washington, D.C.: American Psychological Association.
Sales, B., P. Bricklin, and J. Hall. 1983. *Manual for the identification and continued recognition of proficiencies and new specialties in psychology, August 1, 1983 Draft* (135 pp.). Washington, D.C.: American Psychological Association.

5
Health Psychology and Other Health Professions
Stephen M. Weiss

Introduction

The various subspecialties of psychology have been involved in health and disease issues for several decades (Stone 1979; Schofield 1976, 1979). Until the early 1970s, with the establishment of the American Psychological Association's (APA) Task Force on Health Research (1976), however, little formal recognition was evident for the role of psychologists in areas beyond mental health and illness. The report of this Task Force, the creation of a Section on Health Research in the Division of Psychologists in Public Service of the APA and, finally, the formation of the APA Division of Health Psychology in 1978, provided a conceptual and political framework for the application of psychological principles to physical as well as mental health-illness issues.

In the mid 1970s, another development was taking place which would profoundly affect the role of psychologists in health settings. Frustrated by the inadequacies of the traditional conceptualization of "psychosomatic medicine," a group of disaffected biomedical and behavioral scientists met at Yale in early 1977 to formally establish the field of behavioral medicine (Schwartz and Weiss 1978). A meeting the following year hosted by the Institute of Medicine at the National Academy of Sciences resulted in the formation of the Academy of Behavioral Medicine Research and the Society of Behavioral Medicine (Schwartz and Weiss 1978). Most importantly, it developed a definition for the field which has served to clarify the unique parameters of behavioral medicine: "Behavioral medicine is the interdisciplinary field concerned with the development and integration of behavioral and biomedical science knowledge and techniques relevant to the understanding of health and illness and the application of this knowledge and these techniques to prevention, diagnosis, treatment and rehabilitation."

These events challenged both the behavioral and biomedical science communities to consider ways of capitalizing on the potential synergy of such multidisciplinary interactions. It also placed a new set of responsibilities on all involved disciplines in terms of adequately preparing themselves to enhance existing relationships and to create new ones. If health psychology is truly the contribution of the discipline of psychology to health and illness concerns, then this places particular responsibility on the leaders of this emerging subdiscipline to ensure that health psychologists are properly trained to take full advantage of the interactive opportunities offered by the interdisciplinary field of behavioral medicine.

In the spring of 1983, the Arden House Conference on Education and Training examined the role, functions, and responsibilities of health psychologists in the following health-related venues: basic research, applied research, health care services, health policy and industrial/organizational settings (Stone 1983). It became obvious to the conferees that the breadth of actual and potential opportunities for psychologists to make signal contributions to the vexing disease prevention and control issues facing our nation rested in large measure upon the adequacy and appropriateness of the training they would receive. To a great extent this training would require extensive interaction with and understanding of scientists and professionals from other health-related disciplines (DiMatteo and Friedman 1982).

In this chapter we will briefly review the various health-related disciplines with which psychologists may interact within each venue, as well as the research, application, or policy issues which might encourage such multidisciplinary interaction. Finally, we will consider recommendations for expanding the role of the psychologist in the health system.

Basic Research

There is a long history of basic research within the biomedical and the behavioral sciences, but such developments have occurred along parallel rather than interactive lines until recent times. Classic studies of experimental analogues of human cardiovascular disease, for example, have traditionally neglected behavioral considerations, whereas behavioral studies have rarely considered, for example, the biochemical sequelae of environmental manipulations. The importance of controlling for, if not systematically manipulating, both biological and behavioral variables is becoming increasingly evident to all relevant scientists.

In examining the role of biobehavioral factors at, for example, the "brain-body" mechanism level, one must establish within the relevant scientific communities a reciprocal appreciation for the potential contributions of the neurosciences, physiology, biochemistry, anatomy, and biology as well as those of psychology, anthropology and sociology, among others. Also various "hybrid" specialties have emerged in recent years (e.g., biopsychology, neurocardiology, sociobiology) to focus effort on new emerging areas which crosscut traditional disciplinary lines.

It is essential that health psychologists interested in pursuing careers in basic health research receive both pre- and postdoctoral coursework in and experience with the biomedical sciences to properly equip them to function in these increasingly multidisciplinary settings. To address biobehavioral research issues of common concern to the physiologist, neuroscientist, and the health psychologist, for example, all disciplines must understand both the language and the theoretical perspective of their counterpart disciplines. For health psychologists, combining their behavioral expertise with the knowledge and skills of the physiologist in organ/systems structure and function can be a major step toward addressing a given problem at the level of complexity at which it presents itself. Adding the input of the neuroscientist and the bioengineer further increases both the complexity and the potential of scientific endeavors.

Ideal as this all might sound, it is unlikely to take place unless very careful consideration is given to the development of such activities. Although the concept of behavioral medicine strongly supports this "marriage" of disciplines, how to accomplish this goal is a major challenge, particularly for psychologists. Although the situation is changing (for the better) in many parts of the country, the majority of basic health research activity does not involve psychologists and has yet to see the need for doing so. In other parts of the world, including psychologists on basic research teams is *extremely* rare. Thus, we need to consider the existing obstacles and develop strategies for helping the uninitiated basic biomedical scientists to become more familiar with the potential contributions of psychologists to their efforts.

Although the potential range of options are myriad, there are a few basic points one must keep in mind. For example, pre- and postdoctoral exposure to the training programs of the biomedical sciences is extremely important not only because the content is relevant, but because the *process* is critical to understanding the "gut-level" perspective and approach of the biomedical scientist to a given problem. As one quickly realizes with experience, the amount of variance biomedical scientists will tolerate in their measurement technology as compared to what is considered acceptable among the behavioral sciences is more than a mere "number" difference. There is also a tendency toward reductionistic thinking which strives to answer complex human function questions at the cellular level and an emphasis on attempting to generate single factor theories to explain multifactorial phenomena (psychologists can also be guilty of these predilections, albeit on a different functional level). It is probable that observing such tendencies in others helps us to recognize more readily similar predispositions in ourselves. In this way, gently yet persistently taking every opportunity to increase by one "j.n.d." one's counterpart discipline colleagues exposure to increasing levels of complexity helps both (all) parties to expand their scientific horizons. Although the process is admittedly slow, it is imperative that the psychologist be fully cognizant of the *current* framework and its parameters and limitations within which his or her colleagues feel at ease—and to begin from there, moving at a measured pace toward a more biobehavioral perspective.

Lipid biochemists, for example, are typically concerned with natural observations of lipid metabolism variation, the effects of dietary, structural, genetic and/or biochemical manipulations on lipoprotein subfractions and how such phenomena may relate to the disease of atherosclerosis. Their very success in characterizing the relative contributions of the above factors has led them to broaden the search for other relevant factors to account for still sizable portions of unexplained variance. In those cases where behavioral scientists have been present to recognize such opportunities, timely inputs to their biomedical colleagues have been extremely successful in opening new vistas of research opportunity (e.g., Kaplan et al., 1983; Manuck et al. 1983; Clarkson et al. 1986).

Furthermore, the biobehavioral approach stressing *interaction* among variables producing effects which cannot be obtained by the independent study of those variables (the *synergistic* potential) has collectively broadened our understanding of very complex phenomena. This combining of skills, perspectives, and approaches has led to exciting scientific breakthroughs which would have been impossible to achieve by the biomedical or behavioral scientist working independently of one another.

Finally, there is the hazard of being "too successful" in awakening our biomedical colleagues to the potentials of biobehavioral research. Expectations as to what behavioral scientists can contribute tend to escalate at an exponential rate (the other side of the pendulum), which places us in the uncomfortable position of promising more than we can deliver. Even allowing the appearance of such a situation to persist, once recognized, will inevitably come back to haunt and discredit us. Neal Miller's words, "be bold in what you try, but cautious in what you claim" sum it up very nicely.

Applied Research

As one moves from basic research (e.g., brain-body mechanism issues) to studies directly relevant to disease diagnosis, prevention and control, a new host of health related disciplines come into play. Health educators, physicians (all specialties), nurses, nutritionists, epidemiologists, pharmacologists, sociologists, anthropologists, exercise physiologists—even bioengineers may be involved in addressing research questions that require multidisciplinary attention.

The recent dramatic advances in noninvasive measurement have brought biotechnology into the mainstream of biobehavioral research (Herd et al. 1984). Ambulatory blood pressure monitoring, echocardiography, continuous "exfusion" (blood withdrawal) pumps, nuclear magnetic resonance, to name but a few of the instruments available today, allow us to obtain data undreamed of twenty years ago. Although these technologies have been available for some time, only within the past few years have behavioral scientists begun to incorporate them into their research armamentarium. Only recently, too, has theoretical formulation concerning the impact of environmental stressors upon the functioning of the intact organism reached the point where the hypotheses generated have demanded such sophisticated measurement devices for their testing. It is now incumbent on the biobehavioral research community to continue to actively engage the attention of the bioinstrumentation folk in the pursuit of expanded and more refined tools to explore increasingly complex patterns of brain physiology-behavior interactions.

Having such tools increasingly available has placed additional responsibility on both biomedical and behavioral scientists to use them well and wisely. To avoid the risk that biobehavioral science may become "data driven" (a button in search of a coat), we must formulate cogent theory which simultaneously addresses neural, genetic, physiologic, biochemical, behavioral, and sociocultural dimensions of the issue under study. To understand, for example, the complexity of hypertension differences between blacks and whites, all of the above factors must be considered. Therefore, we are confronted again with the need to become familiar with the language and perspective of the relevant discipline and how interaction among variables can produce a synergistic result that must be addressed at a more complex level than heretofore considered.

Clinical research involving diagnosis and treatment concerns involves various medical specialties, epidemiologists, pharmacologists, and exercise physiologists to name but a few of the relevant health disciplines (e.g., Palinkas and Hoiberg 1982). Health educators, nurses, even health economists have also become directly involved in life-style issues related to health behavior change (Singer and Krantz 1982).

Where does health psychology find itself in this plethora of disciplines? In fact, the health psychologist can make several unique contributions to this area—given proper training and experience. The fact that not all people benefit equally from *any* treatment, behavioral, biomedical, or biobehavioral, suggests issues of individual differences which may have genetic, behavioral, structural, or sociocultural correlates, perhaps in some combination. The study of individual differences has long been of interest to psychologists—this would just be an expansion of that theoretical approach into a multifactorial framework.

Compliance/adherence to medical regimens is another point of fruitful interface between a major biomedical issue and acknowledged expertise in motivation principles (Taylor 1978). Research in this area clearly extends into health care practices. In doing so, a significant bioethical issue for the health psychologist as a health professional arises: when performing compliance research or services in response to requests from the biomedical community, one must also address the ethical question of whether doing so is in the ultimate best interests of the patient. In taking a more holistic, integrated view of the individual, the practitioner, and the sociopolitical issues surrounding health research and health care, one must become "fully informed" of both the risks and benefits of specific treatment approaches, on the clinical as well as public health levels, to assure oneself that the benefits truly outweigh the risks. Where this is uncertain (as is the case many times) one must make a careful analysis of the pros and cons before rendering a professional judgment as to the nature and extent of one's involvement in such research or practice. It is insufficient and unprofessional to disregard these issues by confining one's contribution exclusively to the academic exercise of "pill counts" or number of appointments kept without cognizance of the potential ethical concerns associated with compliance research. Such confinement suggests one is functioning as a technician rather than as a fully qualified health professional.

Although traditionally psychologists have functioned at the clinical or individual level, epidemiologic population research has much to offer in terms of identifying promising leads, particularly in terms of diagnostic and prevention correlates with behavioral factors. Health psychologists need to become more familiar with the strengths and limitations of epidemiologic research to assist in identifying potentially meaningful relationships and interactions among behavioral and biomedical variables which can then be explored more intensively in controlled field or laboratory settings.

Health psychologists also need to become more familiar with public health research strategies involving risk-reduction efforts with large populations. Health educators have been extensively involved with this area for some time but could benefit from combining forces with psychologists who have the methodologic and learning theory expertise necessary to take full advantage of research opportunities, e.g., to assess alternative strategies for influencing behavior in health enhancing directions (Dwore and Matarazzo 1981).

Finally, physician research scientists have become increasingly interested in the potential synergism to be gained in joining forces with health psychologists. Neither group by themselves can adequately address all of the variables that increasingly appear to be involved in the prevention and control of disease. Research cardiologists, neurologists, pediatricians, diabetologists and oncologists, to name but a few are jointly authoring publications with health psychologists in increasing numbers—an objective indicator of research productivity and interdisciplinary activity. I have every reason to expect that this trend will continue to accelerate, providing we continue to provide well-trained health psychologists to meet the needs of the health research establishment.

Health Care Services

The role of health psychologists in the health care arena brings them into contact with a broad range of disciplines, in a wide variety of venues directly and indirectly related to health. (DeLeon et al. 1982; Schofield 1979). The provisions of services involves many diverse settings such as hospitals, HMOs, schools, worksites, clinics, and independent practice rehabilitation centers.

CLINICAL SERVICES

In most instances (including independent practice), the health psychologist will typically be working in close proximity to other health professionals as a member of a team or as a consultant specialist where his or her skills will provide information essential to the diagnostic, treatment, or planning process.

The health psychologist will be involved with such diverse disciplines as dentistry, pharmacology, physical therapy, law, nursing, nutrition, and health education (Dwore and Matarazzo 1981) as well as various specialties in clinical medicine.

Diagnostic issues such as those related to chronic lower-back pain, TMJ (temporomandibular joint syndrome), hypertension, angina pectoris, Raynaud's disease, neuropsychological impairment, and migraine headaches, among others will bring psychologists directly into the decision-making process in medical, legal, insurance, and policy-making arenas. As both consultant and team member/leader, the health psychologist will be asked to render professional opinions on nonmental health related issues which must be conveyed in language tailored to the recipient of this information.

In both diagnostic and treatment activities, the health psychologist must become thoroughly familiar with the prerogatives and responsibilities of the consultant/specialist as practiced in clinical medicine (e.g., Belar 1982). Learning (and scrupulously adhering to) the guidelines and standards of professional consultant/specialist practice in relation to the referring health care provider (usually a physician) will ensure effective working relationships and professional communications between the health professionals involved. Nothing will diminish one's credibility more quickly than disregarding (or being ignorant of) these standards relating to the consultant role (see chap. 9). For example, *prompt,* intelligible, and concise communication concerning highlights of the evaluation, diagnostic judgements, and treatment recommendations will reassure referring physicians that one is cognizant of their role as *primary* health care provider and is mindful of keeping them fully informed. If treatment recommendations involve continued contact with the health psychologist, they should be made in consultation with the referring physician. During the course of such treatment, the health psychologist should periodically advise the primary health care provider of the progress made. Upon completion of treatment, a final summary should be conveyed to the primary referral source. Likewise, when health psychologists are the referring health care providers (as is increasingly common), they can expect reciprocal consideration from consultant physicians or other health care professionals.

During the past several years, the nursing profession has become very interested in behavior modification strategies as applied to patient management and health life-style issues. Nurses are also becoming increasingly involved with health services research, although some of them have experienced problems in developing the methodological aspects of their proposals. As psychologists traditionally are noted for their strengths in learning theory and experimental design, collaboration among members of these two professions could yield benefits from sharing expertise on these issues. Nurses typically have *extensive* patient care experience and can be extremely helpful in facilitating/advising or collaborating on health care research in in- and outpatient settings. As collaborators, their skill in performing invasive measurement procedures can be particularly helpful in biobehavioral research.

A chapter on health psychology's relationship to other health professions would not be complete without mentioning psychiatry. Without belaboring the history of this relationship (see Arnett and Leichner 1982), the most salient issue with respect to health psychology concerns the opportunity (at last) for *direct* collaboration with biomedicine on problems that relate to the unique skills of the psychologist. The responsiveness of biomedicine to these opportunities has been reflected by the rapidly growing number of psychologists in medical settings with primary appointments outside of departments of psychiatry. Departments of medicine, family practice (Bibace and Walsh 1979), pediatrics (Wright 1979), orthopedics, rehabilitation, and surgery, as well as schools of dentistry and nursing are recognizing the desirability of having psychologists dedicating full-time efforts to their needs.

It goes without saying that psychiatry has felt threatened by this "realignment" and in many instances has very actively attempted to oppose such developments (fortunately "unsuccessfully," in most instances). There are a few hopeful signs that recognition by psychiatry of the "new realities" of psychology's role in health has engendered a willingness to consider ways of constructive coexistence in the health care environment. A most welcome development—and long overdue.

As concerns for cost-containment and appropriate utilization of health resources spawn health legislation creating (or supporting) new models of health care (e.g., DRGs, PPOs, HMOs), health psychologists will have long-awaited opportunities to demonstrate their ability to contribute meaningfully to health care problems in a cost-effective fashion (Davis 1982; Dorken and Associates 1986; Wiggins 1976). In the area of hypertension, for example, for which perhaps 40 to 60 million adults in this country may be at risk, the opportunities to work collaboratively with the medical profession in developing blood pressure control strategies using combinations of pharmacologic and nonpharmacologic techniques are becoming increasingly common. Recent research has demonstrated that such techniques hold the promise of developing rational treatment strategies for effective control of this epidemic disorder with significant reductions in medication requirements as compared to standard pharmacologic regimens (Patel et al. 1985; Engel et al. 1983). One can readily see the potential cost savings to the health care system of even minimal per-patient cost reduction when dealing with a health problem of this magnitude (Blanchard 1985).

Disease Prevention/Health Promotion

Although the province of health psychology spans the gamut from basic brain-body mechanism research to public health risk-reduction efforts, special emphasis should be placed on the psychologist's role in modifying health-threatening behaviors caused by life-style choices (Matarazzo 1980, 1982, 1984; Hamburg et al. 1982). Such issues are considered of paramount importance in the prevention of premature morbidity and mortality from chronic diseases and accidents. What we eat, drink, do (exercise), whether we smoke or wear seatbelts all involve habits that are ostensibly modifiable. The national attention now focused on disease prevention and health promotion will bring psychologists into intimate working contact with health educators, teachers, school nurses and administrators, community leaders, state and local health department officials, safety engineers, health economists, occupational physicians, and public policy-makers, among others (Dwore and Matarazzo 1981; Singer and Krantz 1982).

Such research and applied programs will take place at three levels: (1) schools, where the focus will be on health behavior *development;* (2) worksites, where the emphasis will be on health behavior *change* and health behavior *maintenance;* and (3) communities, where all three, health behavior *development, change,* and *maintenance* will be involved.

Health psychologists will be working with a broad variety of health-related personnel in each area. In schools, one will be dealing with school nurses and dietitians, health educators, plus individuals with various teaching and administrative responsibilities relevant to the conduct of the program. Worksite activities will involve occupational health physicians and nurses, nutritionists, exercise physiologists, management and labor "decision-makers," program developers, health economists, personnel specialists, as well as environmental engineers and space planners.

Community programs include most of the above in addition to public health officials; media representatives; community organization specialists; local medical, dental, and pharmaceutical groups; the local offices of the national voluntaries, such as the American Cancer Society and the American Heart Association; community hospitals, including HMOs and PPOs; not to mention the local community spokespersons. In the planning and implementing of community programs, the health psychologist will make heavy use of group process skills in establishing viable working relationships across disciplines and organizations.

Prepaid health care modes, such as health maintenance organizations (HMOs), are becoming increasingly widespread. Considering that the HMOs are the only health care organizations for which there are financial incentives for keeping people well, disease prevention and health promotion programs should be particularly relevant to their mission. Unfortunately, with a few notable exceptions (e.g., Kaiser-Permanente) the HMOs have taken a fairly conservative stance with regard to incorporating such strategies into their programs. Hopefully, research findings, which are gradually becoming available from large-scale industry-supported health promotion efforts, will encourage HMOs to invest more in the long-term implications of maintaining and enhancing health for their subscribers. Health psychologists should take every opportunity to explore such possibilities for program development in the course of their professional consultations with HMOs.

Training

As one considers the role of psychologists in relation to other health-related disciplines, it is also important to consider what these fields can offer to enhance or improve the psychologist's capabilities to function effectively in the health system. For example, when considering disease prevention models, epidemiology and public health typically deal with person-environment interactions at the "population" level rather than at the intra- or interpersonal levels (Singer and Krantz 1982). Such approaches are not only complementary to traditional psychological research but have the potential to expand such areas as attitude change, learning theory, values reorientation, and behavior maintenance to community-wide populations (Coates and De-Muth 1984).

Extern, intern, residency, and research fellowship opportunities in relevant health settings, plus the presence of effective health psychologist role models, will enable our emerging subdiscipline to take its place as a viable and essential discipline dedicated to the maintenance and enhancement of the nation's health (Tanabe 1982; also chap. 24).

To accomplish this, however, requires additional training in fields such as epidemiology, biostatistics, and public health issues (Palinkas and Hoiberg 1982). The same holds true for treatment or rehabilitation efforts. To fully utilize one's skills as a psychologist, one must become well versed in such biomedical areas as cardiovascular physiology and/or neurophysiology, biochemistry, and pharmacology, among others. Although the psychologist need not have the same depth of knowledge in each area as is required of those who represent those disciplines, one needs sufficient background in the theory, concepts, and techniques of each area relevant to a given health-illness issue to be able to "speak the language" on issues which cut across discipline boundaries.

Developing appropriate training opportunities, both for the new graduate as well as the *ancien combattant,* will continue to be a challenge to this new subdiscipline in the coming years. The Arden House Conference has provided an initial framework for this training by elucidating the knowledge and skill requirements in the various research and applied venues (Stone 1983). The emphasis on postdoctoral training as a formal, two-year training program speaks to the extensive body of information and skill development that must be acquired to assure optimal performance as health psychologists.

Health psychologists must also make themselves available in health professional training settings (medicine, nursing, dentistry, public health, etc.) to facilitate familiarity of these professions with health psychology's contribution to health research and practice as well as to public health issues of disease prevention and health promotion (Matthews and Avis 1982; Singer and Krantz 1982). As students of the learning process, psychologists have much to offer the health professions, particularly to medicine as it struggles to incorporate a steadily increasing number of complex issues in its predoctoral curriculum. In addition to content relevant to the practice of medicine, the *process* of acquisition and retention could be facilitated by encouraging more psychologists to contribute their unique skills toward improving the efficiency of medical education. For example, it is commonly accepted that medical students retain relatively little of their basic science studies of their first two years because it is not, in most cases, associated with pragmatic issues of patient diagnosis and care.

Upon reaching the third and fourth years of clinical clerkship, students must "relearn" this material so it can then be incorporated into patient-related decisions—a most inefficient system given the heavy demands placed on the four years of the predoctoral training period. By encouraging psychologists to become involved in this issue, the psychologists in training would become more conversant with the *content* of medical courses; and the efficiency of the learning process would improve.

Summary

Thus far, the development of health psychology holds tremendous potential for the field of psychology as a whole as well as for making signal contributions to the health status of the nation (Matarazzo 1984; Mickel 1982). With judicious guidance and maintenance of the current momentum, there is every reason to believe these expectations will come to fruition in the foreseeable future. Much will depend, however, on the health psychologist's skills on two levels: (a) having the requisite *content* knowledge to collaborate effectively with relevant health disciplines; and (2) having the requisite *process* skills to enhance multidisciplinary team functioning. Combining these capabilities with the generic, unique, contributions of the field of psychology to the critical problems of health and illness facing our world can result in a realignment of perspectives on the part of many disciplines concerning the most effective approach to the detection, prevention, and control of disease and the promotion of health.

REFERENCES

Arnett, J., and P. Leichner. 1982. Attitudes of psychiatry residents toward psychology. *Professional Psychology* 13 : 244 – 51.

Belar, C. D. 1982. Establishing health psychology services in an academic medical center. Paper presented at the annual meeting of the American Psychological Association, August 1982, Washington, D.C.

Bibace, R., and M. E. Walsh. 1979. Clinical developmental psychologists in family practice settings. *Professional Psychology* 10 (4): 441 – 50.

Clarkson, T., S. Manuck, and J. Kaplan. 1986. Potential role of cardiovascular reactivity in atherogenesis. In *Handbook of stress, reactivity, and cardiovascular disease,* edited by K. A. Matthews, S. M. Weiss, T. Detre, T. M. Dembroski, B. Falkner, S. B. Manuck, and R. B. Williams, 35 – 47. New York: John Wiley & Sons.

Coates, T., and N. DeMuth. 1984. An analysis of competencies and training needs for psychologists specializing in health enhancement. In *Behavioral health: A handbook of disease prevention and health enhancement,* edited by J. D. Matarazzo, N. E. Miller, S. M. Weiss, J. A. Herd, and S. M. Weiss, 1196 – 1203. NY: John Wiley and Sons.

Davis, C. 1982. Commitment and cost control in the health care system. *American Psychologist* 37 (12): 1359 – 61.

DeLeon, P. H., M. S. Pallak, and J. A. Heffernan. 1982. Hospital health care delivery. *American Psychologist* 37 : 1340 – 41.

DiMatteo, M. R., and H. S. Friedman. 1982. *Social psychology and medicine.* Cambridge, MA: Oelgeschlager, Gunn, & Hain, Publishers, Inc.

Dörken, H., and Associates. 1986. *Professional psychology in transition: Meeting today's challenges.* San Francisco: Jossey-Bass.

Dwore, R., and J. Matarazzo. 1981. The behavioral sciences and health education: Disciplines with a compatible interest? *Health Education* (May – June): 4 – 7.

Engel, B., M. Glasgow, and K. Gaarder. 1983. Behavioral treatment of high blood pressure: III. Follow-up results and treatment recommendations. *Psychosomatic Medicine* 45 (1): 23 – 29.

Hamburg, D., G. Elliott, and D. Parron. 1982. *Health and behavior: frontiers of research in the biobehavioral sciences.* Washington, D.C.: National Academy Press.

Herd, J. A., A. Gotto, P. Kaufmann, and S. M. Weiss. 1984. *Cardiovascular instrumentation: Applicability of new technology to biobehavioral research.* U.S. Department of Health and Human Services. NIH Publication no. 84 – 1654. Washington, D.C.: U.S. Government Printing Office.

Kaplan, J., S. Manuck, T. Clarkson, F. Lusso, D. Taub, and E. Miller. Social stress and atherosclerosis in normocholesterolemic monkeys. *Science* 220 : 733 – 35.

Manuck, S., J. Kaplan, and T. Clarkson. 1983. Behaviorally induced heart rate reactivity and atherosclerosis in cynomolgus monkeys. *Psychosomatic Medicine* 45:95–108.

Matarazzo, J. D. 1980. Behavioral health and behavioral medicine: Frontiers for a new health psychology. *American Psychologist* 35:807–17.

———. 1982. Behavioral health's challenge to academic, scientific and professional psychology. *American Psychologist* 37:1–14.

———. 1984. Behavioral health: A 1990 challenge for the health sciences professions. In *Behavioral health: A handbook of health enhancement and disease prevention,* edited by J. D. Matarazzo, S. M. Weiss, A. Herd, N. E. Miller, and S. M. Weiss, 1–40. NY: John Wiley and Sons.

Matthews, K. A., and N. E. Avis. 1982. Psychologists in schools of public health: Current status, future prospects, and implications for other health settings. *American Psychologist* 37:949–54.

Mickel, C. 1982. Innovative projects earning psychologists spots on hospital health care teams. *American Psychologist* 37:1350–54.

Palinkas, L., and A. Hoiberg. 1982. An epidemiology primer: Bridging the gap between epidemiology and psychology. *Health Psychology* 1:269–78.

Patel, C., M. Marmot, D. Terry, M. Carruthers, B. Hunt, and M. Patel. 1985. Trial of relaxation in reducing coronary risk: Four-year follow-up. *British Medical Journal* 290:1103–6.

Schofield, W. 1976. The psychologist as a health professional. *Professional Psychology* 7(1):5–8.

———. 1979. Clinical psychologists as health professionals. In *Health psychology: A handbook,* edited by G. C. Stone, F. Cohen, and N. E. Adler, 447–63. San Francisco: Jossey-Bass Publishers.

Schwartz, G. E., and S. M. Weiss. 1978a. *Proceedings of the Yale Conference on Behavioral Medicine.* DHEW Publication no. (NIH) 78–1424. Washington, D.C.: U.S. Government Printing Office.

———. 1978b. Behavioral medicine revisited: An amended definition. *Journal of Behavioral Medicine* 1:249–51.

Singer, J. E., and D. S. Krantz. 1982. Perspectives on the interface between psychology and public health. *American Psychologist* 37:955–60.

Stone, G. C. 1979. Psychology and the health system. In *Health psychology: A handbook,* edited by G. C. Stone, F. Cohen, and N. E. Adler, 47–75. San Francisco: Jossey-Bass Publishers.

———, ed. 1983. National working conference on education and training in health psychology. *Health Psychology* 2: supplement section.

Tanabe, G. 1982. The potential for public health psychology. *American Psychologist* 37:942–44.

Taylor, S. E. 1978. A developing role for social psychology in medicine and medical practice. *Personality and Social Psychology Bulletin* 4:515–23.

Wiggins, J. 1976. The psychologist as a health professional in the health maintenance organizations. *Professional Psychology* 7 (1): 9–13.

Wright, L. 1979. Health care psychology: Prospects for the well-being of children. *American Psychologist* 34:1001–6.

Part Two

The Knowledge Base
Editor: Neal E. Miller

In all fields of science, there are complex symbiotic relationships between research and application (Conant 1947). New knowledge from research provides the basis for new practical applications. Sometimes the steps are rather simple and direct, but often they are unexpected and may occur after a considerable lapse of time. In a monumental study, Comroe and Dripps (1976, 1977) investigated the history of the ten clinical advances in the broad area of pulmonary and cardiovascular medicine that a panel of ninety knowledgeable physicians and surgeons had rated as being of the greatest value to their patients. They found that of the 663 key articles essential for these clinical advances, forty-two percent reported research done by scientists whose goal at that time was unrelated to the later clinical advance. On the other hand, the results of practical applications supply the rationale for supporting both basic and applied research. Furthermore, encounters with the applied situation suggest fruitful new theoretical problems for investigation, and techniques developed during the course of practical applications open up new possibilities for research. The complex interactions among practical applications, basic, and applied research are illustrated in a book on the history of chlorpromazine (Swazey 1974). The rapidly developing area of health psychology is yielding additional examples of such symbiotic interactions (Miller 1983).

The following three chapters illustrate in detail the ways in which in health psychology the requirements for training in basic or applied research in the laboratory or in the field have many more similarities than differences. In chapter 6 on laboratory research, Neil Schneiderman describes the wide range of interdisciplinary training that is useful and the different opportunities for postdoctoral support of such training. He describes the chief sources of support for research in health psychology and the wide range of topics being investigated. The chapter concludes with examples from the author's laboratory of how different areas of social, experimental, and physiological psychology, neuroanatomy, neurophysiology, and other biomedical sciences can be integrated into a research program.

Chapter 7, by Nancy Adler, Shelley Taylor, and Camille Wortman, is on basic field research in health psychology and emphasizes the desirability of incorporating theoretical considerations into applied field research and also of designing basic field research projects so that they also will yield some information of direct practical value. From the wealth of their experience, they present an extremely valuable survey of the many practical problems that are likely to be encountered in either basic or applied field research and of useful ways of dealing with these problems.

Chapter 8 by Jerome Singer, on training for applied research in health psychology, reiterates the need for interdisciplinary training. He points out that investigators conducting applied research frequently have their problems assigned to them rather than being free to choose problems that suit their own personal interests and skills. Therefore, they have, if anything, a greater need for broad training than those in basic research. Since they often have to analyze situations that were designed for other purposes, they also have an especially great need for knowledge of sophisticated techniques of statistical analysis.

Finally, I would like to point out that, as the pressure to contain rapidly increasing medical expenses continues to mount, one increasingly important area of research in health psychology will be that of evaluating the cost-effectiveness of the various behavioral techniques used in medical settings. As the financial pressure on them continues to intensify, legislators and the administrators of health care programs are likely to become increasingly responsive to such data.

REFERENCES

Comroe, J. H., Jr.; and R. D. Dripps. 1976. Scientific basis for the support of biomedical science. *Science* 192:105–11.

Comroe, J. H., Jr.; and R. D. Dripps. 1977. *The top ten clinical advances in cardiovascular-pulmonary medicine and surgery, 1945–1975. Final report, January 31, 1977.* Bethesda, MD: National Heart, Lung, and Blood Institute.

Conant, J. B. 1947. *On understanding science.* New Haven, CT: Yale University Press.

Miller, N. E. 1983. Behavioral medicine: Symbiosis between laboratory and clinic. *Annual Review of Psychology* 34:1–31.

Swazey, J. P. 1974. *Chlorpromazine in psychiatry: A study of therapeutic innovation.* Cambridge, MA: MIT Press.

6

Basic Laboratory Research in Health Psychology

Neil Schneiderman

The National Working Conference on Education and Training in Health Psychology (1983, 9) reached the consensus that "health psychology is a generic field of psychology, with its own body of theory and knowledge, which is differentiated from other fields in psychology." Although a generic field in its own right, health psychology draws upon the traditional areas of biological, clinical, cognitive/learning, developmental/child and personality/social psychology to contribute uniquely to the scientific understanding of how psychosocial and biobehavioral processes influence the prevention, progression, and treatment of physical disorders. By its nature, research in health psychology also contributes to the broad interdisciplinary field of *behavioral medicine,* which is concerned with the integration of biomedical and psychosocial knowledge as it impacts upon the etiology, pathogenesis, diagnosis, treatment, and prevention (including rehabilitation) of physical disorders (Schwartz and Weiss 1978a, 1978b).

This chapter deals with basic laboratory research in health psychology. It is concerned with the training required to be a basic scientist in this field and with the opportunities available for conducting important health-related research. At the outset it must be admitted that it is difficult, if not impossible, to distinguish fixed boundaries between basic and applied research in health psychology because the ultimate objective of all research in health psychology has the applied goal of improving human health. In some instances it is also becoming difficult to distinguish between laboratory and field research in health psychology and behavioral medicine because investigators have begun to find innovative ways to improve stimulus control and manipulate variables in field settings and combine laboratory experimentation and field studies in unique ways.

The primary goal of basic laboratory research is to provide new scientific information about fundamental processes. As such, basic research is usually theoretically driven. In contrast, strictly applied research asks such questions as whether a particular treatment method is effective or whether one therapeutic intervention is more efficacious than another. In practice the distinction can become blurred because thoughtful comparisons between treatments may provide useful insights about fundamental processes.

Basic laboratory research in health psychology differs from other basic laboratory research in psychology only in its emphasis on addressing questions that are relevant to health. Thus, in a health psychology experiment, the independent variable is thought to be health-related and/or changes in the dependent variable are believed to have implications for physical health.

Laboratory research is traditionally distinguished from field research in terms of controlled manipulation of the independent variable. As Singer points out in chapter 8, there is a tradeoff between greater control and precision in the laboratory with greater ecological validity in the field. Increasingly, however, health psychologists have begun to use both methods in complementary fashion. Thus, for example, in their studies of social instability and coronary artery atherosclerosis in cynomolgus monkeys, Manuck, Kaplan, and Clarkson (1983) took animals being observed under field conditions and subjected them to psychosocial reorganization in a controlled manner. The animals were also subjected under experimental control to a behaviorally stressful stimulus. In our own human research, my research group has been using measures of psychophysiological reactivity in the laboratory to predict ambulatory blood pressure measurements in the workplace. Because those interested in basic research problems in health psychology may expect to do some of their work at the interfaces between psychology and medical disciplines, basic and applied research, and laboratory and field studies, there is need for both broad-based research training and an understanding of the research opportunities that are available.

Training

The task group on basic research at the Arden House Conference felt that the unique skills of the health psychologist include those at the interface between traditional areas of psychology and health psychology and those at the interface between psychology and various biomedical disciplines (National Working Conference on Education and Training in Health Psychology 1983, 67–68). It was felt that those desiring to become basic research scientists in health psychology must learn to apply basic behavioral research skills to the study of health and disease and develop relevant models based upon these relationships.

Training of psychologists in research has long required strong emphases on experimental design and statistical analyses. These emphases are particularly relevant to the training of health psychologists because of the practical sampling problems faced and the need to deal with multiple response systems and complex subject variables. Increasingly, within the health psychology literature one notes the extensive use of multivariate statistics, time series analysis, and causal modeling. The use of such quantitative methods, in turn, requires that basic scientists in health psychology acquire considerable statistical and computer skills.

Health psychologists need a firm grounding in the basic principles of psychology, which is the parent discipline. Also needed is an understanding of important relationships between behavior and health as well as detailed knowledge of the vocabulary, concepts, and values of other professionals within the health sciences community. Many basic research problems in health psychology also require an understanding of mechanisms of disease.

Matarazzo (1983) has pointed out that the current leaders in health psychology research received generic training in psychology with predoctoral emphasis on various facets of the field. Thus, the skills and knowledge derived from biological, clinical, developmental, experimental, and social psychology have been applied to basic research into health problems with some degree of success.

Although core training in general psychology and specialized training in the traditional subareas of psychology provide useful preparation for basic laboratory research in health psychology, they provide only a part of the training needed. The basic research task force at the Arden House Conference, for example, pointed out that health psychologists need to take additional coursework in health psychology/behavioral medicine, the physiological bases of health and disease, and computer literacy (National Working Conference on Education and Training in Health Psychology 1983, 68–70). A substantial body of coursework is developing within the field of health psychology itself, and additional coursework in the biomedical sciences, epidemiology, and biostatistics is to be encouraged. The basic research task force felt that the number of years available for predoctoral training in basic research can at most prepare a student for a career that needs to be implemented at the postdoctoral level.

The National Institutes of Health (NIH) have made a strong commitment to research training by means of National Research Service Awards (NRSA). One type of award is the NRSA individual fellowship that offers "health scientists with a doctoral degree the opportunity to receive full-time research training in areas that reflect the national need for biomedical and behavioral research" (National Institutes of Health 1983, 126). A second type of award is made to eligible institutions to develop or enhance pre- and postdoctoral research training opportunities in biomedical and behavioral research. According to MacCanon (1983) the Division of Heart and Vascular Diseases at the National Heart, Lung, and Blood Institute (NHLBI) is currently supporting fourteen behavioral research training programs at a cost of about 1.5 million dollars annually.

In summary, it would appear that as health psychology emerges as a generic field, the academic preparation required for quality basic laboratory research is becoming more rigorous. Basic scientists in health psychology not only need a solid background in their parental discipline and in a specialty such as biological or social psychology, but also a firm grounding in health psychology, computers, quantitative methods, and the physiological bases of health and disease. As the field of health psychology has begun to mature, its expanding knowledge base and opportunities for conducting high-quality research have begun to require that research training be considered at both the predoctoral and postgraduate levels. This is consistent with the training requirements of other biomedical disciplines. As Brendan Maher (1983) has pointed out, the successful emergence of health psychology as a field will depend upon the extent to which we can develop small, selective, high-quality programs with rigorous standards at both the graduate and postgraduate levels.

Support of Basic Research in Health Psychology

Research directly relevant to health psychology is supported by both governmental and nongovernmental agencies. Sources of nongovernmental support range from national organizations such as the American Heart Association, National Cancer Society, and National Parkinson Foundation to large private foundations such as the MacArthur Foundation to a host of smaller foundations. State government support of biobehavioral research related to health is offered through state departments of human resources and through state university systems. By far the largest supporter of such research, however, is the federal government. This includes the Department of Health and Human Services, which is the parent agency for both the NIH and the Alcohol, Drug Abuse, and Mental Health Administration (ADAMHA) where the National Institute of Mental Health is housed. Other sources of federal support include the National Science Foundation, the Department of Defense, Department of Education, Environmental Protection Agency, and the Veterans Administration. The largest single source of funding directly related to health psychology is the NIH.

THE NATIONAL INSTITUTES OF HEALTH

The mission of the NIH is to improve human health through biomedical research. In order to accomplish this mission the NIH supports basic and applied investigations related to the causes, diagnosis, prevention, treatment, and rehabilitation of human diseases and disabilities. In fiscal year 1984 the NIH budget was 4.2 billion dollars of which more than 2.1 billion dollars went for research support at colleges and universities (Sweeney 1984).

In order to carry out their responsibilities the NIH is organized into sixteen separate units. The eleven national institutes included in this organization are:

National Cancer Institute (NCI)
National Heart, Lung, and Blood Institute (NHLBI)
National Institute of Arthritis, Diabetes, and Digestive and Kidney Diseases (NIADDK)
National Institute on Aging (NIA)
National Institute of Allergy and Infectious Diseases (NIAID)
National Institute of Child Health and Human Development (NICHD)
National Institute of Dental Research (NIDR)
National Institute of Environmental Health Sciences (NIEHS)
National Eye Institute (NEI)
National Institute of General Medical Sciences (NIGMS)
National Institute of Neurological and Communicative Disorders and Stroke (NINCDS)

A separate unit within the NIH, the Division of Research Grants, receives and processes grant requests. An initial review group, called a study section, provides the scientific merit review for most NIH applications, including applications for research project grants and individual NRSA awards. Several study sections including Behavioral Medicine, Biopsychology, and Human Development provide peer review for research proposals submitted in areas of interest to health psychologists.

The institutes of the NIH support a large number of biobehavioral and psychosocial programs relevant to health psychology. While it is beyond the scope of this chapter to describe all of these programs, the following discussion is intended to offer a brief overview of a few programs in which health psychologists are able to participate because of their specific training.

The National Institute on Aging (NIA) supports biomedical, behavioral, and social science research and training concerning the aging process as well as the diseases and special needs of the aged. Of particular interest to health psychologists is the program in Behavioral Sciences Research. This includes subprograms in cognitive and biopsychological aging, social psychological aging, older people in the changing society, and older people and social institutions. Descriptions of these and other extramural programs at the NIH can be obtained by consulting the pamphlet *NIH Extramural Programs* (National Institutes of Health 1983) or by writing directly to the individual institutes.

Another NIH institute with large behavioral components is the National Institute of Child Health and Human Development (NICHD). A Social and Behavioral Sciences Branch at the institute supports programs in causes and consequences of population change. The Clinical Nutrition and Early Development Branch has a Nutrition and Endocrinology Section that supports research in nutritional status assessment and the cultural and behavioral aspects of nutrition. A Human Learning and Behavior Branch emphasizes the biological bases of behavioral development, learning and cognitive development, development of communicative abilities, social and affective development, and health-related behaviors. Within the Mental Retardation and Developmental Disability Branch is a section on Behavioral and Social Science Research in Mental Retardation whose concerns include learning, cognition, and memory; studies of family relationships; communication and behavior; and the effects of teratogens on behavior, cognition, and social functioning.

Other institutes that provide strong research support for health psychologists include the National Heart, Lung, and Blood Institute (NHLBI), which has a Behavioral Medicine Branch within its Division of Epidemiology and Clinical Applications, and the National Institute of Neurological and Communicative Disorders and Stroke (NINCDS), which supports biobehavioral research through programs in Communicative Disorders, Fundamental Neurosciences, Stroke, and Nervous System Trauma.

In summary, there are a larger number of opportunities available for health psychologists to conduct high-quality, extramurally supported, basic laboratory research. Funds for such research are available through both governmental and nongovernmental agencies. The NIH in particular, is hospitable to supporting the kinds of basic research of interest to health psychologists.

Basic Laboratory Research Programs

The scope of basic research being investigated in the laboratory by health psychologists is extensive. Topics under investigation range from animal behavior studies of immune responses, tumorigenesis, addiction, obesity, atherogenesis, and hypertension to psychoneuroendocrine studies of human emotional behavior and psychophysiological studies of biofeedback, the Type A behavior pattern, exercise, and sleep. Basic laboratory studies of coping, discrimination, and conflict have helped to elucidate putative relationships between stress and illness. Experimental studies of decision making have provided a basis for examining the manner in which individuals decide upon issues relevant to their health including whether or not to seek treatment. New approaches to cognitive psychology have added increased clarity to the study of health beliefs. Principles of learning have been useful in the study of adherence (compliance) to medical regimens. Behavioral principles derived from the basic research laboratory have also been applied to the modification of physiological processes and health-related behaviors. Research approaches used have been derived from biological, developmental, experimental, and social psychology as well as from anthropology, epidemiology, sociology, and the biomedical sciences. The manner in which basic laboratory research in behavior has led to practical applications of medical significance has been reviewed by Miller (1983).

One important problem faced by physicians and other therapists involves getting patients to adhere to therapeutic regimens. Although hypertension can nearly always be controlled using drugs, only about half of all hypertensive patients are thought to take as much as eighty percent of their prescribed medication (Sackett et al. 1975). Social psychological research into basic processes of communication (Leventhal 1965) and attitude change (Bandura 1977) have had important implications for compliance research. So, too, have basic laboratory studies that have taught us how to shape specific responses. Research programs that have combined laboratory research with field studies are beginning to provide important insights into both adherence to treatment and disease risk reduction (Leventhal, Zimmerman, and Gutman 1984).

Several of the more successful laboratory research programs in health psychology and behavioral medicine have integrated animal behavior studies with human research. Thus, for example, Obrist and his collaborators have examined the effects of emotional stress in the laboratory upon kidney function and cardiovascular reactivity (Obrist 1981). In one study conducted with dogs, both treadmill exercise and avoidance conditioning led to similar increases in heart rate and blood pressure but to different renal responses (Grignolo, Koepke, and Obrist 1982). Exercise led to natriuresis due to an increased filter load; whereas, the antinatriuretic effect induced by the avoidance conditioning situation was apparently due to an increased rate of tubular reabsorption of filtrates. In a subsequent study conducted with humans, participation in a competitive perceptual-motor task resulted in decreases in urinary flow and sodium excretion in saline-loaded young adults with either hypertension or with a family history of hypertension (Light et al. 1983). The decreased urinary flow and sodium excretion did not occur in normotensive subjects without a family history of hypertension. Magnitude of diuresis inhibition was directly correlated with the magnitude of blood pressure and heart rate changes elicited during the experiments. Studies such as those conducted by Obrist, Light, and their collaborators illustrate how basic behavioral research in the laboratory can be brought to bear upon the study of important biomedical disorders such as essential hypertension.

In order to provide further insight into how integrative, multidisciplinary approaches to basic laboratory research are contributing to our understanding of health problems, I would like to describe briefly my own research program. This particular example is not being offered because it is the best, but because it is the one with which I have most familiarity.

Research in my laboratories has been funded by research grants from the American Heart Association, NIH, National Science Foundation, and the pharmaceutical industry. The program is also supported by an NHLBI training grant entitled "Behavioral Medicine Research in Cardiovascular Disease."

Several years ago we began to study the effects of behavioral challenges on cardiovascular reactivity in humans. Previously we had examined autonomic nervous system mediated changes in the circulation during exercise (Gaide et al. 1980) and during conditioning (Fredericks et al. 1974; Klose et al. 1975) in nonhuman primates and rabbits. We had also used intracranial electrical stimulation, coagulative lesions, horseradish peroxidase histochemistry, and extracellular single neuron recording to examine the central neuronal pathways involved in cardiovascular regulation (Gimpl et al. 1976; Kaufman et al. 1979). Thus, for example, we described the medio-lateral functional organization of the rabbit hypothalamus in terms of cardiovascular regulation and behavior (Gellman et al. 1981).

Of particular interest for the present discussion is our finding that stimulation of a pathway passing through the ventromedial hypothalamus elicits defensive behavior, increases in heart rate and blood pressure, preferential release of plasma epinephrine and aortic endothelial damage (Schneiderman 1983a, 1983b). Based upon these findings we become interested in determining whether humans reveal correlations between the same highly integrated patterns of autonomic activity and behavior.

During one experiment conducted with male college students, we examined the effects of harassment, hostility, and the Type A behavior pattern on heart rate and blood pressure reactivity during a competitive arcade-type video game (Diamond et al. 1984). The study had four major objectives. First, the effects of competition alone or in conjunction with either goal-blocking or harassment were compared in terms of heart rate and blood pressure reactivity. Second, the physiologic reactivity of interview-defined As versus Bs was compared as a function of experimental conditions. Third, the role of hostility in the Type A pattern was examined by comparing the reactivity of high versus low hostile As. Fourth, anger and hostility were assessed by component analysis of the structured interview and by psychometric instruments in order to examine their relationship to cardiovascular reactivity.

The results of the experiment proved interesting. Harassment in conjunction with competition elicited significantly greater elevations in systolic blood pressure and heart rate than those elicited either by competition alone or in conjunction with goal blocking. Type A subjects had significantly greater systolic blood pressure increases than Type Bs *only* in the harassment condition. Finally, significant positive correlations occurred between Buss-Durkee scores and systolic blood pressure for Type As, those classified as hostile in a component analysis of the structured interview, and people characterized as anger-out using the Framingham Anger-in versus Anger-out questionnaire.

Based upon our human laboratory experiments such as those by Diamond et al. (1984) and Lake et al. (1985) and our previous studies relating autonomic nervous system physiology to behavior, we responded to an NHLBI request for applications concerning biobehavioral factors affecting hypertension in blacks and received funding for the project. Our working hypothesis was that racial differences in renal function, an elevated intake of sodium, and high levels of psychosocial and socioecologic stress interact to produce a higher prevalence of hypertension in blacks than in whites. Our hypothesis about the interaction of sodium and emotional stress in producing hypertension was in part derived from the results of animal experiments by the health psychologist, David Anderson (1984).

In order to test our hypotheses concerning the prevalence of hypertension in blacks, we have been examining cardiovascular (heart rate, blood pressure) and hormonal (plasma epinephrine, norepinephrine, renin, cortisol) responses to standardized laboratory challenges (bicycle ergometer, competitive video game, cold pressor test, Type A structured interview). The cardiovascular and hormonal responses to the biobehavioral challenges are specifically being compared as a function of race, sex, socioeconomic status, and normal blood pressure versus borderline hypertension. The results are being further analyzed as a function of dietary (sodium, potassium, and calcium intake), genetic (family history of hypertension), organismic (urinary sodium, potassium, calcium; plasma renin, cortisol, catecholamines; aerobic fitness; obesity), and psychological (alienation; anger expression; chronic anxiety) variables. Extent to which the reactivity findings obtained in the laboratory generalize to everyday life are being examined using ambulatory heart rate and blood pressure monitoring.

A brief description of some of the project investigators illustrates the range of skills required to conduct this type of research. One co-principal investigator is in the Department of Epidemiology and Public Health. His experience as a director of intervention in the NHLBI Multiple Risk Factor Intervention Trial has provided us with the expertise required to assess dietary factors and ensure subject compliance to our protocol. A second co-principal investigator, an MD-Ph.D. who is Chief of Clinical Pharmacology, has medical responsibility for the conduct of our research.

Another active collaborator on the project is a personality/social psychologist who has guided us in our choice of psychosocial instruments. Expertise in this area is particularly useful because of the need to obtain information from subjects differing widely in cultural background and literacy. Professor Theodore Dembroski has also helped us in this area and has trained our personnel in the administration of the Type A interview and its component scoring. Other personnel associated with the project have strong backgrounds in critical care nursing, computer programming, statistics, and biochemical analysis.

Standardized psychophysiological experimentation such as that used in our laboratory offers the advantages of comprehensive measurements and precise stimulus control. The disadvantage of an approach that is restricted only to the laboratory, however, is that the experimental manipulations are necessarily contrived and somewhat removed from the ongoing, continuous adjustments that occur daily in real life. Thus, there is a need to relate the comprehensive findings observed in tightly controlled laboratory settings to cardiovascular and hormonal adjustments that occur in more natural settings. In recent years, advances in noninvasive ambulatory monitoring of blood pressure have made this procedure a useful one. Thus, for example, when blood pressure readings were compared with echocardiographic estimates of left ventricular hypertrophy in mild hypertensives, it was found that hypertrophy was much more highly correlated with ambulatory monitored blood pressure in the workplace than it was with blood pressure readings in a clinician's office (Devereux et al. 1983). It appears likely that in the future increased emphasis will be placed on relating psychophysiological and neurohormonal responsiveness observed in the laboratory to reactivity observed in more naturalistic settings.

In summary, the range of basic science investigations being carried out by health psychologists is growing rapidly. Several of these studies overlap into applied areas and in some cases extend beyond the confines of the laboratory. The skills required by some of these studies presently require extensive intradisciplinary as well as interdisciplinary collaboration. While training programs such as our own may decrease the number of active collaborators required to mount comprehensive studies in the future, the thrust of much of the research conducted by health psychologists is likely to remain interdisciplinary. A major goal of health psychology for the future is to conduct increasingly sophisticated, high-quality research.

REFERENCES

Anderson, D. E. 1984. Interactions of stress, salt, and blood pressure. *Annual Review of Physiology* 46:143–54.

Bandura, A. 1977. Self-efficacy: Toward a unifying theory of behavioral change. *Psychological Review* 84: 191–215.

Devereux, R. B., T. G. Pickering, G. A. Harshfield, H. D. Kleinert, L. Denby, L. Clark, V. Preibgon, M. Jason, B. Kleiner, J. S. Borer, and J. H. Laragh. 1983. Left ventricular hypertrophy in patients with hypertension: Importance of blood pressure response to regularly occurring stress. *Circulation* 68:470–576.

Diamond, E. L., N. Schneiderman, D. Schwartz, J. C. Smith, R. Vorp, and R. D. Pasin. 1984. Harassment, hostility and Type A as determinants of cardiovascular reactivity during competition. *Journal of Behavioral Medicine* 7:171–90.

Fredericks, A., J. W. Moore, F. U. Metcalf, J. S. Schwaber, and N. Schneiderman. 1974. Selective autonomic blockade of conditioned and unconditioned heart rate changes in rabbits. *Pharmacology, Biochemistry, and Behavior* 2:493–501.

Gaide, M. S., K. J. Klose, W. Gavin, N. Schneiderman, T. Robertson, M. Silbret, and M. Faletti. 1980. Hexamethonium modification of cardiovascular adjustments during combined static-dynamic arm exercise in monkeys. *Pharmacology, Biochemistry, and Behavior* 13:851–57.

Gellman, M., N. Schneiderman, J. Wallach, and W. Le Blanc. 1981. Cardiovascular responses elicited by hypothalamic stimulation in rabbits reveal a medio-lateral organization. *Journal of the Autonomic Nervous System* 4:301–17.

Gimpl, M. P., A. L. Brickman, M. P. Kaufman, and N. Schneiderman. 1976. Temporal relationships during barosensory attenuation in the conscious rabbit. *American Journal of Physiology* 230:1480–86.

Grignolo, A., J. P. Koepke, and P. A. Obrist. Renal function, heart rate, and blood pressure during exercise and avoidance in dogs. *American Journal of Physiology* 242 : R482–R490.

Kaufman, M. P., R. B. Hamilton, J. H. Wallach, G. K. Petrik, and N. Schneiderman. 1979. Lateral subthalamic area as mediator of bradycardia responses in rabbits. *American Journal of Physiology* 236 : H471–H479.

Klose, K. J., J. S. Augenstein, N. Schneiderman, K. Manas, and B. Abrams. 1975. Selective autonomic blockade of classically conditioned cardiovascular changes in rhesus monkeys. *Journal of Comparative and Physiological Psychology* 80 : 810–18.

Lake, B. W., E. C. Suarez, N. Schneiderman, and N. Tocci. 1985. The Type A behavior pattern, physical fitness, and psychophysiological reactivity. *Health Psychology* 4 : 169–87.

Leventhal, H., R. P. Singer, and S. Jones. 1965. Effects of fear and specificity of recommendations upon attitudes and behavior. *Journal of Personality and Social Psychology* 4 : 137–46.

Leventhal, H., R. Zimmerman, and M. Gutmann. 1984. Compliance: A self-regulation perspective. In *Handbook of Behavioral Medicine*, edited by W. D. Gentry, chap. 10. New York: Guilford.

Light, K. C., J. P. Kooepke, P. A. Obrist, and P. W. Willis. 1983. Psychological stress induces sodium and fluid retention in men at high risk for hypertension. *Science* 220 : 429–31.

MacCanon, D. 1983. Research training interests of the Division of Heart and Vascular Diseases of the National Heart, Lung, and Blood Institute. *Health Psychology* 2 (5) : 63–65, supplement section.

Maher, B. 1983. The education of health psychologists: Quality counts—Numbers are dangerous. *Health Psychology* 2 (5) : 37–48, supplement section.

Manuck, S. B., J. R. Kaplan, and T. B. Clarkson. 1983. Social instability and coronary atherosclerosis in cynomolgus monkeys. *Neuroscience and Biobehavioral Reviews* 7 : 485–91.

Matarazzo, J. D. 1983. Education and training in health psychology: Boulder or bolder. *Health Psychology* 2 : 73–113.

Miller, N. E. 1983. Behavioral medicine: Symbiosis between laboratory and clinic. *Annual Review of Psychology* 34 : 1–31.

National Institutes of Health. 1983. *NIH extramural programs: Funding for research and training*. U.S. Department of Health and Human Services. NIH Publication no. 83–33.

National Working Conference on Education and Training in Health Psychology. 1983. *Health Psychology* 2 (supplement to no. 5), p. 153.

Obrist, P. A. 1981. *Cardiovascular psychophysiology*. New York: Plenum.

Sackett, D. L., E. S. Gibson, D. W. Taylor, R. B. Haynes, B. C. Hackett, R. R. Roberts, and A. L. Johnson. 1975. Randomized clinical trial of strategies for improving medication compliance in primary hypertension. *Lancet* 2 : 1205–7.

Schneiderman, N. 1983a. Behavior, autonomic function, and animal models of cardiovascular pathology. In *Biobehavioral bases of coronary heart disease— Behavioral approaches to a twentieth-century epidemic*, edited by T. Dembroski, T. Schmidt, and G. Blumchen. Karger: Basle.

————. 1983b. Animal behavior models of coronary heart disease. *In Handbook of psychology and health,* edited by D. S. Krantz, A. Baum, and J. E. Singer, vol. 3, Cardiovascular disorders and behavior. Hillsdale, NJ: Lawrence Erlbaum Associates.

Schwartz, G. E., and S. M. Weiss. 1978a. Yale conference on behavioral medicine: A proposed definition and statement of goals. *Journal of Behavioral Medicine* 1:3–12.

————. 1978b. Behavioral medicine revisited: An amended definition. *Journal of Behavioral Medicine* 1:249–51.

Sweeney, J. 1984. Federal contract tips. *Federal Research Report* 20:39.

7

Basic Field Research in Health Psychology

Nancy E. Adler, Shelley E. Taylor, and Camille B. Wortman

This chapter addresses issues involved in the conduct of basic field research in health psychology, although many of the problems considered and suggestions made are applicable to any field research. Our first step is to define what is meant by basic field research. The basic-applied differentiation is commonly made in psychology, with the former generally referring to theory-testing research and the latter to studies addressing real-world problems. The terms are often polarized and associated with other, similar dichotomies such as "rigor" versus "vigor" (Kelman 1968) and "scientism" versus "clinicalism" (Chein 1966). Similarly, the distinction is frequently made between laboratory and field research, with the former often assumed to be theory-testing research and the latter, the examination of problems as they occur in natural settings. The terms "laboratory" and "field" are also often polarized and associated with dichotomies such as "experimental" versus "quasi-experimental" or "non-experimental" (cf. Cook and Campbell 1979).

In the context of these distinctions, the concept of basic field research might appear to some to be inherently contradictory. Increasingly, however, psychologists are realizing that the polarized distinctions referred to above are no longer appropriate. Laboratory and field as qualifiers of "research" connote only the setting in which either basic or applied research may be done. Theoretically inspired work can be conducted in the field as well as in the laboratory and still be oriented toward elucidation of real-world problems. Indeed, the singular advantage of testing basic research in field settings is the two-way exchange this process creates. When real-world problems are addressed through a theoretically inspired perspective, the theory and/or hypotheses provide a way of looking at the problem that the problem itself might not suggest. For example, in applying learned helplessness theory to hospital settings, Taylor (1979) suggested an alternative way of thinking about "good patient behavior." In most cases, the "good patient" is highly regarded by the staff because he or she is compliant, noncomplaining, and generally nondemanding. Taylor suggested that, in fact, patients manifesting "good patient behavior" may be in a state of helplessness—a state that is not conducive to a speedy recovery. In addition to shedding light on practical problems, the application of theories to applied health settings can provide a healthy dose of feedback concerning the adequacy of the theory. Silver and Wortman (1980) discovered this when they tried to apply learned helplessness theory to understand how people react to uncontrollable life events, such as acute illness or injury. Learned helplessness theory suggests that loss of control will result in passivity and depression. Yet the literature suggests that other emotional reactions, particularly anxiety, are even more prevalent than depression among individuals who experience acute illness or injury. Silver and Wortman (1980) suggested that perhaps the learned helplessness model should be broadened to incorporate other emotional reactions to loss of control if the model is to be truly useful in predicting behavior in field settings.

Historically, basic field research on real-world problems has not been the norm. Rather, investigators have tended toward either a focus on theory or a focus on problems, but not both. There are risks in both extremes. Some programs are implemented in health settings primarily to address a particular problem, and whatever implications the program may have for basic theory are serendipitous byproducts of the investigation. For example, much of the work on the relationship of Type A behavior to heart disease was done with no explicit theory of personality (Matthews 1982). Similarly, there are many studies linking social support to particular health outcomes such as recovery from surgery or compliance with treatment for hypertension (see Mumford, Schlesinger, and Glass 1982; or Levy 1983, for reviews). Almost without exception, however, these studies have not been based on theories of support processes and have not been designed to elucidate the mechanisms through which support may influence health (see Wortman and Conway 1985; or Wortman 1984, for a more detailed discussion).

If a researcher's interest is primarily in a target behavior, he or she may fail to examine theoretical literature that could provide important insights to the problem. The problems faced by patients and providers in the health system are often insistent and compelling, and it is tempting to conduct research that will provide immediate guidance or improvement of the situation or of individuals who are suffering. Thus, it is reasonable, from an applied perspective, to try to find something that will work, even if one does not have a rationale for why it should be effective. For example, some researchers have taken a technique like biofeedback, which has proven useful in treating one disease, and tried it in relation to another disease without any underlying rationale (Rittenhouse 1984). If something holds out the promise of an immediate solution, investigators may fail to see if this is the best solution, to understand why it is effective, and to understand the parameters of the situation that would influence when and how the solution would work.

There are other practical reasons why researchers interested in specific problems may not conduct research that addresses basic theoretical questions. If the chief goal of the research is the improvement of patients' status, it makes sense to develop an intervention that is as potent as possible. This will usually entail drawing from several sources and combining a number of different efficacious interventions. For example, studies with surgery patients designed to improve their functioning following surgery may provide patients with information about the sensations associated with surgery, exercises the patient can engage in to improve ambulation, and cognitive coping techniques that can be used to distract oneself from discomfort (see Johnson 1983 for a review). The theoretical purist may be understandably distressed by such a design because if it works, it is impossible to know why. A deliberately confounded design may be appropriate in the early stages of research. Thus, an intervention with many components may be compared with no treatment or standard care. Such a beginning study can then lay the groundwork for more careful exploration of the particular variables that contributed to the change. In most cases, however, it is unusual for such intervention studies to be followed up in this way.

At the opposite extreme are researchers who are primarily interested in basic processes of theoretical issues that are relevant to health which are only loosely tied to real-world problems. For example, researchers interested in the impact of fear on behavior may select a particular target behavior such as tooth flossing or wearing seat belts as a convenient attitude object. In many cases, the primary interest of such researchers may be in the theoretical questions, not in the target behavior. But unless the researcher is able to develop a full understanding of the behavior, the research may be limited in important ways. For example, suppose a researcher interested in the theoretical sequelae of sudden loss decides to focus on the health and mental health consequences of bereavement. The investigator may conceptualize social activity on the part of the bereaved as a sign of good social functioning. However, those with a detailed knowledge of the bereavement experience would know that the matter is more complex. They would be aware that the bereaved frequently engage in social activities because the loss is so painful that they cannot stand to be alone. Thus, investigators who use the context of bereavement to examine basic theoretical notions may produce misleading findings if they lack a detailed understanding of the bereavement experience.

How can the necessary knowledge of problem areas be obtained? First, researchers must look beyond the psychological literature; literature about particular health settings or problems may be scattered in a variety of journals from disciplines such as nursing, medicine, dentistry, and public health.

Second, the researcher may establish an interdisciplinary research team that includes health care providers working on the problem as well as basic researchers whose interests are primarily theoretical. Because of the complexity of the social context, some problems can only be studied through an extensive interdisciplinary effort. All three authors of this chapter are involved in research with co-investigators from different disciplines.

Another way that investigators can gain insight about a problem is to organize a series of "focus groups" and "feedback groups" comprised of individuals who are experiencing the problem. A focus group is a group discussion centered around the impact of the problem on the respondents' lives. In such groups, participants are given an opportunity to discuss the issue as they see it, while the researchers listen in order to learn about the most important facets of the problem from the point of view of those who are experiencing it. Focus groups are sometimes followed by feedback groups in which researchers attempt to articulate their understanding of the problem or their attempts to assess certain constructs related to the problem and individuals who are experiencing the problem provide feedback about whether the researchers are on target.

A final approach has elements of the last two but is less formal. This approach involves the establishment of an "advisory council" of individuals who are experiencing the problem and/or who are knowledgeable about it. These individuals can provide valuable information about sensitive aspects of research (e.g., the appropriate time for interviews during a crisis period) as well as on recruitment, follow-up, or interview procedures.

An exciting challenge of health psychology is the potential for combining theory and application by conducting basic research in field settings. To do so, as we have implied in the previous discussion, requires a thorough knowledge of the relevant theoretical vantage points as well as a thorough conversance of the health problem to be addressed. This may seem like a demanding load for the researcher. However, many existing studies have done precisely this. For example, Bandura's (1977) self-efficacy theory has been applied to a variety of health problems, including the control of pain in childbirth (Manning and Wright 1983), exercise behavior in patients with chronic obstructive pulmonary disease (Kaplan, Atkins, and Reinsch 1984), and patients who have suffered a heart attack (Ewart et al. 1983). Each of these studies has not only clarified the particular problem to which it has been addressed but has provided an opportunity for testing critical hypotheses within the theory. Similarly, research by Smetana and Adler tested aspects of Fishbein and Ajzen's theory (Ajzen and Fishbein 1980) of reasoned action (Smetana and Adler 1980) and simultaneously identified issues that are salient for women deciding to continue or terminate a pregnancy (Smetana and Adler 1979).

The remainder of this chapter addresses some of the special issues that arise in attempting to do theoretically inspired research in health settings. These problems will be divided into four general categories: developing research settings, establishing a relationship with respondents, communicating research results, and resolving ethical dilemmas.

Special Problems of Research in Health Settings
DEVELOPING RESEARCH SETTINGS

In the conduct of basic research, a researcher generally starts with conceptual variables and then seeks the best setting for examining those variables. Ideally, the setting selected should allow for the best test of one's hypotheses and enable one to rule out alternative plausible explanations in order to establish causal relationships among the variables (Ellsworth 1977). Unfortunately, this ideal situation is difficult to achieve in many health settings.

Because health care settings are designed for care-giving there may be resistance to any disruptions that proposed research introduces. Most settings place a heavy demand on staff, and there is not much time for them to participate in research projects. One might, for example, want to have a provider make a rating of patients' adjustment immediately after visits, but the schedule of visits and unforeseen complications with individual cases may make this a time-consuming, unrealistic task. Similarly, one may wish to administer questionnaires to patients immediately after their visit to a physician, but some patients may wish to leave the office immediately following their visit. Alternatively, one might question patients before their physician visit, but if so, one runs the risk that results will be influenced by anxiety about the forthcoming visit or the protocol may not be completed if the patient is called for his or her appointment.

Except in special cases, patients do not have to participate in research investigations, and consequently, studies are conducted on volunteers. The bias that can be introduced by volunteers (Rosenthal and Rosnow 1975) needs to be evaluated to determine if factors influencing willingness to participate might also influence the variables under investigation. For example, a study of patient satisfaction with physicians would be biased indeed if subjects who had been seen promptly and who were therefore contented with their visit were more likely to stay to answer the researcher's questions than patients who had been kept waiting a long time and were anxious to get on with their daily activities.

Establishing a good relationship with the health care setting not only provides access to appropriate respondents but also helps insure that the project will be carried out smoothly and efficiently. Before identifying and approaching key personnel to introduce the project, it is important to become as fully informed as possible about the health-care setting.

In most cases, obtaining access to patients in a health setting requires the approval and/or cooperation of a great many people. Health systems are often hierarchical, and one may need to gain cooperation from each level. At the top, administrators in charge of the facility are generally concerned with the financial, legal, and practical functioning of the facility. Below them is usually a ward administrator or chief physician in charge of a specific clinic or ward, then nurses, receptionists, and practitioners who are in most direct contact with the patients. Permission to conduct the research may need to be solicited from each of these individuals who will have varying degrees of interest in research and different concerns regarding it. A study can be undermined or even halted by any of these individuals. For example, the chief physician may support the study and give it his or her full endorsement, yet the receptionist who must ask each patient to complete a questionnaire may fail to do so as he or she becomes overloaded with daily tasks. Alternatively, clinic staff may be more than happy to cooperate, but an administrator may veto the study because of fears that it will create too much disruption in the clinic without providing any clear advantage. While a researcher must consider all levels of the hierarchy, there are often particular individuals who could be instrumental to the success or failure of the study and to whom more attention should be paid. For example, the researcher should identify individuals who may be most burdened or threatened by the research. Similarly, there may be individuals who can facilitate the research even in the face of lack of support from other levels.

We have found several techniques to be helpful in negotiating with the agency for approval of the project, soliciting cooperation, and in laying the groundwork for the smooth conduct of the research. In presenting the research to the agency, the investigator will naturally want to stress the potential knowledge to be derived and its applicability to the target population and the agency itself. In deciding whether to approve the project, administrators often weigh these potential benefits against costs to the institution, such as staff time and the disruption of routines. By showing sensitivity to such costs, and by making a conscious effort to minimize them, the researcher may increase the likelihood that the project will be approved. The researcher who is knowledgeable about routines can propose procedures that are minimally disruptive. Similarly, the investigator may want to consider offering some service to the organization in exchange for staff time. For example, it may be possible to add a few items to the questionnaire or interview schedule that are of special interest to the agency or help the agency evaluate a particular service. Alternatively, the investigator can offer to compensate staff members in some way for the time that must be spent on the research project.

In planning the presentation to personnel in the health-care setting, the researcher needs also to show sensitivity to the needs of the respondents. Agency personnel are often suspicious of researchers, viewing them as unconcerned outsiders more interested in publication than in the welfare of the respondents (Fairweather and Tornatzky 1977). Some of the approaches described earlier for increasing the researcher's familiarity with the problem can be indicative of the researcher's good intentions.

We have seen many projects fail because the researcher has not considered the needs or concerns of the staff members who are asked to collect the data and has relied only on the approval from an administrator or supervisor. Staff may resent the extra duties that have been foisted upon them. Those on the front lines who will actually become involved in the data collection will want to know exactly what is demanded of them and whether these demands are in addition to their usual workload. If so, they will need to feel sufficiently invested in the research to make it worth their efforts. One possible way to increase the staff's involvement in the project, as well as to strengthen the research itself, is to draw on their practical experience in designing the study or in providing a critique of the questionnaire or interview schedule. For example, in a study of factors influencing high-risk pregnancy outcomes (Nethercut and Adler 1983), the researchers shared their purpose with the nurses, solicited their clinical intuitions, and included these ideas in the study so that they could be tested. Because the research promised to enlighten the facility about these issues, the nurses solicited participants and distributed questionnaires for almost two years. Such efforts not only help to strengthen agency personnel's commitment to the project, but may be highly useful in their own right.

Even when staff members are willing to cooperate with the research project, problems may still emerge. Particularly in health settings where personnel are accustomed to assuming a helping role, staff may have difficulty administering experimental manipulations or collecting data in the objective, standardized manner required in research. In one study, for example, the ward nurse was asked to give each cancer patient who met the eligibility criteria a letter describing the project. Subsequently, the researchers learned that the nurse had made a judgment about whether the patient would like to be in the study and gave letters only to those patients. In another study, nurses were recruited to help administer an experimental manipulation. Patients recovering from their first heart attack were given exercises designed to facilitate their feelings of control. The nurses were so impressed with these exercises that they surreptitiously taught them to control patients as well. A way to avoid misunderstandings and problems once the agency has approved the research is to spell out the responsibilities of both the researcher and the agency staff in a written agreement signed by all parties. The agreement not only delineates the researcher's expectations regarding hospital personnel and vice versa, but may be helpful in insuring cooperation from the organization throughout the investigation. Such an agreement should clarify the rights and responsibilities of all parties and should include a detailed discussion of the study procedures, selection of respondents, and plans for dissemination of the data (Fairweather and Tornatzky 1977).

ESTABLISHING A RELATIONSHIP WITH RESPONDENTS

The success of any study conducted in a health care setting depends not only on gaining access to the setting, but on obtaining respondents' consent to participate, maintaining their participation throughout the study, and encouraging them to provide data that are reliable and valid. What steps can the health researcher take to facilitate these goals?

Unless the vast majority of the respondents who are approached to participate agree to do so, the generalizability of the results will be suspect. In our judgment, the best way to increase the likelihood of participation is to provide a clear and informative introduction to the project. In introducing our studies, for example, we attempt to build rapport with our respondents. We try to explain why their participation is important to us. We also try to work out arrangements with staff personnel to obtain as much information as possible about all respondents who are approached to participate. This information makes it possible to conduct analyses on those who agree to participate and those who refuse in order to determine whether there are any systematic differences among them in the extent of their illness, in demographic variables, etc. (Adler 1976).

It is important that respondents be told why they are being selected for the study. Particularly in studies on coping and adjustment, respondents may assume that they have been chosen because the staff thinks they are having problems. It is important to alleviate this anxiety by explaining that all patients who meet certain criteria are being approached for participation in the study.

Longitudinal studies, in which participants are interviewed several times over a period of months or years, are becoming increasingly common in health-care settings (Kessler et al. 1985). In introducing such studies one may want to stress the importance of a longitudinal approach, include an explanation of the problems that are created when respondents drop out of the project, and ask the respondent to make a commitment to participate in subsequent interviews. Obtaining the addresses and phone numbers of a few family members and friends will also enhance the likelihood that one can recontact them in the future. In many studies, problems in being unable to locate respondents have contributed more to attrition than the refusal of respondents to contribute their participation. Riecken et al. (1974) provide several practical suggestions for locating respondents who have moved since the last interview, such as contacting the post office, utility companies, schools, and neighbors.

COMMUNICATING RESEARCH RESULTS

Once research questions have been addressed, there arises a question as to how results of the study should be communicated. As noted earlier, basic researchers tend to report their results in psychological journals and health practitioners in health journals. The consequence is that research results may never reach the full range of their appropriate audience. Therefore, articles that stress the theoretical findings of the research should be published in psychological journals, providing insights regarding the basic health problem as a secondary goal. Very different publications emphasizing the health problem itself may be appropriate for medical journals. As a secondary goal, these articles should try to communicate the importance of theoretical insights so that the audience of practitioners may see the implications that the results of a specific investigation have for other treatment settings.

Let us take a specific example. Recently psychologists have exposed patients awaiting noxious medical procedures to interventions designed to enhance feelings of control (e.g., the provision of information). Such investigations are generally beneficial and reveal that patients adjust more successfully to a procedure when they feel they have some control over it (e.g., Anderson and Masur 1983; Taylor and Clark, forthcoming). Reports of such research addressed to practitioners should note not only the value of the specific intervention for this particular procedure, such as an endoscopic examination, (Johnson and Leventhal 1974), but point out the potential generalizability of the intervention as well, so that practitioners may come to think of the control concept as a general strategy for helping patients cope with painful medical events.

Because there is such a demand for information in the health area, investigators may find that their results generate more interest than expected. This can be troublesome when research is translated prematurely into actions or interventions that may have health and mental health consequences. For example, Bulman and Wortman (1977) published a paper suggesting that patients with spinal cord injuries who blamed themselves for their accident coped better than those who blamed others. As mentioned in the article, they regarded this as a preliminary investigation in the area and in need of replication from other researchers. Subsequently, the researchers were contacted by health care providers at rehabilitation institutes who wanted to apply the research findings by assessing the attributions of patients with spinal cord injuries and making treatment decisions for them on the basis of the patients' choices. There is a burden on researchers working in the health area to be particularly clear about the limits on the generalizability of one's findings, the degree to which causal relationships have been demonstrated, and the power of the effects found.

An important aspect of reporting results is to communicate them back to the research setting in which the data were collected. Indeed, a chief complaint of health care providers is that researchers come into a setting, collect their data, and are never heard from again. Psychologists have an obligation to report their results back to those in the setting and to do so in a way that is helpful to that audience. Clearly, practitioners and patients are less interested in theoretical implications of results than in practical implications for treatment. It is useful to think through, prior to data collection, the kinds of results one may be able to report back at the conclusion of the study. The researcher should not promise too much, lest he or she be placed in an awkward position if the results do not show clear or easy solutions to the problems faced by patients or practitioners. Alternatively, the conclusions reached by a researcher may be awkward for the facility. For example, physicians tend to attribute patient noncompliance to personality dispositions in patients (e.g., DiMatteo and DiNicola 1982). From a study of noncompliance, the provider may expect to see a profile of patients who are likely to be noncompliant. A researcher who finds provider variables and/or patient-provider interaction variables that contribute to the compliance problem may find it uncomfortable to report back to providers that their own behaviors have contributed to the problem. Clearly, these ethical and practical problems demand advance planning.

ETHICAL ISSUES

A major strength of field settings for research is that the researcher is dealing with naturally occurring, often powerful events. These events frequently involve phenomena that could not be ethically studied in a laboratory. Thus, for example, critical studies of stress and coping have been conducted with patients facing surgery (e.g., Cohen and Lazarus 1973; Janis 1958). Ethical issues arise from the fact that one is studying people who may be in the midst of an intense and difficult situation.

One such ethical issue concerns whether patients perceive themselves as volunteers in the research. In field settings, the researcher may be mistakenly viewed as a member of the health care team and, in some studies, may be introduced as such. Patients may feel vulnerable and fear that they will not receive good care from the providers if they do not participate in the research. Special care must be taken to assure them that their care will in no way be affected by their participation.

Another issue that arises is what one can reasonably demand of people who may be sick, under stress, or otherwise taxed. A study that might be easy and acceptable with a population of healthy people may not be justifiable with individuals who are ailing and facing difficult choices or unpleasant outcomes.

Researchers in health settings may also encounter another ethical problem: the dilemma of what to do with information that has implications for a patient. A patient may tell a researcher information that relates to a life or health-threatening situation but which is unknown to the patient's physician. For example, a male hypertensive patient may reveal that he is not taking his medication but that the physician thinks he is. Or, a breast cancer patient on chemotherapy may confide that she is drinking to avoid her chemotherapy sessions; the physician may know only that her white count is too low for her to tolerate chemotherapy but may not know the reason (Lichtman, Taylor, and Wood 1985).

There are no easy rules for resolving the dilemma between confidentiality on the one hand and the need to protect the health of the patient on the other. The patient, after all, has chosen not to tell his or her provider the information and has agreed to participate in the research with the assurance of confidentiality and/or anonymity. In some cases, the researcher may feel compelled to intervene and inform the provider. In other cases, the researcher may need to break out of a neutral role and urge the patient to confide in the provider.

The emotionally charged issues often investigated by researchers in health psychology present many challenges for the interviewer. What should the interviewer do if the respondent begins to cry during the interview? What if the respondent asks whether his or her feelings of anxiety and depression are normal? In such settings, interviewers may feel compelled to shift from a data collector to a helper role—a role for which they may not be adequately prepared or trained. Such dilemmas should be reviewed during an extensive period of interviewer training. Interviewers should receive guidance about responding to different crises and on the conditions under which they should attempt to refer the respondent for psychological help.

Almost any researcher involved in health care settings will need a plan to refer subjects who need psychological help. In even the most benign study, there may be subjects who participate because they see it as an opportunity for contact with a psychologist. They may use this opportunity to reveal serious problems or pathology which have not been shared with others. Studies may also place patients in physical stress situations that require access to competent medical help. Both physical and psychological emergencies, then, must be planned for when conducting research in health settings.

Research in field settings usually has to be reviewed by ethics panels not only from the researcher's home institution but also within the health care setting. Each of these committees may address their attention to different factors. In the health setting, the research may be reviewed by a committee that is used to dealing primarily with biomedical research and which may have few if any social scientist members. Such committees often raise questions about the effects of standardized psychological measures on patients. Unfortunately, psychologists have little data on which to base assessments of patients' responses or to rebut fears that patients will become embarrassed or upset. In many cases, this issue is resolved by employing a consent form that alerts patients in advance that some items may be embarrassing or upsetting. Such a solution can create an unnecessarily negative introduction to the study and may raise defenses. However, it is also possible that psychologists who are comfortable with psychological questions and who are used to studying them on articulate, nonthreatened college students may underestimate the effects of these questionnaires on older, sicker, lower socioeconomic status individuals. We need to undertake more systematic collection of data regarding the effects of our research on patients so we can better gauge the impact of our studies and address these concerns more effectively with our medical colleagues.

The reverse problem can occur when one must have one's research protocol reviewed by committees used to dealing with laboratory data collection. Healthy academicians may have little sense of the questions that ill individuals will be able, and even desire, to answer. They may fear that questions about coping, fears, and surgeries will raise anxiety to a point that it overwhelms the patient and makes him or her unable to cope with the disorder. Their lack of experience with such populations may make them unable to see that such patients often welcome and actually profit from the ability to talk about these seemingly sensitive issues. For example, Mitchell and Glicksman (1977) report that eighty-six percent of the cancer patients they studied wished that they could discuss their situation more fully with someone. Perhaps for this reason, our own experience and that of other researchers indicate that individuals who have experienced a life crisis are generally quite eager to discuss their experiences and concerns and readily cooperate with an interviewer (e.g., Bulman and Wortman 1977; Hinton 1963; McCubbin, Hunter, and Metres 1974; Schwab et al. 1975). Thus, the basic researcher who would address questions in health settings might also want to collect documentation to demonstrate that patients often welcome and benefit from investigations that would seem, to an outsider, to be insensitive violations of private and frightening matters.

Conclusions

In the previous pages, we have provided a brief glimpse into some of the issues that arise when the researcher conducts basic research in field settings involving health and illness. In particular, we have highlighted the difficulties involved in developing research settings, communicating research results, and resolving ethical issues. Conducting basic field research in health psychology is not an easy task. It combines the problems of theory-guided research with the difficulties of field research. Nonetheless, it also provides a unique set of challenges and opportunities. It enables the researcher to bring theoretical guidance to some of the most significant research problems a psychologist faces and to refine theoretical tools on the basis of feedback from these same challenging settings.

REFERENCES

Adler, N. E. 1976. Sample attrition in studies of psychosocial sequelae of abortion: How great a problem? *Journal of Applied Behavioral Science* 6:240–59.

Ajzen, I., and M. Fishbein. 1980. *Understanding attitudes and predicting social behavior.* Englewood Cliffs, NJ: Prentice-Hall.

Anderson, K. O., and F. T. Masur, III. 1983. Psychological preparation for invasive medical and dental procedures. *Journal of Behavioral Medicine* 6:1–40.

Bandura, A. 1977. Self-efficacy: Toward a unifying theory of behavioral change. *Psychological Review* 84(2): 191–215.

Bulman, R. J., and C. B. Wortman. Attributions of blame and coping in the "real world": Severe accident victims react to their lot. *Journal of Personality and Social Psychology* 35:351–63.

Chein, I. 1966. Some sources of divisiveness among psychologists. *American Psychologist* 21:333–42.

Cohen, F., and R. S. Lazarus. 1973. Active coping processes, coping dispositions, and recovery from surgery. *Psychosomatic Medicine* 35:375–89.

Cook, T. D., and D. T. Campbell. 1979. *Quasi-experimentation: Design and analyses for field settings.* Chicago: Rand McNally.

DiMatteo, M. R., and D. D. DiNicola. 1982. *Achieving patient compliance: The psychology of the medical practitioner's role.* New York: Pergamon Press.

Ellsworth, P. C. 1977. From abstract ideas to concrete instances: Some guidelines on choosing natural research settings. *American Psychologist* 32:604–13.

Ewart, C. K., C. B. Taylor, L. B. Reese, and R. F. DeBusk. 1983. Effects of early postmyocardial infarction exercise testing on self-perception and subsequent physical activity. *The American Journal of Cardiology* 51:1076–80.

Fairweather, G. W., and L. G. Tornatzky. 1977. *Experimental methods for social policy research.* New York: Pergamon Press.

Hinton, J. M. 1963. The physical and mental distress of the dying. *Journal of Family Practice* 6:985–89.

Janis, I. L. 1958. *Psychological stress: Psychoanalytic and behavioral studies of surgical patients.* New York: Wiley.

Johnson, J. E. 1983. Psychological interventions and coping with surgery. In *Handbook of psychology and health,* edited by A. Baum, S. E. Taylor, and J. E. Singer, vol. 4. Hillsdale, NJ: Lawrence Erlbaum and Associates.

Johnson, J. E., and H. Leventhal. 1974. Effects of accurate expectations and behavioral instructions on reactions during a noxious medical examination. *Journal of Personality and Social Psychology* 29:710–18.

Kaplan, R. M., C. J. Atkins, and S. Reinsch. 1984. Specific efficacy expectations mediate exercise compliance in patients with COPD. *Health Psychology* 3(3): 223–42.

Kelman, H. C. 1968. *A time to speak.* San Francisco: Jossey-Bass.

Kessler, R. C., R. H. Price, and C. B. Wortman. 1985. Social factors in psychopathology: Stress, social support, and coping processes. *Annual Review of Psychology* 36:531–72.

Levy, S. M. 1983. Host differences in neoplastic risk: Behavioral and social contributors to disease. *Health Psychology* 2:21–44.

Lichtman, R. R., S. E. Taylor, and J. V. Wood. 1985. Research on the chronically ill: Conceptual and methodological perspectives. In *The handbook of environmental psychology,* edited by J. Singer and A. Baum, vol. 5. Hillsdale, NJ: Lawrence Erlbaum and Associates.

Manning, M. M., and T. L. Wright. 1983. Self-efficacy expectancies, outcome expectancies, and the persistence of pain control in childbirth. *Journal of Personality and Social Psychology* 45:421–31.

Matthews, K. 1982. Psychological perspectives on the Type A behavior pattern. *Psychological Bulletin* 91:293–323.

McCubbin, H. I., E. J. Hunter, and P. J. Metres. 1974. Adaptation of the family to the prisoner of war and missing in action experience: An overview. In *Family separation and reunion: Families of prisoners of war and servicemen missing in action,* edited by H. I. McCubbin, B. B. Dahl, P. J. Metres, E. J. Hunter, and J. A. Plag. Washington, D.C.: U.S. Government Printing Office.

Mitchell, G. W., and A. S. Glicksman. 1977. Cancer patients: Knowledge and attitudes. *Cancer* 40:61–66.

Mumford, E., H. J. Schlesinger, and G. V. Glass. 1982. The effects of psychological intervention on recovery from surgery and heart attacks: An analysis of the literature. *American Journal of Public Health* 72(2): 141–51.

Nethercut, G., and N. E. Adler. 1983. *Anxiety, stress and social support: Prenatal predictors of obstetrical outcomes.* Paper presented at the American Psychological Association Meetings, Anaheim, California.

Riecken, H. W., R. F. Boruch, D. T. Campbell, N. Caplan, T. K. Glennan, J. W. Pratt, A. Rees, and W. Williams. 1974. *Social experimentation: A method for planning and evaluating social interventions.* New York: Academic Press.

Rittenhouse, J. August 1984. Discussion on the current status and future of health psychology. American Psychological Association Annual Meeting, Toronto, Canada.

Rosenthal, R., and R. L. Rosnow. 1975. *The volunteer subject.* New York: John Wiley & Sons.

Schwab, J., J. Chalmers, S. Conroy, P. Farris, and R. Markush. 1975. Studies in grief: A preliminary report. In *Bereavement: Its psychosocial aspects,* edited by B. Schoenberg, I. Gerber, A. Weiner, A. H. Kutscher, D. Peretz, and A. C. Carr. New York: Columbia University Press.

Silver, R. L., and C. B. Wortman. 1980. Coping with undesirable life events. In *Human helplessness: Theory and applications,* edited by J. Garber and M. E. P. Seligman. New York: Academic Press.

Smetana, J., and N. E. Adler. 1979. Decision-making regarding abortion: A value x expectancy analysis. *Journal of Population* 2:348–57.

———. 1980. Fishbein's value x expectancy model: An examination of some assumptions. *Personality and Social Psychology Bulletin* 6:89–96.

Taylor, S. E. 1979. Hospital patient behavior: Reactance, helplessness, or control? *Journal of Social Issues* 35:156–84.

Taylor, S. E., and L. F. Clark. Forthcoming. Does information improve adjustment to
    noxious events? In *Advances in applied social psychology,* edited by M. J. Saks
    and L. Saxe, vol. 3. Hillsdale, NJ: Lawrence Erlbaum and Associates.
Wortman, C. B. 1984. Social support and the cancer patient: Conceptual and meth-
    odological issues. *Cancer* 53(10): 2339–60.
Wortman, C. B., and T. Conway. 1985. The role of social support in adaptation and
    recovery from physical illness. In *Social support and health,* edited by S. Cohen
    and L. Syme. New York: Academic Press.

8

Training for Applied Research in Health Psychology

Jerome E. Singer

Both modern art and obscenity have been defined as a field that no one can define exactly, but people know it when they see it. Applied research in health psychology is cast from this same mold except that people don't always know it when they see it. Nancy Adler, Shelley Taylor, and Camille Wortman (in chap. 7) have pointed out the difficulty of distinguishing basic field research in health psychology from basic laboratory research (discussed by Neil Schneiderman in chap. 6). They conclude that the laboratory-field distinction is one of setting only; both research sites may contribute equally well to theory and to application. How then is applied research in health psychology to be further separated from this continuum of basic studies?

One of the major definitional issues can be illustrated by accepting that the concept of setting—field vs. laboratory—is independent of the concept of referent—basic vs. applied. Logically, then, there should be a fourfold table of basic research in laboratory and field and applied research in laboratory and field. In reality, the amount of applied research in the laboratory conducted in areas of health psychology is small in amount and rather specialized. Such research does occur. For example, some investigators do assays as part of an evaluation or service; others may use the laboratory to develop or refine techniques for use in applications of one or another kind. Even if it is assumed that these laboratory procedures are so atheoretical as to not draw claims for inclusion from the community of basic health psychology researchers, it is possible that the laboratory setting requires the same proficiency of all researchers, basic and applied. The techniques of conducting these applied studies, or the training necessary for the preparation to conduct them, does not differ very much from that needed for basic laboratory studies. This similarity of training may not hold for basic and applied field research, which will be discussed briefly later.

The majority of applied health research is conducted in the field with respect to the formal characteristics of the research—the methods, the rigor, etc. Much of it is indistinguishable from basic field studies in health psychology. Indeed, for most field studies, the ideal outcome would be a contribution to both the conceptual-theoretical domain and the practical-applied domain. Most of the differences are matters of degree and probability. Applied research is more likely to utilize patient populations, to focus on program evaluation, and to accept the study conditions as a given rather than to manipulate or change them. However, none of these debatable differences of degree are very useful in conceptualizing the implications of a set of training procedures for doing applied research in health psychology.

One possible way of delineating applied health psychology research is through the purpose and control of the research rather than its mode of conduct. These purposes are often seen more clearly in a sequence or set of investigations than in a single study. Although still a matter of degree, applied research is more likely to have been initiated by people other than the investigator; it is more likely to have a well-defined objective generated by someone other than the investigator; its results are more likely to be framed and intended for publication in technical bulletins and sponsor reports than scientific outlets; the findings are more likely to be proprietary; and, in general, applied research is less likely to be under the investigators' discretionary control. A prototypic applied project in health psychology would be a study in which a psychologist was asked to evaluate the success of a treatment program. The aim of the study would be to supply information to the dispensers of the treatment, who may or may not include the health psychology researcher. The nature of the evaluation, the characteristics to be evaluated, and the variables to be considered are not for the investigator alone to decide. The investigator may wish to incorporate some additional measures or to interpret the mandated ones in a way that addresses some issue other than the outcome desired, but the success of research is not determined or affected by the investigator's ability to do this. The purpose and goal of an applied study is to answer the sponsor's question. Other questions may or may not be encouraged or even allowed.

Other aspects of applied health psychology research may involve the study of treatment delivery or types of regimen as in the comparison of several modes of stress management or, more likely, stress management programs. Even here, purely applied research is usually overlaid with theoretical considerations. There is likely to be a rationale for the choice of stress management programs in the first place, and even if there isn't, some theoretical basis is required to be able to select a pertinent control group against which to assess program success. Whether research is basic or applied is also a matter of the disciplinary affiliation of the investigator. Just as basic engineering science is often indistinguishable from applied physics, so applied health psychology is often indistinguishable from basic epidemiology. Both are relatively problem-focused, atheoretical, eclectic, and hypothesis seeking. The point, of course, is to underscore that the research dimension of applied versus basic is a continuous one. Not only are there no seams in the continuum, but it is not even clear that the dimension is a linear one with basic clearly at one end and applied at the other. As has been discussed previously (Singer and Glass 1975), it is arguable that what is often called applied research makes as much a contribution to basic theoretical understanding as what is often called basic research.

While there is a tradeoff between greater control and precision in the laboratory opposed to a greater ecological validity in the field, the generalizability of either type of research seems to be a matter of personal preference and adjudication of the utility of the study on a case by case basis. A large fraction of precise, well-controlled laboratory studies languish in back copies of journals, never to be cited by other studies and never incorporated into whatever theory they were intended to illumine. Similarly, much field research, clearly relevant to the point at issue, is sufficiently lacking the precise controls necessary to rule out alternative explanations and thus fails to realize its full potential to contribute.

Applied Psychology and Applied Research

One distinction should be emphasized. Most applications of psychology, even health psychology, are not research. The application of health psychology primarily involves the delivery of services. The provision of support groups for various diseases, the initiation and conduct of stress management regimens, weight control programs, smoking cessation, and addiction control programs of various sorts represent just a fraction of the ways in which applied health psychology can contribute to society. Other areas of application include providing of liaison services to the ill and all those areas in which health psychology overlaps with other areas of psychology, such as traditional clinical, counseling, and neuropsychology. The range of activities spans such aspects of health and disease as health education, prevention, treatment rehabilitation, pain management, etc.

The vast majority of health psychology applications do not involve research. To be sure, all of them lend themselves to one or another study, but such studies are the exception not the rule. Routine statistics of how many people were seen for what kinds of treatment do not constitute research; without some framed research question and a minimum of management, the compendia of facts do not qualify as research reports. Similarly, although it is not infrequent for particular psychologist interactions with clients or patients to be examined for quality control assurances, these, too, fail to qualify as research reports. Most instances of applied health psychology are cases of service delivery, provided by psychologists with varying kinds of training, different levels of competence and experience, and having a spectrum of outcomes from success to failure. Occasionally, some of these activities will be included in an evaluation study, more rarely in a clinical trial. Most often, they will be provided as service with their outcomes and effectiveness noted only by the provider and the client or patient—appraisals that need not be congruent.

Just as most applied health research is only a small faction of applied health psychology, so too are applied health researchers only a small faction of those in the service delivery area. With all due regard to the Boulder model of the scientist-practitioner, most of those trained to provide service have been either inadequately prepared to conduct independent research, have little inclination or incentive to do so, or practice psychology in settings that do not foster or permit the routine arrangement of conditions necessary for research nor provide the psychologist with the time, resources, or permission to engage in studies. For applied health psychologists in academia or research institutes, the blending of application and research seems a natural combination. But this is not the case in those far more common settings in which most applications and service delivery occurs. The psychologists in academia, whose careers are marked by publications, are already a selected set, skimming off the most research oriented of the scientist-practitioner cohort. The rest of their colleagues work in situations where either a consultantship, a salary, or a fee for service is the basis of remuneration. Research generated publications do not contribute to either the financial basis under which the service is provided or the criteria by which the service provider is remunerated. In fact, for most applied psychologists, the conduct of research is extraneous to their job requirements. And many who were trained as researchers lose those skills through disuse, disinterest, and lack of time, resources, and encouragement.

It is probably unlikely that any revision of training or education programs will alter this situation. Most psychologists trained as scientist-practitioners will serve their careers as practitioners: this is neither good nor bad, simply a recognition that if there is a societal need for services, service providers will be engaged to provide those services and not for ancillary activities such as research. Whether people who will function as service providers should be trained as scientists and the extent to which research methodology and experience complement and synergistically enhance their didactic and clinical training is a separate issue—one that need not be addressed in this chapter. The parallel question, to what extent do scientists planning for applied research careers need to be trained as practitioners, is one of a series of such questions. The germane larger issue is what are the training needs of applied researchers?

Before examining that topic, a brief recapitulation is in order. One dimension on which research can be ordered is the setting in which it is conducted—whether in the field or in the laboratory. The other dimension, basic versus applied, cuts across that of setting. While it is clear (cf., chap. 7) that basic research can be conducted in the field, it is equally true that applied research can be conducted in the laboratory. For example, pharmaceutical firms have psychopharmacology units in which experimental psychologists in laboratory settings assess the effects of various drugs on the behavior and performance of laboratory animals and use well-calibrated animal behaviors to screen drugs. These activities are clearly research, are conducted in laboratories, and most frequently are applied to questions of marketing, manufacturing, and safety raised by the firm rather than to a basic scientific issue raised by the investigator. Both applied and basic research occur in a variety of settings.

Without reiterating the original caveats against forced distinctions (although they still apply), it is possible to list some of the salient characteristics that distinguish applied from basic research. Overall, applied research is more likely than basic research to:

1. Have its purpose and problems selected by someone other than the investigator
2. Go from one to another problem rather than follow a thread of interest from study to study
3. Be directed to goals set by a sponsor with less opportunity for the researcher to explore other questions as they arise
4. To be framed in ways that do not match traditional disciplinary training and skills, necessitating a team of investigators

5. Be interwoven with the delivery of a service or product, with there being limited control over the circumstances of that product or service delivery

6. Select the techniques to fit the problem, rather than frame the problem to a form amenable to the investigator's skills and interests

7. Be directed by someone other than the investigator.

Aphoristically, basic research is usually directed toward the understanding of a process; applied research is directed toward solving a problem.

The discussion of basic and applied research has been simplified. Many investigators seek both to understand the process and to solve the problem. Often, when research is conducted by a group or team of investigators, some will be problem oriented, others process oriented. Many of the best investigators wish to achieve both goals. It frequently happens that a basic investigator in one field needs a technique, a finding, or a skill from another field—only to find that the crucial need for her or his basic research is regarded as an applied contribution from the other field. Psychologists engaged in basic health research may wish to have a particular statistical technique, a pertinent epidemiological or demographic analysis, a specific neurochemical assay, or bit of physiological knowledge. They are, in effect, asking other basic fields to do applied work for them. In parallel fashion, investigators in other fields may call upon psychological researchers for a specific bit of knowledge; the request may be for an application, but may be addressed to a basic researcher. All of these complexities are well known and make the separation of basic and applied research difficult. Indeed, the same piece of research may be basic or applied (or both) depending on the motives, interest, and intentions of the investigator.

The question of why one should bother characterizing basic and applied research if they are so interwoven may be legitimately raised. After all, the complexities are great, the reservations numerous, and the clear-cut distinctions few. Why bother with another seemingly interminable discussion of the ineffable? There are two salient reasons why it is worth laboring through the separation and identification of these two modes of research. First, although basic and applied are not separated at their margins and many investigations are unclassifiable as a pure example of either type, there are many other research endeavors that clearly fall into one or another camp. These are evaluated, judged, funded, adopted, and used by different criteria. In the 1940s, Charles Fort, a science fiction writer, coined a graphic metaphor to describe those situations in which, although precise definitions failed to distinguish between two classes, common sense had no problems. He said, "Just because a scientist looking at a cell in a microscope cannot tell whether it is animal or vegetable does not mean that I will send my wife a bouquet of hippopotami." There are real differences between much of basic and applied research. This leads to the second consideration. These real differences, albeit not easily characterized by formal definitions, have implications for training. In designing a training program for students who intend to do primarily one or the other type of research, the nature of the research will affect the priorities of the constituent elements of the program.

Training for Research

All training and education is continuous. All but the most recently graduated of us, whether researchers or service providers, are using techniques, tools, and theories that did not exist when we were going through our formal education. Formal continuing education in the learned professions was a minor component of professional education a decade or two ago. Now it is a major educational component, firmly established with accreditation procedures, its own associations, and licensure laws that sanction and require it. To the trainee, the sequence of undergraduate, graduate, postdoctoral, and fellowship training must seem never ending. And, it would appear no less so to the parent, spouse, or bank loan officer underwriting or subsidizing the costs of the training. As the knowledge base has grown exponentially, the demands it places on training seem to indicate that training is likely to increase in length rather than shorten or even remain constant.

When curricula are developed, it is comparatively easy to design a complete modern course of studies as long as time, money, and number of courses are no objects. For example, in the 1950s, training programs were developed in the behavioral sciences which sought to produce investigators with familiarity in a spectrum of disciplines: e.g., anthropology, economics, philosophy of science, political science, psychology, sociology, and statistics. Many of these programs collapsed of their own weight. As each discipline contributed what it judged to be the minimum amount necessary for provisional proficiency in its domain, the demands on the curriculum and the students proved intolerable, and the substitution of intensive training in one (or two) disciplines became an increasingly attractive training alternative. The situation has parallels in contemporary training, only now within each discipline. In a reasonable amount of time with a feasible appraisal of possible human effort, it is probably no longer possible to master the breadth of a single field. The many jokes about increasing medical specialization accurately reflect a trend in medical training, but they also point out that the length and density of the current medical curriculum, now stretched to the breaking point, are still not sufficient to span the wealth of knowledge necessary. Specialization is not an economic necessity or a one-upmanship ploy, it is a concerted attempt to circumscribe an unmanageable mass of material. And, as has already been indicated, even extreme specialization must be continually supplemented by continuing education. Such specialization must ultimately also come to health psychology with specific training regimens for those planning careers as applied health researchers.

Implications for Training

The gist of the previous sections leads to the conclusions that applied health researchers are less likely to be in control of their choice of problems, issues, and the techniques to be used than are basic researchers. If one is a basic health researcher—whether in lab or field—one can select those problems that match one's interests, proclivities, and skills as a researcher. The choice of problems within a domain of research gives the investigator great control over what might be studied and more importantly narrows the range of techniques that must be employed in order to investigate the issue. In contradistinction, the applied researcher often is assigned a problem and assigned it in such a way that he or she has little control over the methods to be used. It is not rare that the study to be done is part of a larger program involving delivery of services or healing techniques, rehabilitation, or prevention, and the basic structure of the study has been determined for reasons other than the research. For instance, if the team of physicians is attempting a new technique for a surgical procedure, they may contrast this technique with several controls and assign subjects in a particular way. The applied researcher called in as an evaluation expert or to assess psychosocial components starts with the fixed treatment plan and must utilize whatever techniques can be located, given the experimental design.

This often means that the applied researcher must in many ways be more sophisticated, more technically adept, and engage in more subsidiary analyses than the basic researcher who has control over the assignment of conditions and design of the study. The issues involved in an after-the-fact study or evaluation of a project have been discussed by Campbell and Stanley (1966) and illustrated in a popular article by Moses and Mosteller (1971). It is clear that it is necessary for applied researchers—often called in after the fact and who usually are not in complete control of their study—to have more rather than less training in general methodology and statistics and quantitative methods in particular.

Unfortunately for the hopes of a simple training plan, a similar line of reasoning also suggests that those who are trained as applied researchers and intend to primarily practice in this domain must also need more extensive and broader training in a substantive field. A basic researcher has some liberty to select the kinds of problems he is working on whether they are in diabetes, coronary disease, nutrition and health, or whatever. Such a person does not necessarily need deep knowledge into all areas of those fields that can be classified as parts of health psychology. To be sure, the more one knows, the better one will be as a researcher, and there is considerable crossover and cross-fertilization from one area to another, but disease or problem-specific education and training in one area is not necessary for one to do high-quality research in a different specific area of health psychology. As with all sorts of specialized training, the danger is that if one moves outside the specialty one may not be prepared to undertake further research. This danger is greater for the applied researcher than it is for the basic one because the applied researcher, subject to having problems assigned, circumscribed, or directed, may not have the choice of problem selection that the basic researcher does.

In addition, there is a kind of education which relates to administrative and organizational knowledge of the setting in which the research is to be carried out. Health research can be done in a variety of locales and institutional bases: universities, research institutes, hospitals, medical schools, free-standing clinics, and many other places—all of which provide settings where appropriate health research can be carried out. While it is not exhaustive, the diversity even among this small list of possible settings suggests that the way in which researchers get cooperation, assistance, permission, clearances, and the way they function will vary greatly. It is already generally agreed that some type of training—formal or informal, structured or unstructured—should be provided as part of the health psychology preparation program so that people who will work in settings that are different from those in which they were trained will understand the organizational prerequisites and the ways in which their settings will operate. Knowledge of the health care delivery system, the organization of hospitals, the structure of nursing homes, the relationship of free-standing, self-help groups to proprietary health advice organizations, all require some advance preparation if a researcher participating as an employee, consultant, or just as a requester of assistance is to function effectively. And, once again, while this sort of training is equally pertinent to the entire spectrum of basic and applied health psychology, the applied researcher must prepare for a wider range of experiences and settings than the basic researcher. Put another way, the applied researcher may be assigned to a setting as opposed to having some of the basic researcher's mobility to choose settings.

Finally, there is training necessary for service delivery. Much of applied research, as we have stated, takes place in the context of applied health psychology (i.e., the delivery of a particular service or part of a team that delivers a particular service). Many of the settings in which this occurs require that even the researchers on the team or within the setting be able to provide some sort of service for fee or compensation, either to raise money for their own salary, or to provide part of the general health care delivery the setting gives to its clients, or both. It is unclear whether training for health service delivery is more incumbent upon the basic or applied researcher. As basic health researchers take jobs in a variety of different settings, they too may be called upon to provide such services. The ability to generate money— whether for oneself or the organization—is not the only reason for health service training. To the extent that people are concerned with evaluation or health of a service delivery program, the ability of the researcher to provide such service gives an insight which goes beyond the mere entree into those settings. Even if the applied researcher needs this no more than the basic researcher, they need it no less, as they too must understand the nature of the service that their group, or team, or project to be evaluated, is providing.

To recapitulate, the four components of training for applied health psychology research are: (1) general methodological, (2) health psychology substantive content, (3) organizational and setting information, and (4) service delivery. It is possible to expand these four general areas into a large laundry list of subareas, each of which could be given its own crucial importance in the training, but the focus still suggests that training in applied health psychology is not more delimiting or narrow than training for a basic researcher. Quite the contrary, it seems to be at least equally broad with a strong suggestion that it may have to be even broader than that for the basic researcher. It is, of course, possible to get breadth by sacrificing depth of knowledge in any area, but even that is a perilous venture. If the applied researcher is to function as a member of a team, such a person must specialize in order to have a unique place and be worth maintaining on the research group. Overall, training in applied health psychology must convey both breadth and depth in each of the four areas.

Given that the period of formal education is limited by a variety of time and economic constraints, it is not sufficient to outline the components of an educational program. Some priority arrangement must also be provided so that when the ideal training regimen—one that takes ten years to cover all aspects—is pruned back to a reasonable length, there is a basis for the decisions. My subjective preferences are as follows:

1. Training in methodology must be preeminent. This should include statistics, experimental design, psychometrics, evaluations, meta-analyses, quasi-experimental procedures, and any other classes of techniques that can be exported to research teams.
2. Substantive knowledge in some areas of health psychology is necessary. If care is taken to build that knowledge on a core of more basic aspects of psychology such as learning, cognition, social processes, and physiology, then other specific applications can be acquired, as needed or wanted, after the completion of formal training. Substantive knowledge is not regarded as less important than methodological fields, rather additional areas of psychological inquiry are more likely to be acquired by self-study on the part of psychologists than are technical ones from fields outside of psychology.
3. General health delivery systems and knowledge of specific organization structures are vital to the conduct of research in health psychology. It is not known whether all, or even most, training venues can provide the faculty or curriculum or provide this knowledge on a structured basis. Without minimizing its importance, it is likely that instruction in this component of applied health researcher's education would be limited to one or two courses.
4. It is imperative that an applied health psychology researcher have some service delivery skill. It is less important that the researcher be a complete clinician or master a gamut of techniques. The ability to do something professionally, e.g., run a smoking cessation clinic, organize a disease specific support group, outline a stress management program, etc. serves several purposes. It gives the researcher clinical credibility in settings where such credibility is necessary. It provides a means of raising revenue, often a *sine qua non* of settings in which applied health psychology research is conducted. It gives the researcher insight into the nature of the service delivery setting and patient-client population.
5. The widely held bias that basic research is intellectually superior to applied research, which still lingers in university training centers, has a pernicious filtering effect on the choices of trainees. Such prejudices must be modified so that the caliber of students electing applied health psychology research careers remains equal to that of the students choosing basic

health psychology research careers. Applied research in health psychology is worth doing. It is worth doing well. Doing it well requires a cadre of bright, well-trained practitioners. Second-class status and a déclassé attitude on the part of basic researchers may impede the growth of an applied research cadre in health psychology.

Conclusion

Overall, training for applied research in health psychology differs from basic research training only in emphasis. The same elements of the training situation are necessary. If the training is to be mastered in a feasible amount of time, then it is recommended that, in comparison to basic researchers, there be a somewhat greater accent on methodological training and the acquisition of a service delivery skill. These emphases are deemed desirable in order to prepare the applied health psychology researcher to function in settings with a restricted range of choice and control.

REFERENCES

Campbell, D. T., and D. T. Stanley. 1966. *Experimental and quasiexperimental designs for research*. Chicago: Rand McNally.

Moses, L. E., and F. Mosteller. 1971. Safety of anesthetics. In *Statistics: A guide to the unknown*, edited by J. M. Tanur, F. Mosteller, W. H. Kruskal, R. F. Link, R. S. Pieters, and G. R. Rising. San Francisco: Holden-Day.

Singer, J. E., and D. C. Glass. 1975. Some reflections on losing our social psychological purity. In *Applying social psychology*, edited by M. Deutsch and H. A. Hornstein. Hillsdale, NJ: Lawrence Erlbaum and Associates.

Part Three

Applications of Health Psychology

Editor: Michael J. Follick

The current problems faced by the health care system have created a number of opportunities for the application of health psychology. Most of the conditions facing modern medicine today are chronic illnesses and by definition are incurable. Health planners have argued that prevention programs are the best way to improve the health status of the population and control health care costs. Since many chronic illnesses have been shown to be related to lifestyle, health psychologists have become involved in primary and secondary prevention programs. Furthermore, health psychologists, through their attention to psychological and social factors, have attempted to maximize functional capacity and facilitate adaptation and quality of life in patients suffering from chronic illness. With the increasing emphasis on containing health care costs and the need for a cost-effective health care delivery system, health psychologists must demonstrate that a multidisciplinary focus to health care delivery, based on a biopyschosocial model, will not only be more effective in improving the health status of the population but will also help control health care costs. If we are to meet this challenge and establish our place in the health care system of the future, we must identify how to best prepare health psychologists.

Part 3 deals with the application of health psychology from a number of perspectives. These chapters review the applications of health psychology as they presently exist and the training future health psychologists will need to meet both current and future demands. In addition, this part discusses how health psychology might utilize or interface with other areas of psychology to maximize its contributions to the health care system.

The first chapter, by Steven Tulkin, reviews the application of health psychology in a general health care setting. He covers a range of services provided and some specific medical conditions for which health psychology can have a significant impact on either the occurrence, course, or outcome of the condition. He also discusses what he sees as the necessary knowledge base for health psychologists who will be working in health care settings. In addition, he identifies barriers to the integration of health psychology into the health care system in general.

Chapter 10, by Michael Follick and his colleagues, discusses the application of health psychology in the workplace. The workplace is seen as a setting where preventive efforts, through health-related behavior change, may be effectively implemented because it offers accessibility to a broad range of the population. The authors review not only the various approaches that have been identified to date, but also critically evaluate the present status of worksite health promotion. They identify what they feel is needed if prevention programs are to be successful at the worksite.

Chapter 11, by Edison J. Tricket, follows from the previous chapter and discusses the value of drawing on the models and knowledge base of community psychology. He discusses the ecological model as it applies to health psychology and community settings. There is potentially much to be gained by considering preventive efforts within a social context. He also notes the utility of drawing on the knowledge base of community psychology with respect to community intervention and program evaluation.

Ruth Faden, in her chapter on health psychology and public health, addresses the substantial overlap between health psychology and public health. She identifies not only common areas of interest such as life-style change but also areas of concern within public health, such as hazard control, which she believes represent areas with enormous promise for the application of health psychology. Similarly, she cites the need and opportunities for health psychology in the allocation of health care resources. She convincingly argues the need for an interface between health psychology and public health.

The final chapter, by Patrick DeLeon and Gary VandenBos, discusses health psychology and health policy. They contend that health psychology is both influenced by health policy and can influence the formation of health policy. They note specifically how health psychology can influence the development of health policy and point to the need for training institutions to assist health psychologists in appreciating the complexities of health policy. They also inform them of how they may participate in the process and identify specific roles for health psychologists in the policy-formation process. Clearly, this is an area of application that we cannot overlook if we are to establish a place for health psychology in the health care system of the future.

9

Health Care Services

Steven R. Tulkin

The purpose of this chapter is to describe the scope of direct patient care services that are currently being offered by psychologists in health care settings. This overview will be used to generate a discussion of training needs for psychologists delivering health care services in the future. Several specific questions will be addressed: (1) What do health care psychologists actually do with patients? (2) What are the training needs for fully licensed health psychologists? (3) What are some of the barriers to providing psychological services in health-care settings, and how might they be overcome? (4) Is there a place for specialized health psychology service providers who are not clinical psychologists to offer limited services to the public?

The Practice of Health Psychology

Although medical psychology and psychosomatic medicine have an extensive history, practitioners of health psychology hope to add a significant new dimension to patient care. Currently in most settings, health care services are provided by psychologists who were originally trained in clinical or counseling programs with an emphasis on helping clients with various types of emotional problems. These psychologists discovered—through the research literature and through their own experiences—that specific interventions could have an impact on the course and outcome of many "physical" diseases. This discovery coincided with the emphasis on biopsychosocial models of health and illness that were gaining acceptance among other health care service providers (Engel 1977).

As the practice of health psychology is accepted by the health care establishment, it is likely to become a legitimate specialty in its own right; but for

I would like to thank the following people for their ideas and assistance in writing this chapter: Michael Follick, Gerald Frank, Melinda Ginne, Stewart Proctor, Lorinda Sheets, and Norman Weinstein. Author's address: Kaiser-Permanente Medical Center, 27400 Hesperian Blvd., Hayward, CA 94545.

the present, the mode of entry in most settings is through the services we can offer as clinical or counseling psychologists. As requests for health care services increase and the contributions of health psychology are defined more clearly, practicing health psychologists will obtain credibility and establish specific job description and credentialing procedures. These developments will have to be coordinated with groups such as the National Register and Division 38 of the American Psychological Association. In this chapter, however, the focus will be on what psychologists will need over the next five to ten years for successful employment in health care settings; the requirements may change once health psychology is accepted as a unique area of specialization.

Scope of Services

The range of services provided by psychologists in health care settings is broad, and readers are referred to several recent books which describe these services in detail (Ferguson and Taylor 1980; Millon, Green, and Meagher 1982; Prokop and Bradley 1981; and Taylor 1986). Health care services provided by psychologists can be classified roughly in seven categories: (1) prevention and health-related behavior change; (2) nonpharmologic alternative treatment approaches; (3) psychological treatment as a primary intervention; (4) psychological treatment as an ancillary intervention; (5) coping with acute medical crisis; (6) adaptation to chronic disease; and (7) compliance. Each category will be described briefly below.

PREVENTION AND HEALTH-RELATED BEHAVIOR CHANGE

This category covers primary and secondary prevention and thus relates to the general population as well as to specific high-risk groups. Services include programs related to healthy behaviors in areas of nutrition, exercise, coping with stress, and misuse of chemicals such as nicotine, alcohol, and drugs. The goal is to reduce risk factors associated with cardiovascular diseases, respiratory diseases, and other conditions where life-style variables have significant impact (for example see Krantz, Baum, and Singer 1983).

NONPHARMOLOGIC ALTERNATIVE TREATMENT APPROACHES

Several conditions for which drugs are commonly prescribed can often be relieved without the use of medication. Because these medications often cause side effects, alternative interventions are highly desirable. Hypertension (Shapiro 1983) and migraine headache (Bernstein and Deltredici

1983; Cinciripini, Williamson, and Epstein 1981) are examples of conditions in which patients have responded positively to dietary and behavioral interventions.

Psychological Treatment as a Primary Intervention

Many disorders that have continually frustrated physicians and other health care providers respond favorably to behavioral interventions. Included in this category are conditions diagnosed as "chronic benign intractible pain" (Fordyce 1976; Steger and Fordyce 1982) and various gastrointestinal disorders including fecal incontinence, rumination syndrome, and irritable bowel syndrome (Whitehead and Bosmajian 1982). Treatment usually involves a range of behavioral interventions and environmental contingency management. Before suggesting this type of treatment, it is important to be sure that all possible medical interventions have been ruled out.

Psychological Treatment as an Ancillary Intervention

Many conditions are exacerbated by stress even though psychological components may not be primary etiological factors. Asthma is one of the conditions commonly described under this heading. A variety of psychological interventions have been used with asthmatics (Alexander and Solanch 1981), including relaxation and biofeedback to alter pulmonary function and systematic desensitization to reduce the anxiety and panic associated with asthma attacks.

Coping with Acute Medical Crisis

How patients respond emotionally to the crisis of a major medical procedure can affect the course of recovery. Psychologists in medical settings have helped patients cope with procedures including chemotherapy, bone marrow transplants, cardiac catheterization, endoscopy, and surgery (Moos 1984). In most cases, interventions are brief, focus on a specific problem, and involve education, desensitization, behavioral rehearsal, and other techniques which attempt to increase the patients perception of control (see Taylor 1986).

Adaptation to Chronic Diseases

Chronic diseases such as diabetes, arthritis, and multiple sclerosis present ongoing management problems for patients and their families. Interventions typically include strategies for pain and stress management, group support for development of coping mechanisms and adaptive behaviors, and techniques to improve medical compliance. Clinicians and researchers in health psychology continue to emphasize that in order to appeal to patients and be successful, interventions need to address the patient's physical condition as opposed to "mental health needs" because such patients do not have primary psychological problems (Achterberg-Lawlis 1982). One disease in which attention to the psychosocial issues has increased in recent years is cancer, and interested readers are referred to a recent review of clinical literature in this area by Goldberg and Tull (1984).

COMPLIANCE

Compliance may be an issue in each of the above categories, but it also represents a unique area of practice for health psychology. Nonadherence to medical regimens is a serious problem in the practice of medicine, and various techniques have been developed by psychologists to increase compliance (Epstein and Cluss 1982). Clinical populations have included diabetic, hypertensive, and depressed patients, among others.

A wide variety of psychological interventions have been used with patients in all of these seven categories. Some are fairly specific (e.g., dealing with a particular type of pain) while others are more general (e.g., helping families cope with chronic illness). Many of the techniques are behavioral, but the overall approach requires a biopsychosocial perspective in order to understand the interrelationship of behavior, physiology, emotions, and environment.

Training Goals

Obviously no one person can specialize in all of the above areas. It is necessary, however, that a psychologist trained to deliver health care services have some general medical knowledge of one or two medical conditions, including pathophysiology and epidemiology of the diseases. Although most health psychologists will practice collaboratively with physicians and thus will not need to make a medical diagnosis, it is necessary for health psychologists to understand diagnostic issues related to the conditions being treated. For example, what kinds of medical problems are likely to mimic psychological symptoms (Hall 1980)? When does a pain complaint of a chronic pain patient merit further evaluation by a physician? When does a patient's drinking or drug history indicate that abrupt cessation is likely to lead to dangerous withdrawal symptoms? Some of this education can come in the form of coursework. Health psychologists need courses such as physiology and pharmacology, as well as public health courses such as epidemiology and health education. Much of this knowledge, however, will come from on-the-job internship and residency experiences at the predoctoral and postdoctoral levels.

What types of professional skills will be needed? Will it suffice for a psychologist delivering health-care services to be an expert in biofeedback and stress reduction techniques without more basic knowledge and experiences in personality and general clinical theory? There is debate about the extent of the need for training in clinical psychology (see Perry 1983; Sechrest 1983), and this issue will be addressed further below. There is no debate, however, about the need for a fully trained health psychologist to have a broad understanding of personality and psychopathology *as related to health and disease*. Millon (1982) has argued that the ability of the professional health psychologist "to function effectively in diverse clinical settings will demand a broader array of technical skills than . . . behavioral" and that health psychologists "must acquire a sensitivity to the psychological complexities that often underlie what appear ostensibly to be 'simple' behaviors" (p. 21).

This need is especially strong because in the foreseeable future most health-delivery settings will not have specific job descriptions for health psychologists and will expect all "clinicians" to provide a broad range of clinical interventions, (e.g., emergency or crisis coverage). Until such time as the specialty of health psychology is accredited by the APA and recognized by the National Register and state licensing boards, students without a degree in clinical or counseling psychology are likely to have difficulty finding employment in clinical settings.

Specific clinical skills in short-term, cognitive-behavioral, group, and crisis therapy would make a candidate desirable for employment. Being skilled in *short-term therapy* is necessary because reimbursements are likely to be limited; *cognitive-behavioral therapy* because this approach is the most relevant for dealing with the life-style issues relating to medical conditions; *group therapy* because programs are likely to have a greater impact if they can make use of the increased motivation which comes from peer support; and *crisis therapy* because medical settings need to be able to respond to patients in crisis, and every mental health professional is expected to carry his or her share of the load in this difficult area. The practicing health psychologist also needs to be familiar with assessment procedures for medical patients. These include behavioral assessments, neuropsychological assessments, and paper-and-pencil tests such as the Millon Behavioral Health Inventory.

In addition to familiarity with medical conditions and clinical interventions, psychologists delivering health services need to understand the *systems* in which health care services are delivered. Knowledge of the economics and politics of health care services as well as the social and interpersonal issues which lead to acceptance or rejection of change in an established system is needed. Psychologists involved with health policy have addressed the former issues (see chap. 13), and community and organizational psychologists have addressed the issue of barriers to changing systems. This topic will be discussed more fully in part 4. Of primary importance is that psychologists are not currently in power in the health care system. Psychological expertise is central to the functioning of *mental* health service delivery but has only begun to be accepted in other areas of the health care delivery system.

In order to function effectively in the health care delivery system, survival skills are necessary. These skills include everything from managing professional relationships to basic business management issues. Professional relationship issues revolve around being a member of a team. Membership on the health-delivery team requires an understanding of the expectations of team members. For example, what response is expected to a consultation request? If one wants to be consulted again, the response should not be a theoretical statement of personality or psychopathology but a concise statement of *s*ubjective and *o*bjective observations, followed by *a*ssessment (diagnosis) and *p*lan ("SOAP" is the common acronym which physicians use for the above outline).

Another expectation is that team members have familiarity with life and death issues faced by health care professionals. Psychologists working in a neonatal intensive care unit or a hospice face life and death issues daily, and every practicing health psychologist will face some ethical questions in the course of practice. These issues are developed further by Swencionis and Hall (see chap. 15) and need to be a part of both the academic training and practical experiences of psychologists who deliver health care services.

Business issues are similar to those faced by other professional psychologists: how to start a practice, fee setting, third-party reimbursement, and hospital privileges. Professional health psychologists, however, need to be more attentive to legal constraints than colleagues dealing strictly with emotional problems. Working with medical problems increases the risk of legal liability, and practicing health psychologists need to be cautious about the limits of practice. These issues are also developed further in chapter 16 by Frohboese and Overcast.

Finally, the importance of research in the delivery of health care services needs to be emphasized. Miller (1983; and chap. 1) and others have discussed the importance of the "scientist/practitioner" model and argued that all health psychologists need a basic background in the issues that are important for research and clinical practice. Even though research may not occupy a major portion of time in the daily activities of a practicing health psychologist, it will play a critical role in the acceptance and development of health psychology services in applied settings. The unique contribution of health psychology services is that they are more than technical interventions; they derive from and are supported by ongoing research. As issues of effectiveness and cost/effectiveness assume greater importance in health care, administrators will look more toward psychologists not only because of the expertise in changing behaviors but because of the training at a conceptual level. This training enables psychologists to accurately assess patient needs, to understand what current research has to say about those needs, to develop programs which can then be evaluated, and to maintain an openness to expand or contract services as needs change and as evaluation indicates that changes are necessary.

Brendan Maher (1983) emphasized this point when he stated that a competent health psychologist "will need to understand the bases of measurement in the areas in which he or she is to work—but will need to do so in a context sufficiently broad to prevent risk of the kind of permanent attachment to outmoded techniques that still characterizes the work of many clinical psychologists in the field of psychiatric disorder" (p. 45). This flexibility, said Maher, comes from methodological expertise, which "provides the basis for a true professional autonomy for the health psychologist . . ." (p. 46).

Thus training needs for the practicing health psychologist include: (1) medical knowledge about specific disorders as well as about the health care delivery system; (2) knowledge of basic psychology as well as personality and psychopathology as they apply to health; (3) knowledge of broad-based approaches to assessment and intervention emphasizing the biopsychosocial model; (4) real-life experiences in the delivery of health services as part of an interdisciplinary staff; and (5) understanding of research methods which will allow an ongoing assessment of the services being provided. More details of the proposed content of predoctoral and postdoctoral programs appear in part 6.

Institutional Barriers to the Practice of Health Psychology

Integration of health psychology into the existing health-care delivery system presents a multitude of challenges. People in positions of power in most systems are invested in retaining the status quo, and community psychologists who have studied system change have issued warnings about naive expectations about the acceptance of psychology. One of the strong advocates of a systems approach in community psychology has been Murray Levine, who in 1974 suggested some "Postulates of Community Psychology Practice." These postulates are relevant for the practice of health psychology as well, especially for understanding some of the barriers that can be expected over the next decade as psychologists become more active in health care delivery. The postulates will be presented and discussed in terms of what health psychologists can do to overcome some of the obstacles to system change.

> *Postulate I. When a problem arises in a setting or in a situation, some factor in the situation either causes, triggers, exacerbates, or maintains the problem.*

This postulate is familiar to health psychologists. It suggests that the health care system itself is responsible for some of the problems in health care delivery. Recent critics of our health care system have enumerated some of these contributions.

First, our medical system is based on a disease model; a medical complaint is needed to gain entry. People who want to discuss their health or any aspect of their well-being cannot easily do so. Specifically, the health care system does not typically provide for systematic health counseling, which could include everything from nutritional evaluations to training in breast self-examinations. These educational experiences may be available, but generally they are not reimbursed by third-party insurance and are not always advocated by primary-care physicians. Thus, patients are likely to perceive them as having minor importance.

A more serious complaint about the health care system is that symptomatic treatment, which often does not attack the etiologic condition needing attention, keeps patients in a state of ill health and in need of ongoing medical attention. Treatment of chronic pain, stress, and anxiety with drugs alone are prime examples.

Hospital administrators are aware of the literature reporting that a significant percentage of physician visits and hospitalizations are related to life stress or bad health habits. As the health care delivery system becomes more cost conscious (especially through the increased emphasis on HMOs and preferred provider groups), attempts will be made to utilize treatment approaches that are appropriate and effective for the problems being presented. Health psychologists are a logical choice of a professional group to develop and deliver these services, but for these programs to be accepted, it is important to keep in mind that many people in places of power in the system are likely to resist the change. Postulate II is relevant to this issue.

> *Postulate II. A problem arises in a situation because there is some element(s) in the social setting that blocks effective problem-solving behavior on the part of those charged with carrying out the functions and achieving the goals of the setting.*

Most physicians would probably agree that it is important to prevent disease and promote health, but their training limits their skills and understanding of how to do so. Physicians are trained to see themselves as the dispensers of a cure which they give to their patients. They are also trained to see disease only in terms of dysfunction of the body's physical and chemical systems. As dispensers of a cure, there is little need to establish a working alliance with the patient. Although much has been written about patients' contributions to their own health and illness (e.g., Vickery and Fries 1976), physicians rarely utilize this alliance to its full potential.

Levine mentions that if a system is failing to solve an important problem, the failure "will involve more than simply a lack of skills or knowledge on the part of the people in the setting." He suggests that failure often relates to the needs of the system to maintain what it sees as its essential functions. In the case of a health care system, the introduction of self-care programs directing patients to diagnose and treat various problems or the referral of patients suffering from chronic stress or pain to a health psychologist would dramatically change the physician's role as "dispenser-of-cure." In the current climate, this could seriously affect the self-concept of the medical profession—which may be a part of the reason that effective health psychology programs will be difficult to establish. To overcome this barrier, attention must be paid to Postulate III.

> *Postulate III. Effective help has to be located strategically, preferably in the very situation involved at the time at which the problem manifests itself.*

This is perhaps the most controversial idea to be discussed. It suggests that for health psychology to be effective, it needs to be integrated into the health care system. Integration does not simply mean that the program be located in the same physical structure; there are programs that exist in medical centers unbeknownst to the primary care physicians practicing there. What the postulate means is that the primary providers must work collaboratively with health psychologists for these programs to be maximally effective.

At the Kaiser-Permanente Medical Center in Hayward, California, this model has been used in the development of several programs including treatment for alcoholism, smoking cessation, and chronic pain. The conclusion from these experiences is that the most effective way to integrate health psychologists into the health care system is through a behavioral medicine unit that operates in a fashion similar to other specialty clinics in the medical center. In this model, health psychologists direct the programs in consultation with medical personnel. Physician involvement and endorsement provides the necessary liaison with primary care departments, and physicians also attend group meetings and participate in educational and behavior change processes. In addition to physicians providing useful medical information, their endorsement enhances patient commitment to the program. Finally, physician involvement serves an important credibility function throughout the medical center. An example of such a program will be presented below.

> *Postulate IV. The goals or values of the helping service must be consistent with the goals or the values of the setting in which the problem is manifested.*

If psychology is to have a role in the health care system, it is necessary to understand the values of the system as it exists, and to work within those values. Levine states that ". . . the setting will act to expel or otherwise isolate or make ineffective those helping agents who promote goals or values at variance with the major goals and values of the setting." There are numerous examples from school, prison, and self-help systems in which psychologists and other program innovators have been told to leave. The health care system is now presenting a tentative invitation for an alliance, but practicing health psychologists need to proceed with caution and with an understanding that, at the present time, psychologists are the "guests" in a health care delivery system in which others are in charge.

> *Postulate V. The form of help should have the potential for being established on a systematic basis, using the natural resources of the setting, or through introducing resources which can become institutionalized as part of the setting.*

This postulate again emphasizes the need for health psychology to be an integrated part of a biopsychosocial health care delivery system. The "natural resources" of the setting are practitioners of several different disciplines including medicine, nursing, health education, social work, physical therapy, and others. The structure of the team may differ from setting to setting, and flexibility is important. The only stipulation is that psychology's status as an autonomous profession cannot be compromised.

Who Is an Eligible Provider?

The question of who can provide health psychology services is an important one. Economics, ethics, and egos are all involved. At the recent Conference on Education and Training in Health Psychology, no agreement was reached on whether a psychologist needed to be trained in clinical psychology in order to be eligible to offer health psychology services. Two major points of view were raised. On the one hand, Perry (1983) presented the view that "dealing for a fee with distressed and vulnerable persons" is only appropriate for psychologists who are fully trained clinicians. On the other hand, Sechrest (1983) argued that "delivery of health services (should not) be predicated on completion of a Ph.D. in clinical psychology." He especially pointed to "circumscribed but valuable health services [such as] . . . stress management, habit control, and compliance" as areas where psychologists trained in social psychology, personality, and applied behavior analysis can make contributions.

These views need not be contradictory. State laws require that all psychologists offering services to the public be licensed, and licensing is, in most cases, generic. Psychologists offering "specialized" services need not be *clinical* psychologists but would need to be licensed and trained comprehensively in the service being practiced. Obviously, the criteria for what constitutes comprehensive training will need to be defined for the various types of services which health psychologists might offer.

One criterion which might be used to specify how "comprehensive" one's clinical training should be is the extent to which the people being served are psychologically "distressed and vulnerable." Perry's experience is that many people asking for help quitting smoking, reducing stress, etc. *are* vulnerable and have shown considerable psychological disturbance. Sechrest and his colleagues have seen a very different type of person in their program—people who are basically healthy and are simply seeking information and guidance about changing specific behaviors. Experiences with these different populations have convinced each group of the validity of its position.

One approach to resolution would be to differentiate educational and clinical services. Clinical services would only be offered by fully trained clinical psychologists; educational services would not have that requirement. Health psychologists providing educational services *would* be expected to be familiar with signs and symptoms which reflect greater emotional distress, to screen those people out of their programs, and to refer them to appropriate practitioners. An example of such a two-tiered system is the collaborative stop-smoking program developed by the Departments of Health Education, Medicine, and Psychiatry at Kaiser-Permanente in Hayward (Tulkin and Frank 1985) which will be described briefly below.

Interdisciplinary Stop-Smoking Program[1]

The history of the program began in 1980 when the Health Education Department initiated a stop-smoking program based on the model of smoking as a substance dependency (Harrup, Hansen and Soghikian 1979). A masters-level smoking cessation counselor was hired and supervised by a licensed psychologist. While the program was still in its early stages, it became clear that smoking cessation viewed as a substance dependency was different from smoking cessation viewed as a health education problem. The program which was developed emphasized individual assessments and intense interventions. After an individual intake interview, patients attended a 13-session group which incorporated hypnosis, guided imagery, discussions of family relationships and personal feelings in addition to the behavior change suggestions found in most smoking cessation programs. Waiting lists built up, and the staff spent many hours in discussions of divergent philosophies of health education and behavioral medicine.

After a series of meetings with an organizational development specialist, a proposal was developed. The Health Education Department was given responsibility for administration of primary and secondary prevention programs while tertiary programs were to be jointly administered by the departments of psychiatry and medicine as part of the jointly administered Substance Dependency Clinic. Tertiary prevention was defined as "the rehabilitation of patients who have manifested symptoms; in order to decrease the impact of the symptoms on patients' lives and to prevent recurrence" (see Caplan 1964; Strain 1982). This decision resulted in the development of two stop-smoking groups. The smoking cessation counselor was transferred to the Substance Dependency Clinic where she developed a tertiary stop-smoking group for patients with significant medical or psychological problems related to smoking. The Health Education Department initiated an

---

1. This program was developed and directed by Melinda Ginne.

"educationally oriented" group for "smokers who would like information and support to stop smoking." A new health educator was hired to develop this group. Considerable effort was expended to specify triage criteria for these two groups. Briefly, the tertiary group was defined as being for patients expected to have more difficulty quitting: (1) patients who continued to smoke despite medical problems related to cigarettes (and thus could be labeled as addicted); and (2) patients with significant psychological problems (psychosis, depression, other addictions, etc.) which also required specialized attention. It was decided that all patients who were not physician-referred to the tertiary group would be screened by the health educator who would then refer appropriate patients. The two group leaders consult with each other frequently and hold monthly meetings with the internist who serves as medical coordinator for smoking cessation.

The two groups differ in some significant ways. The health education group meets for seven 90-minute sessions and covers topics including awareness of cues for smoking, discussion of healthy behaviors to substitute for smoking, redefining self as a nonsmoker, managing urges, and relapse prevention (defined as "behavioral techniques for coping with stressful and high-risk situations"). In addition, the medical coordinator for smoking cessation attends one of the group sessions to discuss "health aspects of smoking and nonsmoking."

In contrast to the seven sessions in the health education group, the tertiary group meets for 13 sessions, and the content is more psychologically oriented. The groups are also smaller (ten to twelve in contrast to between twenty and thirty), and more individualized interventions can be developed. Before patients are admitted to the group, they have screening appointments with the medical coordinator and the smoking cessation counselor. An assessment is made of the potential psychological risks of smoking cessation. Patients in emotional crises or patients whose coping skills are extremely limited are seen individually to bolster their internal resources before admission to the group. Once in the group, specific psychological issues are emphasized: (1) the psychological aspects of the addictive process (feelings of deprivation, abandonment, etc., upon giving up smoking); (2) the need for new coping skills to deal with negative feelings; (3) the role of smoking in interpersonal power struggles; and (4) individualized programs for relapse prevention which analyze stressful events and / or feelings which are likely to increase the risk of smoking. Alternatives to smoking in these situations are discussed and practiced (e.g., self-hypnosis, guided imagery, exercise, etc.).

The model of sharing responsibilities for programs involving health and behavior change is likely to be used again as specialized programs are developed for other problems such as obesity and stress. The model has already been used to help define professional boundaries in the area of educational and psychological interventions in chronic disease. As suggested by Levine's postulates, the program is consistent with the goals and values of the setting and has the potential for being established on a systematic basis using the natural resources of the setting.

Conclusions

Psychologists' roles in health care delivery are increasing, and the potential exists for psychology as a profession to have an impact on health care. By looking at the types of services that psychologists are now delivering, requirements for the training of the health psychologists of the future become more clear. In addition to a knowledge base in psychology and medical sciences, future health psychologists need experience both with patients and with the health-care delivery system. Appreciation of system barriers to the acceptance of health psychology is critical, and the experience of community psychologists in working with systems may be valuable. Interdisciplinary collaboration is a skill which needs to be nurtured from the beginning days of graduate school through the ongoing years of professional practice.

REFERENCES

Achterberg-Lawlis, J. 1982. The psychological dimensions of arthritis. *Journal of Consulting and Clinical Psychology* 50:984–92.

Alexander, C. B., L. S. Solanch. 1981. Introduction to bronchial asthma. In *The comprehensive handbook of behavioral medicine,* edited by J. M. Ferguson and C. B. Taylor, 1:3–40. Jamaica, NY: Spectrum Publications.

Bernstein, A., and A. Deltredici. 1983. Migraine in children. *Headache* 23:142.

Caplan, G. 1964. *Principles of preventive psychiatry.* New York: Basic Books.

Cinciripini, P. M., D. A. Williamson, and L. H. Epstein. 1981. Behavioral treatment of migraine headaches. In *The comprehensive handbook of behavioral medicine,* edited by J. M. Ferguson and C. B. Taylor, pp. 207–27. Jamaica, NY: Spectrum Publications.

Engel, G. L. 1977. The need for a new medical model: A challenge for biomedicine. *Science* 196:129–36.

Epstein, L. H., and P. A. Cluss. 1982. A behavioral medicine perspective on adherence to long-term medical regimens. *Journal of Consulting and Clinical Psychology* 50:950–71.

Ferguson, J. M., and C. B. Taylor, eds. 1980. *The comprehensive handbook of behavioral medicine.* Jamaica, NY: Spectrum Publications.

Fordyce, W. E. 1976. *Behavioral methods for chronic pain and illness.* St. Louis: C. V. Mosby.

Goldberg, R., and R. Tull. 1984. *The psychosocial dimension of cancer: A guide for health care providers.* New York: The Free Press.

Hall, R. C. W. 1980. *Psychiatric presentations of medical illness: Somato-psychic disorders.* Jamaica, NY: Spectrum Publications.

Harrup, T., B. A. Hansen, and K. Soghikian. 1979. Clinical methods in smoking cessation: Description and evaluation of a stop-smoking clinic. *American Journal of Public Health* 69 : 1226–31.

Krantz, D. S., A. Baum, and J. E. Singer, eds. 1983. *Cardiovascular disorders and behavior.* Hillsdale, NJ: Lawrence Erlbaum and Associates.

Levine, M. 1974. Some postulates of community psychology practice. In *The psychoeducational clinic,* edited by F. Kaplan and S. B. Sarason. Boston: Massachusetts Department of Mental Health.

Maher, B. 1983. The education of health psychologists: Quality counts—Numbers are dangerous. *Health Psychology* 2 (5) : 37–48, (supplement).

Miller, N. E. 1983. Some main themes and highlights of the conference. *Health Psychology* 2 (5) : 11–14, (supplement).

Millon, T. 1982. On the nature of clinical health psychology. In *Handbook of clinical health psychology,* edited by T. Millon, C. Green, and R. Meagher. New York: Plenum Press.

Millon, T., C. Green, and R. Meagher, eds. 1982. *Handbook of clinical health psychology.* New York: Plenum Press.

Moos, R., ed. 1984. *Coping with physical illness: New perspectives.* New York: Plenum Press.

Perry, N. 1983. Majority position in favor of health service delivery by fully trained psychologists. *Health Psychology* 2 (5) : 115–16, (supplement).

Prokop, C. K., and L. A. Bradley, eds. 1981. *Medical psychology: Contributions to behavioral medicine.* New York: Academic Press.

Sechrest, L. 1983. Minority position in favor of health service delivery by clinical and non-clinical psychologists. *Health Psychology* 2 (5) : 117–18, (supplement).

Shapiro, A. P. 1983. The non-pharmologic treatment of hypertension. In *Cardiovascular disorders and behavior,* edited by D. S. Krantz, A. Baum, and J. E. Singer. Hillsdale, NJ: Lawrence Erlbaum and Associates.

Steger, J., and W. Fordyce. 1982. Behavioral health care in the managment of chronic pain. In *Handbook of clinical health psychology,* edited by T. Millon, C. Green, and R. Meagher, pp. 467–97. New York: Plenum Press.

Strain, J. 1982. Collaborative efforts in liaison psychiatry. In *Handbook of clinical health psychology,* edited by T. Millon, C. Green, and R. Meagher, pp. 251–76. New York: Plenum Press.

Taylor, S. 1986. *Health psychology.* Westminister, MD: Alfred A. Knopf.

Tulkin, S. R., and G. W. Frank. 1985. The changing role of psychologists in health maintenance organizations. *American Psychologist* 40 : 125–30.

Vickery, D. M., and J. F. Fries. 1976. *Take care of yourself: A consumer's guide to medical care.* Reading, MA: Addison Wesley.

Whitehead, W. E., and L. S. Bosmajian. 1982. Behavioral medicine approaches to gastrointestinal disorders. *Journal of Consulting and Clinical Psychology* 50 : 972–83.

10

Health Psychology at the Worksite

Michael J. Follick, David B. Abrams, Rodger P. Pinto, and Joanne L. Fowler

Despite a dramatic increase in health-related expenditures between 1950 and 1980, overall health status has remained virtually constant since 1955 (Michael 1982). However, there is a strong relationship between life-style and chronic diseases, and health planners have argued that health promotion efforts will lead to improvements in health status, decrease the incidence of disease, and reduce health care costs. Consequently, there is increased emphasis on primary prevention (Stamler 1979). Because most health-risk factors involve life-style or specific behavior patterns (e.g., cigarette smoking, diet, exercise patterns), health psychology's emphasis on understanding and modifying health-related behaviors can potentially play a major role in this relatively new and important aspect of health care. However, to justify the inclusion of health psychologists and our procedures in comprehensive health-promotion efforts, we must unequivocally demonstrate that behavior change programs are effective with a broad segment of the population.

The worksite has been identified as a setting where health-promotion programs might best be implemented because it offers accessibility to a broad segment of the population (Abrams and Follick 1983; Orleans and Shipley 1982; Stunkard 1976). Industry has expressed significant interest in worksite-based health promotion and has strong economic motives as a result of their large health care expenditures and the costs related to absenteeism and lost productivity.

This brief review focuses on worksite programs designed to modify cardiovascular risk; coronary heart disease (CHD) is the leading cause of death and disability in this country. Selected studies, issues, and future directions are highlighted for smoking, hypertension, obesity, physical fitness, and stress management. A number of approaches to the modification of cardiovascular risk are reviewed and outcome evaluation is discussed in terms of behavior change, health status, non-health-related outcomes, and cost-effectiveness. The role of health psychology in worksite-based, public, health-promotion programs is also discussed.

Screening and Health Education

Screening procedures are simple tests carried out on large numbers of people to identify those who are at risk of physical illness. Several studies have utilized screening procedures to aid in identifying and treating individuals with hypertension (Schoenberger 1976; Foot and Erfurt 1976; and Murphy 1976). While these studies detected large numbers of hypertensive employees, they demonstrated only marginal success in encouraging these employees to seek treatment. Although screening is a convenient and economical way to detect hypertension in large numbers of people, it does not necessarily lead to improved control of blood pressure (Alderman, Green, and Flynn 1982). However, when screening is used as part of a more comprehensive treatment approach, results are considerably better (Murphy 1976). Increasing emphasis is being placed on comprehensive step-care that includes detection as well as follow-up and compliance-enhancing components (Chadwick, Chesney and Jordan 1977).

Health education refers to the use of persuasive methods to encourage people to change their behavior, usually by means of increased knowledge and altered attitudes about health and illness. Worksite health-education programs have been employed by a number of corporations, including the American Hospital Association, American Telephone & Telegraph Company, Campbell Soup Company, and the Ford Motor Company (Parkinson et al. 1982). Like screening programs, these educational methods can reach large numbers of people relatively inexpensively. In one comparison study of high-risk individuals, health education plus limited counseling fared better than no treatment in reducing the risk of heart disease, as measured by biochemical parameters and the multiple logistic function (Kornitzer, De-Backer, Dramaix, and Thilly 1980).

The assumption underlying health education is that changing knowledge and attitudes will lead to behavior change. However, outcome is usually measured by assessing changes in awareness, knowledge, and attitudes rather than behavior or physiological mediators of CHD. Unfortunately, knowledge does not necessarily lead to lasting behavior change (Thompson 1978). While increasing awareness via education is an important motivational component of a health-promotion program, the majority of individuals require more explicit behavioral skills training and social support to produce and maintain changes in health-related behaviors (cf., Abrams et al. 1986).

Direct Risk Factor Interventions

SMOKING

Many industries are beginning to offer smoking cessation programs to their employees (McDougall 1978; Rosen and Lichtenstein 1977; Cathcart 1977). Small-group behavioral treatments, health counseling, physician's advice, self-help programs, smoking restrictions, and videotape smoking clinics have all been utilized. Orleans and Shipley (1982) review these programs in detail and report on at least five controlled evaluations of worksite smoking cessation programs (Meyer and Henderson 1974; Bauer 1978; Danaher 1982; Rogers 1977; and Kanzler, Zeidenberg, and Jaffe 1976). While many studies lack methodological rigor, the data suggest that behavioral treatment methods are the most effective, and the results of worksite-based programs are similar to those obtained in clinic settings. Thus, it is reasonable to expect that six months after treatment, approximately twenty to thirty percent of the participants will be nonsmokers (Danaher 1982). Orleans and Shipley (1982) suggest that worksite programs should: (1) incorporate protocols known to be effective in other settings; (2) evaluate the programs and their interaction with population and setting characteristics; and (3) capitalize on unique elements present at the worksite, such as social support networks and various organization-wide incentive or environmental change components. One major challenge for worksite smoking cessation programs is to reach the "hard-core" (especially blue-collar) smokers who have not been able to quit on their own despite exposure to massive education campaigns. These individuals may be far more physiologically and/or psychologically dependent on cigarettes and require environmental change and social support procedures which are more adaptable to the work setting.

OBESITY

There have been few empirical evaluations of behavioral weight-loss interventions in industrial settings. Trials have been conducted with employees of the Ford Motor Company, General Foods, and Kimberly Clark, as well as with the military and the federal government (Foreyt, Scott, and Grotto 1980). However, the absence of control groups and the nonrandom assignment of participants to groups makes meaningful evaluation of these programs difficult. Two reasonably well-controlled research programs have recently been reported (Stunkard and Brownell 1980; Abrams and Follick 1983). The data from these studies suggest that at the six month follow-up, an average weight loss of 1.2 kilograms to 4.1 kilograms per person can be expected. However, these studies report extremely high attrition rates, up to eighty-two percent. More recently, in an effort to develop strategies to curb the attrition problem, Follick, Fowler, and Brown (1984) successfully utilized an incentive procedure to increase adherence to a behavioral, worksite, weight loss program. They found that sixty percent of the participants in the incentive group completed treatment compared to twenty percent in the control group.

Some worksite, weight loss programs have also included innovative approaches such as organizational behavior modification (e.g., goal setting, incentive systems, and feedback to the entire worksite) and social psychology principles (e.g., within group co-operation and intergroup competition) to augment the traditional small-group behavioral approach (Abrams and Follick 1983). These components may improve treatment effectiveness by capitalizing on the unique potential inherent in the nature of the organizational structure. Brownell et al. (1983) recently conducted a weight loss program employing intergroup competition between banks and found significantly improved treatment effectiveness and reduced attrition.

The problem of attrition in worksite weight loss programs, combined with less than desirable maintenance of weight loss, seriously challenges the overall cost-effectiveness of clinic-based procedures in this setting. The simple transfer of existing clinical programs to worksite settings may be of limited value. There may be important population differences between worksite and clinic settings which necessitate innovative approaches to weight loss at the worksite.

HYPERTENSION

Several studies have been conducted in the area of hypertension at the worksite (Haynes et al. 1976; Sackett et al. 1975; Chadwick, Chesney, and Jordan 1977; and Drazen, Nevid, Pace, and O'Brien 1982). Most of these studies utilized strategies aimed at increasing compliance with antihypertensive medication. Chadwick, Chesney, and Jordan (1977) used a "step-up" program to increase compliance of hypertensive employees at Lockheed Missiles. Those individuals whose behavior did not change as a result of a low-cost intervention received a more rigorous behavioral intervention. Haynes et al. (1976) and Sackett et al. (1975) demonstrated that behavioral interventions in work settings are successful in improving compliance rates. However, they note iatrogenic effects such as increased absenteeism.

A few studies have employed nonpharmacologic interventions for the treatment of hypertension at the worksite. One such study was reported by Drazen et al. (1982). Results of this study provide encouraging but limited support for the use of behavioral-based blood pressure reduction procedures. The study by Drazen et al. (1982) has important implications for individuals with "borderline hypertension" who are not necessarily candidates for antihypertensive medication but who may benefit from reductions in blood pressure.

CARDIOVASCULAR FITNESS

Although lack of physical fitness is not a CHD risk factor in and of itself, fitness has many beneficial effects that cut across most cardiovascular risk factors. Fitness can be used as a maintenance procedure for exsmokers or as part of a weight loss or blood pressure reduction program. Several studies have demonstrated that an active worksite-based exercise program can have a beneficial effect on productivity and reduce the amount of sick leave utilized by the participants (Durbeck et al. 1972; Laporte 1966; Petrushevskii 1966; Bjurstrom and Alexion 1978; Linden 1969; and Yarvote et al. 1974). Additional positive effects include ability to work harder than before, both mentally and physically, and an increase in job satisfaction. However, Yarvote et al. (1974) reported that employees who chose not to participate in an employee exercise program were older, smoked more, had higher serum cholesterol levels, higher blood pressure, and poorer treadmill performance. Thus, those who might benefit most from an exercise program elected not to participate. This suggests that recruitment and compliance are also important issues that need to be addressed in worksite-based exercise programs.

STRESS MANAGEMENT

Considerable research has been directed at occupational stress, and work stress has been linked to physical illness (cf. Chesney and Feuerstein 1979). Stressors implicated include job dissatisfaction, underutilization of skills and ability, job insecurity, and poor social support. Furthermore, because the Type A coronary-prone behavior pattern has been identified as a CHD risk factor, theories about occupational stress have incorporated Type A into their models (cf. Chesney and Rosenman 1980; Davidson and Cooper 1980).

Due to the relationship between work stress and both physical illness and occupational performance, various industries have provided stress management interventions for their employees. Most of these programs have primarily employed educational procedures, and a few have utilized screening procedures accompanied by referral to professional services. Several controlled evaluations of stress management at the worksite have recently been reported. Peters, Benson, and Porter (1977) investigated the effects of fifteen-minute relaxation breaks during each workday on 126 volunteers from the corporate offices of the Converse Rubber Company. One group was taught Benson's relaxation response, the second group was instructed to sit quietly, and the control group received no instructions. Following an eight-week experimental period, the group receiving relaxation response training showed the greatest mean improvement in work performance and reductions in physical symptoms and illness days. The group instructed to sit quietly showed intermediate improvement, and the control group showed the least change. In a related study, Peters, Benson, and Peters (1977) found mean decreases in blood pressure of 6.7 mm hg systolic and 5.2 mm hg diastolic in the group receiving specific relaxation training. These changes were significantly greater than the changes observed in the other two groups.

Manuso (1980) investigated the effects of a biofeedback and stress management procedure on a group of employees suffering headaches ($n=15$) and a group of employees reporting general anxiety ($n=15$). The experimental procedure included frontalis EMG feedback, muscle relaxation, breathing exercises, and imagery techniques. Both groups reported significant improvement in physical symptoms, reductions in visits to the health center during three-month follow-up, and improvements in work-related satisfaction and effectiveness. Manuso (1980) further analyzed the cost-effectiveness of this program by computing the cost associated with health center utilization, time away from the job, and work interference due to symptoms. His computations indicated a 1.0 / 5.52 cost-benefit ratio. While these figures may be somewhat optimistic, they suggest a substantial return on investment for stress management services provided to symptomatic employees. Patel, Marmot, and Terry (1981) examined the effects of a stress management program that consisted of education regarding health-risk factors, deep muscle relaxation, breathing exercises, meditation training, and GSR feedback. At the end of treatment and at eight-month follow-up, the intervention group showed significantly greater reductions in systolic and diastolic blood pressure, plasma renin activity, and plasma aldosterone than the control group.

While there are a limited number of empirically evaluated stress management programs in industrial settings, and most suffer from methodological weaknesses, the data suggest that relaxation procedures may be effective for modifying cardiovascular risk and improving job satisfaction and performance. Chesney and Feuerstein (1979) suggest that future research should focus on assessing the interaction between characteristics of the stressor and person-specific characteristics such as cognitive style, personality, and habitual behaviors. This should facilitate the development of stress management procedures and may lead to the identification of the best strategies for different individuals under different types of stress.

Comprehensive Health Promotion Programs

Multicomponent programs are designed to impact on several cardiovascular risk factors at once. Several of these ambitious programs have recently emerged (Parkinson, et al., 1982) and two, Johnson & Johnson's "Live for Life" and Control Data's "Stay Well" program, have recently reported preliminary data on their initial efforts. Both programs utilize nutrition education, weight control, stress management, fitness, and smoking cessation. The "Stay Well" program also includes employee self-help participation groups which are composed of employees and spouses who are interested in taking a more active leadership role in the program.

Multicomponent programs usually have a "wellness" philosophy emphasizing the interaction between various life-style habits, emotional well-being, and job satisfaction. These programs have great potential for enhanced generalization and maintenance of life-style change. Individuals who quit smoking or lose weight are more likely to join a fitness or stress management program and vice-versa. A growing social movement is created in the entire organization, thus influencing everyone via incentives, role modeling, and changes in the environmental and social climate (Abrams et al. 1986).

Preliminary data from these programs suggest that at one-year follow-up, a significant number of participants have lower blood cholesterol, exercise more, have lower blood pressure, and smoke less as compared to pretreatment levels. While these programs are generating significant interest, it is premature to draw any firm conclusions at this time. The programs are expensive and may be applicable only to larger and more affluent industries. In addition, they are very complex so that traditional research designs will be hard to implement within them.

Evaluation of Worksite Health Promotion Programs

While there has been much interest recently in the implementation of worksite-based health promotion programs, little attention has been devoted to the systematic evaluation of outcome. Outcome evaluation of worksite health promotion programs should be considered on four levels. First, is the evaluation of *behavior change*. Specifically, does the intervention result in specific behavior changes such as reduction or cessation in smoking, weight loss, or increase physical exercise? An assessment of the extent of change needs to be conducted as well as a determination of the maintenance of that behavior change. In addition, it is also imperative that programs evaluate attrition rates. Some programs appear to have limited applicability because of large dropout rates.

Second, *health-related* outcomes must also be evaluated. Health related outcomes can be divided into two subcategories: (1) disease specific criteria such as cholesterol or blood pressure levels, and (2) general health criteria such as the amount of medical utilization, absenteeism, and disability or sick leave (e.g., Moos 1977). Traditionally, research on health promotion has focused on either the extent of behavior change (Drazen et al. 1982) or general health criteria (Petrushevskii 1966; Linden 1969). Perhaps of greatest importance, however, are changes in the hypothesized physiological mediating mechanisms. While it is important to demonstrate that a program changes behavior and results in weight loss, it is equally important to determine the effect of the intervention on factors that influence the risk of CHD, such as plasma lipoproteins (cf. Brownell and Stunkard 1981; Follick et al. 1984).

The third level of outcome criteria is *non-health-related* and includes such factors as employee satisfaction, job turnover rates, productivity level, and safety or accident rates. These outcome criteria may be of only secondary importance to the health promotion researcher, but they have great relevance to industry and can be important variables in a cost-effectiveness equation. As health psychologists continue to develop and refine worksite health promotion procedures, it is important that we do not adversely affect non-health-related outcome criteria. If anything, we should attempt to maximize the impact of our programs on these important secondary outcomes. In fact, it can even be argued that variables like job satisfaction and productivity are critically important outcome variables in that they relate to job stress levels.

The final area of outcome criteria is related to *cost*. The combination of program costs and outcome have often been ignored, or even scorned, by professionals who have been primarily concerned with the well-being of clients and quality services (Sorensen and Binner 1979). However, an evaluation of a worksite health promotion program is inadequate if it does not consider the resources required to achieve the outcome (Sorensen and Binner 1979). Thus health psychologists must devote increased attention to cost factors and systematically include them in outcome evaluations.

Conclusions and Future Directions

There are several conclusions that seem to be evident from this brief review of the area. First, it would appear that the value of screening and health education is significantly enhanced when they are incorporated into more comprehensive programs. They are usually not sufficient in isolation to produce behavior change. Second, programs designed to modify risk factors directly have certain advantages. Individuals who participate in direct behavior interventions can achieve behavior change, improve health status, and reduce the risk of CHD. Third, it is clear that the worksite in and of itself is not a solution to many of the problems encountered in clinic settings (e.g., maintenance). Some worksite programs have been accompanied by very large attrition rates and less than satisfactory maintenance. In addition, a number of unexpected iatrogenic effects (e.g., increased absenteeism) have also been reported following worksite interventions (Haynes et al. 1976). This suggests that the worksite is a unique setting and that the simple transfer of existing programs may not be possible. It is also likely that the population encountered in the worksite is significantly different from that encountered in a traditional clinic setting, and therefore, worksite-based interventions may need to be tailored to the specific population and setting characteristics.

Worksite health promotion programs mandate an integration of various disciplines and techniques (i.e., social psychology, organizational psychology, health education, behavioral methodology, etc.). While multicomponent programs and techniques derived from organizational and social psychology (cf. Abrams and Follick 1983), appear to offer potentially promising solutions to the problems of generalization and maintenance of health-related behavior change, the use of these procedures in health promotion programs is of such recent origin that any conclusion would be premature at this time.

Unfortunately, there are few methodologically rigorous studies of worksite health promotion at this point in time. What is needed is a standardized set of outcome criteria with specific dependent measures to be employed in future worksite health promotion studies. Perhaps of greatest importance, however, is to examine the effects of behavioral interventions on hypothesized physiological mediating mechanisms. This information is necessary to justify the inclusion of weight loss and other behavior change procedures in health promotion and disease prevention programs. In addition, outcomes other than those related to health risk, such as job satisfaction, absenteeism, work stress, and social climate (e.g., Moos 1977), are of importance but are frequently overlooked.

Although some promising results of behavioral health promotion in the worksite have recently been reported, we believe that a very cautious interpretation of the data is indicated at this time. At best, we have been able to duplicate results typically obtained in clinic settings, and more frequently, worksite health promotion programs have fallen far short of clinic-based programs because of large attrition rates.

It appears that worksite health promotion programs will be best advanced by the integration of various disciplines and techniques. Health psychologists must come to understand the roles and functions of other disciplines involved in health promotion programs such as health education, occupational nursing, and occupational medicine. Health psychologists will also need to draw upon other bodies of knowledge within psychology such as social psychology, organizational psychology, and behavioral psychology. Worksite health promotion programs may be significantly enhanced when combined with other procedures and techniques derived from these other areas (cf. Abrams and Follick 1983).

Health psychologists must focus on the systematic evaluation of worksite-based health promotion programs. This implies that health psychologists may need special training in research procedures applicable to large-scale clinical trials, such as quasi-experimental designs and survey techniques. Furthermore, they need training in mass media and other health education technologies, as well as in program and cost-effectiveness evaluation methods. They need a thorough understanding of the specific relationship between life-style habits, physiological mediators, and disease endpoints for the chronic diseases that are preventable. The role of health psychology in large-scale, public, health-promotion programs may be doomed if we do not provide empirically derived programs and procedures. If we work effectively with other disciplines and establish the utility of our interventions, health psychology may fulfill a current need and occupy an important role in the health care system.

REFERENCES

Abrams, D, J. Elder, R. Carlton, T. Lasater, and L. Artz. 1986. A comprehensive framework for conceptualizing and planning organizational health promotion programs. In *Behavioral medicine in industry,* edited by M. Cataldo and T. Coates. New York: John Wiley & Sons.

Abrams, D. B., and M. J. Follick. 1983. Behavioral weight loss intervention at the worksite: Feasibility and maintenance. *Journal of Consulting and Clinical Psychology* 51:226–33.

Alderman, M., L. W. Green, and B. S. Flynn. 1982. Hypertension control programs in occupational settings. In *Managing health promotion in the workplace,* edited by R. S. Parkinson and Associates, 62–172. Palo Alto, CA: Mayfield Publishing Company.

Bauer, R. B. 1978. Bell laboratories helps employees quit smoking. *American Lung Association Bulletin* (July/August), 11–14.

Bjurstrom, L. A., and N. G. Alexion. 1978. A program of heart disease intervention for public employees. *Journal of Occupational Medicine* 20:521–31.

Brownell, K. D., and A. J. Stunkard. 1981. Differential changes in plasma high-density lipoprotein-cholesterol levels in obese men and women during weight reduction. *Archive of Internal Medicine* 141:1142–46.

Brownell, K. D., A. Stunkard, P. E. McKeon, and M. Felix. August 1983. Cooperation vs. competition: Four studies in department stores and banks. Paper presented at the annual convention of American Psychological Association. Anaheim, CA.

Cathcart, L. M. 1977. A four-year study of executive health risk. *Journal of Occupational Medicine* 19:354–57.

Chadwick, J. H., M. A. Chesney, and S. C. Jordan. May 1977. High blood pressure education in industrial setting. Paper presented at the annual High Blood Pressure Education Research Program meeting. Washington, D.C.

Chesney, M. A., and M. Feurerstein. 1979. Behavioral medicine in the occupational setting. In *Behavioral medicine,* edited by J. McNamara, 267–90. New York, NY: Plenum Press.

Chesney, M. A., and R. H. Rosenman. 1980. Type A behavior in the work setting. In *Current concerns in occupational stress,* edited by C. L. Cooper and R. Payne, 187–212. New York: John Wiley & Sons.

Danaher, B. G. 1982. Smoking cessation programs in occupational settings. In *Managing health promotion in the workplace,* edited by R. S. Parkinson and Associates, 162–72. Palo Alto, CA: Mayfield Publishing Company.

Davidson, M. J., and C. L. Cooper. 1980. Type A coronary-prone behavior in the work environment. *Journal of Occupational Medicine* 22:375–83.

Drazen, M., J. S. Nevid, N. Pace, and R. M. O'Brien. 1982. Worksite-based behavioral treatment of mild hypertension. *Journal of Occupational Medicine* 24:511–14.

Durbeck, D. C., F. Heinzelmann, J. Schacter, W. L. Haskell, et al. 1972. The National Aeronautics and Space Administration vs. Public Health Service Health Evaluation and Enhancement Program. *American Journal of Cardiology* 30:784–90.

Follick, M. J., D. B. Abrams, T. W. Smith, L. O. Henderson, and P. N. Herbert. 1984. Behavioral intervention for weight loss: Contrasting acute and long-term effects on lipoprotein levels. *Archives of Internal Medicine* 144:1571–74.

Follick, M. J., J. L. Fowler, and R. A. Brown. 1984. Attrition in worksite weight loss interventions: The effects of an incentive procedure. *Journal of Consulting and Clinical Psychology* 1: 139–40.

Foot, A., and J. Erfurt. October 1976. A model system for high blood pressure control in the work setting. In *High blood pressure control in the worksetting: Issues, models, resources*. Proceedings of the National Conference, Washington, D.C.

Foreyt, J. P., L. Scott, and A. M. Grotto. 1980. Weight control and nutrition education programs in occupational settings. *Public Health Reports* 95: 127–36.

Haynes, R. B., D. L. Sackett, E. S. Gibson, D. W. Taylor, B. C. Hackett, R. S. Roberts, and A. J. Johnson. 1976. Improvement of medication compliance in uncontrolled hypertension. *Lancet* 1: 1265–68.

Kanzler, M., P. Zeidenberg, and J. H. Jaffe. 1976. Response of medical personnel to an on-site smoking cessation program. *Journal of Clinical Psychology* 32: 670–74.

Kornitzer, M., G. DeBacker, M. Dramaix, and C. Thilly. 1980. The Belgian heart disease prevention project: Modification of the coronary risk profile in an industrial population. *Circulation* 1: 18–25.

Laporte, W. 1966. The influence of a gymnastic pause upon recovery following post office work. *Ergonomics* 9: 501–6.

Linden, V. 1969. Absence from work and physical fitness. *British Journal of Industrial Medicine* 26: 47–53.

Manuso, J. 1980. Corporate mental health programs and policies. In *Strategies for public health*, edited by L. K. Y. Ng and D. Davis. New York: Van Nostrand Reinhold Co.

McDougall, A. K. 1978. Smoking ban at workplace; a fiery issue. *The Los Angeles Times*, 1 September, pp. 21, 22, 23.

Meyer, A. J., and J. B. Henderson. 1974. Multiple risk factor reduction in the prevention of cardiovascular disease. *Preventive Medicine* 3: 225–36.

Michael, J. M. 1982. The second revolution in health: Health promotion and its environmental base. *American Psychologist* 37: 936–44.

Moos, R. H. 1977. *The human context: Environmental determinants of behavior.* New York: John Wiley and Sons.

Murphy, A. F. October 1976. The Burlington Industries industrial hypertension program. In *High blood pressure control in the worksetting: Issues, models, resources*. Proceedings of the National Conference. Washington, D.C.

Orleans, C. S., and R. H. Shipley. 1982. Worksite smoking cessation initiatives: Review and recommendations. *Addictive Behaviors* 7: 1–16.

Parkinson, R. S., and Associates, eds. 1982. *Managing health promotion in the work place.* Palo Alto, CA: Mayfield Publishing Company.

Patel, C., M. G. Marmot, and P. J. Terry. 1981. Controlled trial of biofeedback—aided behavioural methods in reducing mild hypertension. *British Medical Journal* 282: 2005–8.

Peters, R. K., H. Benson, and J. M. Peters. 1977. Daily relaxation response breaks in a working population: II. Effects on blood pressure. *American Journal of Public Health* 67: 954–59.

Peters, R., H. Benson, and D. Porter. 1977. Daily relaxation response breaks in a working population: I. Effects on self-reported measures of health, performance, and well-being. *American Journal of Public Health* 67:946–53.

Petrushevskii, I. 1966. Increase in work proficiency of operators by means of physical training. *Voprosy Psikhologii* 2:57–67.

Rogers, J. 1977. *You can stop: A smoke-enders approach to quitting smoking and sticking to it.* New York: Pocket Books.

Rosen, G. M., and E. Lichtenstein. 1977. A worker's incentive program for the reduction of cigarette smoking. *Journal of Consulting and Clinical Psychology* 45:957.

Sackett, D. L., R. B. Haynes, E. S. Gibson, B. C. Hackett, D. W. Taylor, R. S. Roberts, and A. J. Johnson. 1975. Randomized clinical trial of strategies for improving medication compliance in primary hypertension. *Lancet* 1:1205–7.

Schoenberger, J. A. October 1976. Heart disease in industry: The Chicago Heart Association Project. In *High blood pressure control in the work setting: Issues, models, resources.* Proceedings of the National Conference. Washington, D.C.

Sorensen, J. E., and P. R. Binner. 1979. Cost, cost-outcome and cost-effectiveness. In *Evaluation in practice: A sourcebook of program evaluation studies from mental health care systems in the United States,* edited by G. Landsberg, W. Neigher, U.S. Department of Health, Education, and Welfare. DHEW Publications, no. (ADM) 78–763.

Stamler, J. 1979. Research related to risk factors. *Circulation* 60:1575–87.

Stunkard, A. J. December 1976. Obesity and the social environment. Paper presented at the Bicentennial Conference on Food and Nutrition in Health Disease. Philadelphia, PA.

Stunkard, A. J., and K. D. Brownell. 1980. Worksite treatment for obesity. *American Journal of Psychiatry* 137:252–53.

Thompson, E. 1978. Smoking education programs, 1960–1976. *American Journal of Public Health* 68:250–58.

Yarvote, P. M., J. McDonagh, M. E. Goldman, and J. Zuckerman. 1974. Organizations and evaluation of a physical fitness program in industry. *Journal of Occupational Medicine* 16:589–98.

11

Community Interventions and Health Psychology: An Ecologically Oriented Perspective

Edison J. Trickett

The extension of health psychology into community settings and the interest in environmental contributions to health problems and health promotion provides some potential points of overlap between health psychology and community psychology. Community psychology has traditionally been interested in understanding community processes and community settings, as well as accumulating extensive experience in conducting research and intervention programs in the community (see Cowen 1973; Munoz, Snowden, and Kelly 1979; and Iscoe 1984 for reviews and examples of social and community interventions). From these interests a number of models relevant to health psychology have been developed, including prevention strategies (e.g., Price et al. 1980), organizational assessment and change, social action, and ecological approaches (see Mann 1977 for an elaboration of these contrasting models). As a community psychologist at the National Training Conference on Education and Training in Health Psychology, I was impressed at how many issues arising in discussions among conference participants involved themes central to community psychology. Conducting research in community settings such as schools, designing prevention interventions which last over time, making a systemic difference—these themes which combined the commitment to scholarship with the intent to be useful suggested areas of common cause with community psychology.

The intent of this paper is to build on some of these themes from the conference by discussing how one particular paradigm in community psychol-

This article was facilitated by a grant from the University of Maryland's General Research Board and was completed while the author was on leave at Yale University's Institute for Social and Policy Studies. Appreciation is expressed to both these institutions. Trudy Vincent, Judith Albino, Gary Schwartz, Irving Janis, and Jerome L. Singer provided ideas and feedback on aspects of this paper, though the author is solely responsible for its contents. Thanks to Grace Petro and Jacqueline Asmussen for typing and editorial assistance.

ogy approaches them. At least two important provisos are in order, however. First, the paradigm to be described is but one of several in community psychology and thus should not be seen as representing the broader field. Second, because the author is not a health psychologist, this paper represents an effort to outline some more generic issues stimulated by the conference rather than an effort to integrate current work in health psychology within a community psychology paradigm. That latter approach represents a worthy future task, but one that is beyond the scope of the present paper.

An Ecological Orientation for Health Psychology in Community Settings

While the term "ecology" has been used in many different ways, here it refers to a particular perspective within community psychology developed and elaborated by James Kelly and his colleagues (Kelly 1966, 1969, 1970, 1971; Kelly and Associates 1979; Trickett, Kelly, and Todd 1972; Trickett, Kelly, and Vincent 1985). Its basic intent is to serve as a heuristic for understanding human communities, using principles drawn from field biology, the study of naturally occurring biological communities. Within community psychology, it has been applied to such topics as the role of the high school in adolescent socialization (Kelly and Associates 1979), community consultation (O'Neill and Trickett 1983), ecological assessment of individuals (O'Neill and Trickett 1973), and the research relationship between scholar and citizen (Trickett, Kelly, and Vincent 1985).

An ecological metaphor directs attention to two overarching issues relevant to health psychology research and intervention in community settings. First is the importance of understanding the social context in which research and intervention occurs. Here an ecological approach advocates the study of how contextual factors in settings affect the incidence and prevalence of health-relevant behaviors. It further argues for understanding how social setting factors affect the design and durability of interventions. The second issue involves assumptions made about individuals; namely, that individual behavior is embedded in a sociocultural matrix which shapes perceptions, preferred coping styles, and most fundamentally, the meanings that individuals attach to a variety of behaviors, particularly those involving health issues. Thus, the positive value of cultural pluralism as it relates to research assumptions and intervention efforts is stressed.

Implications of these two issues for research and intervention in health psychology will be presented later. First, however, it is necessary to specify the ecological principles from which these larger issues emerge. Briefly, the ecological metaphor derives from four interrelated principles designed to understand different aspects of the social context. While their implications are presented at greater length elsewhere (e.g., Trickett, Kelly, and Todd 1972; Trickett, Kelly, and Vincent 1985), short descriptions can provide the reader with at least the contours of an ecological mind-set.

ADAPTATION

The principle of adaptation addresses the "substance" of the environment; those norms, values, processes, and policies which constitute the demand characteristics of the setting. Demand characteristics of settings constrain some kinds of attitudes and behaviors while supporting others. Behavior of individuals is seen as transactional; that is, individual behavior in social settings is seen as an effort by persons to cope with the demands of the setting in terms of their own skills and interpretations of the situation.

INTERDEPENDENCE

The principle of interdependence, a cornerstone of systems theory, focuses on the interactive nature of the component parts of a social setting. Change in one aspect of the setting, whether it results from the introduction of a research project or a planned intervention, it thus assumed to ripple in some fashion throughout the setting. The behavior of individuals in one setting is viewed within the context of the other settings that the individual must deal with. Thus, school behavior may reflect in part how the individual responds to the home environment (see Bronfenbrenner 1979 for a thorough treatment of this interdependence perspective on behavior).

CYCLING OF RESOURCES

The principle of cycling of resources, in field biology, refers to the ways in which biological communities develop, distribute, and use nutrients, or energy. The focus is on what is needed to sustain the survival and development of the community. In like fashion, a resource perspective on social settings focuses on those aspects which promote their development. Resources can assume a variety of forms, including technology (e.g. computers), persons central to some aspect of the setting, discrete settings within the larger environment which are influential in making policy, and events which help the setting crystallize its identity and values. An assessment of resources is particularly important in deciding how to promote the adoption of a research or intervention program in the setting.

Succession

The principle of succession focuses on the time dimension of settings, including both the institutional history and the hopes for the future development of the setting. It serves as a reminder that traditions and core strategies for survival develop over time along with the setting; like individuals, groups intimately bound to a setting are likely to perceive current events with an eye toward their potential long-range implications for the setting. How people who are intimately bound to a setting conceive of and process researchers and research is part of this historical development. Thus, the researcher uses the succession principle to assess how an institution, or part thereof, has dealt with researchers in the past and how the institution thinks the research and the researchers will fit into long-range goals.

The four principles of this ecological metaphor have implications for *what* the research looks at and *how* the researcher might relate to the community setting. The remainder of the paper elaborates on three implications of this metaphor for health psychology research and intervention in community settings. The first section discusses the two overarching paradigmatic themes of level of analysis and cultural pluralism. Next, the focus shifts to the relationship between the researcher and the community. Here, the emphasis is on the *process* of conducting research in community settings. The final section elaborates on the idea that research in community settings *is* intervention, thus heightening the importance of looking for side effects or unanticipated consequences of research.

The Social Context and Cultural Pluralism: Complementary Foci for an Ecologically Oriented Health Psychology

Various writers have commented over the last decade about how person-centered and acultural the research traditions of psychology have been. Sarason (1981), for example, makes the bold assertion that psychology has been fundamentally "misdirected" through its reliance on research paradigms which imply that individuals can be understood without reference to culture or context. Caplan and Nelson (1973) have reminded us of the relationship between person-based research and "blaming the victim" in their analysis of research on black Americans. They assert that the preponderance of research on blacks is person-based and that the policy momentum from this work tends to swing in the direction of fixing the individual rather than attending to systemic factors and cultural embeddedness as policy issues. Within the area of health psychology, Schwartz (personal communication) has affirmed that there exists an inverse relationship between the level of analysis and the availability of empirical data, in the direction indicated by the preceding comments.

An ecological metaphor, however, argues for different research programs in terms of level of analysis and a differentiated, culturally embedded conception of individuals. There is not a great deal of research emanating from either a more system-oriented focus or pluralistic approach to individuals within health psychology. However, the value of both approaches has been stressed. Moos (1979), for example, summarizes a great deal of relevant data on the impact of the broader social context on the development of health problems. He outlines an integrative conceptual framework for studying the relationship between the social context and health, including both "environmental system" variables such as physical and organizational characteristics, and "personal system" variables, such as socioeconomic status (SES), ways of coping with stress, and impairment factors.

Moos also discusses ways of changing the social context *and* changing individuals to help them cope more successfully. On the environmental level, he offers a framework for examining and changing small social contexts such as psychiatric wards and high school classrooms based on survey feedback techniques (see Pierce, Trickett, and Moos 1971; Moos 1979). On the individual level, he offers such strategies as providing people with information on the demand characteristics of settings of importance to them and developing programs to enhance environmental competence. Moos's social ecological framework differs in many respects from the ecological metaphor described earlier, and these differences are presented elsewhere (Vincent and Trickett 1983). Both, however, share a primary emphasis on the role of the social context as a powerful determinant of behavior.

The emphasis on the relationship of the social context to individual coping is further stressed by Albino (1983), who provides one of the few efforts explicitly linking health psychology to community psychology. She proposes four areas of research and intervention consistent with an ecological orientation: (1) the identification of risk factors in health maintenance and the development of educational and support services for reducing risk; (2) adherence to health recommendations, such as life-style changes and avoidance of environmental contributions to illness; (3) coping with threats to health, including stressors of everyday life; and (4) the development and evaluation of effective systems for health care delivery, including program planning and quality assurance evaluation.

Albino discusses how each of these areas can be enriched by attention to the social context and, in so doing, highlights the issue of level of analysis. With respect to the area of coping with stress, for example, she clarifies how fundamentally different it is to focus on changing the stressor itself (e.g., a work environment whose aversive organizational processes cause stress in workers) as contrasted with the development of a program to enhance workers' competence in dealing with the stressor. The first approach links health psychology to primary prevention and a systemic level of analysis; the second links it to a secondary or tertiary prevention emphasis and an individual level of analysis. These are, of course, not pure cases. The former, for example, may result in an intervention program which includes individual behavior change on the part of workers, while the latter may result in a decision on the part of the workers to meet with their supervisors about altering some of the harmful conditions of their work. The basic emphases, however, are very different.

Albino further underscores the importance of attending to system factors when designing intervention programs. With particular reference to risk factor research and adherence to health regimens, she states that "In the final analysis our efforts to identify and educate people about risk factors and to induce adherence to recommended health regimens will not succeed if the structures to support and maintain them are not in place. This means building social and environmental support, as well as competence within individuals" (1983, 231).

Issues of cultural pluralism, though not represented well in existing literature, cut across all aspects of the previously described research emphases. While there are many aspects to pluralism, a core "exemplar" of the implications is raised in the form of a question by Schneider (1983). "What happens when a dietary regimen is given to a black adolescent from the rural south who suffers from hypertension or juvenile diabetes? How prepared is the health system generally to deal with cultural context and the habits of daily life that will need some modification if treatment is to be successful?"

Thus, the ecological perspective includes the following: that sociocultural context *does* define the meaning of such health-related behaviors as smoking, drinking, and eating various foods; that understanding individuals' sociocultural context is thus *directly related* to the design of successful intervention programs; and that such high-impact systems as school and health care delivery systems need to consider how their norms and ways of providing services mesh with the views of their consumers.

The four principles of the ecological metaphor can, in a chapter of this scope, only highlight a framework for suggesting questions of relevance: *adaptation* of persons to their communities, environments, and life-styles; *interdependence* between the health care delivery system and the preferred norms of varied clients; *cycling of resources* as health psychologists attempt to increase influence for raising consciousness in regard to health promotion in local settings and systems; *succession* as the appreciation of the historical significance of such attitudes as racism and black mistrust of whites as expressed in the execution of intervention programs. The basic thrust is not specific but paradigmatic: to push for the usefulness of a level of analysis and intervention which focuses on systemic contributions to health issues and dignifies the community—embeddedness of persons of varying backgrounds.

THE ECOLOGICAL PERSPECTIVE AND RESEARCH DESIGN: ISSUES OF SITE SELECTION AND IMPLEMENTATION

In an effort to concretize some of the implications of an ecological perspective for research, two examples of how community settings can affect data will be presented. The first involves the selection of research sites per se; the second deals with the way the research is implemented in the community setting. As will be seen, both have implications for the interpretation of data and generalizability of findings.

Ecological Considerations in Selecting Research Sites

Understanding the nature of community research sites is important not only when the research questions center on how social context factors affect health-related issues, but also when one is conducting more individually oriented research in community settings. There are different emphases, however, connected with these different kinds of research strategies. When one is concerned with how the social context contributes to a health-related issue, research sites are selected *because* they vary on the systemic variables of interest. This requires both a conceptual framework for assessing social contexts and an active, community-based assessment of potentially relevant settings.

In individually oriented research and intervention efforts, attention to site selection is necessary to counteract self-selection biases which may influence the ecological validity of the data. Campbell and Stanley (1972, 19) frame the issue in the following way: "Consider the implications of an experiment on teaching in which the researcher has been turned down by nine school systems and is finally accepted by a tenth. This tenth almost certainly differs from the other nine, and from the universe of schools to which we would like to generalize, in many specific ways. It is, thus, nonrepresentative and the effects we find, while internally valid, may be specific to such schools." Thus, the generality of data gathered on individuals is potentially constrained by the larger ecology in which it is gathered.

Ecological Considerations in Implementing Research Programs

In addition to attending to the selection of research sites per se, an ecological perspective suggests that *how* a research or intervention program is implemented will affect the nature of the data gathered. A useful example of how implementation may affect outcome is found in Ransen's (1981) study entitled "Long-term Effects of Two Intervention Programs with the Aged: An Ecological Analysis." The article reviews the short-term and long-term results of two similar intervention programs with the aged (Langer and Rodin 1976; Schulz 1976). Both programs were designed to test the "perceived control" hypothesis through enhancing residents' perceptions of personal control over aspects of their institutional lives. Both had similar and positive short-term effects in stopping and, indeed, reversing aspects of physical and psychological decline. However, follow-up showed marked differences between the two intervention programs. One study found that eighteen months after termination of the program, residents in the experimental group remained happier, more socially active, and had a lower mortality rate than residents in the control group. In the other study, however, follow-up at twenty-four, thirty, and forty-two months revealed a markedly different picture. Mean scores for the experimental group on indices of physical and psychological status were *lower* than those for the controls, and mortality was higher. "In sum," stated Ransen, "those residents who had benefitted most from the intervention in the short run seemed to have suffered the greatest declines in the long run" (p. 18).

In an effort to understand these patterns, Ransen undertook a post hoc analysis of how the intervention programs were implemented in the two different settings. Several differences emerged, including whether or not the actual deliverers of the intervention were insiders (e.g., the activities director) or outsiders (e.g., visiting college students), whether or not the intervention disrupted the ongoing social network of residents or kept it intact, and whether or not the project was designed to affect a broad or narrow range of expectancies about one's institutional life. On the basis of these analyses, Ransen drew the tentative conclusion that the differential long-term results reflected the different ways in which the programs were implemented. Thus, to account for the results, it was necessary to examine not only the theory of "perceived control" underlying the research but also the way the research was implemented. Ransen's analysis suggests that the same basic research program which is implemented differently in different settings is not, conceptually, the same program. This suggests that how the research is coupled with the host environment becomes a salient topic in its own right.

A Community Development Approach to the Research Relationship

Research in community settings is mediated by the nature of the research relationship between researcher and research site. Recently, a group of us sought to understand how we—professionals involved in research in community settings—were perceived by persons in those settings (Billington, Washington, and Trickett 1981). We were interested not only in discovering the truth behind the so-called "horror stories" involving research relationships between scholar and citizen (e.g., Eron and Walder 1961) but also in discovering what kinds of research relationships were seen as beneficial to the sites where the research occurred. We were aware of how social systems can intentionally or inadvertently disrupt or undermine research efforts through how responsive they are toward the research and equally aware of how this aspect of the research process seldom finds its way into published writings, leaving the impression that it has no tangible influence over the substance of results. Our interviews—carried out with a sample of inner-city public school principals—suggested that the dominant paradigm carried by psychologists and other social scientists when they go "into the field" is predominantly an extension of the paradigms used "in the laboratory." The school is a place to run an experiment, and when the study is over, it is debriefed. The setting, in short, is a subject.

The ecological metaphor underlying the present paper takes a different perspective, however. Because it is concerned with systemic impact, and because it values community development as an intervention goal, the ecological metaphor places great emphasis on the structure of the research relationship. The intent is to couple the research with the host environment in such a way that it enhances the work and the setting. Elsewhere, we state:

> The field of psychology, with its emphasis on technique and method, can unwittingly give the impression that preventive interventions such as community research are freestanding techniques and methods which can be transported across settings and over time with minimal regard for local circumstances of history. Often both research paradigms and interventions are seen as primary, and their relation to the site of work as secondary. The ecological paradigm

rejects the premise of a dichotomy between method and setting. Instead, it asserts that community research must strive to be embedded in a social setting, for it is the social setting that provides the resources, energy, and power for the research to develop into a preventive intervention. In fact, the goal of this work is to create connections between the intervention and the setting which are strong and durable enough to enable the intervention to endure over time. (Trickett, Kelly, and Vincent 1985, 301)

The goal of coupling the research with the host environment includes both environmental reconnaissance as a prelude for doing the work and developing mechanisms of feedback and accountability for how the work is going. It advocates a collaborative relationship with persons in the setting. The ecological principles of adaptation, interdependence, cycling of resources and succession provide an orientation to understanding how to proceed with such a task (see Trickett, Kelly, and Vincent 1985 for a more complete description.)

Attention to the research relationship as a collaborative undertaking can have positive consequences far beyond generating good will. It can allow the researcher to draw on the local expertise in thinking about how best to integrate the research with the particular constraints of the setting. This, in turn, can heighten the awareness of the researcher to contextual factors which may influence the data and its interpretation. With respect to the previously cited example, Ransen (1981) concluded that the differential long-term effects of two conceptually similar intervention projects could be traced to how they were coupled with the setting. We do not know, from the research reports, what kind of conversations occurred between researcher and people who were part of the setting concerning the structuring of these programs. We are told, however, that in the study with negative long-term outcomes, the subjects in the same informal networks could be receiving different interventions. It is plausible that informal conversations among these friends may have included a discussion of this fact and that service providers close to the subjects had some awareness of this topic of conversation. How can researchers remain informed about how the local ecology is affecting the research? What kind of relationship between researcher and participant increases the participant's commitment to devote energy to the research? And what kind of resources can the researcher contribute to the setting in return for the participant's commitment of support? Attention to questions such as these becomes a critical component of community research within an ecological paradigm.

Community Research is Intervention:
Attending to the Side Effects of Community Research

The final topic deriving from an ecological metaphor is the notion that community research *is* intervention in the sense that it disrupts the ongoing life of the community setting where it occurs. As such, it is important for the researcher to seek out the side effects and after effects of the research in the setting. There are many reasons why such a proactive concern is important.

The first is simply to acknowledge that what constitutes a "side effect" from the perspective of the research project may indeed constitute a "main effect" from the perspective of the community setting.[1] Community research does intrude into the ongoing life of the community setting, and general concern over its impact must occupy a central place in the execution of the research. More specifically, a search for side effects may uncover positive feelings, attitudes, and behavior of persons as a result of involvement in the research which clarify its value and provide ideas for future efforts. In addition, side effects may offer new opportunities for the researcher to investigate new phenomena of conceptual and pragmatic importance.

Side effects, of course, can also have negative consequences, which can threaten the validity of the data and, indeed, the very continuance of the research itself. For example, it is plausible to think that health-related intervention programs with high-risk children in schools may potentially raise the anxiety of children *not* at risk and arouse the curiosity of parents about what is happening. Perhaps the school begins receiving phone calls from parents inquiring about the work. The example need not be elaborated, except to state that, particularly when one is trying to prevent some unhealthy condition in at-risk children, the potential for fear, misunderstanding, and negative impact on aspects of the local community is great.

Being on the lookout for side effects and after effects is also an affirmation that the researcher cares about the local setting where the work occurs. It enhances the credibility of the researcher in the eyes of participants in the setting because it acknowledges that the researcher knows what the participants know: namely, that there is often a difference between the paradigm-defined *intent* of the research project and the *consequences* of that project for the ongoing life of the community settings. Community research *is* an intervention and the ecological metaphor a vehicle for assessing its systemic impact.

1. The author wishes to thank an anonymous reviewer for framing the issue in this particularly useful way.

Summary

In a brief paper one can hope at best to present the flavor and the general contours of a point of view. The intent has been to focus on touchpoints between community-oriented research in health psychology and an ecological perspective evolving from community psychology. The vehicle for this interface is a series of recurrent and, in the judgment of the author, central intellectual and value questions at the National Working Conference on Education and Training in Health Psychology. The bottom line stresses the importance of conceptual attention to the social context, the sociocultural embeddedness of individuals, and the relationship of the researcher to the community setting.

REFERENCES

Albino, J. E. 1983. Health psychology and primary prevention: Natural allies. In *Preventive psychology: Theory, research, and practice,* edited by R. D. Felner, L. A. Jason, J. N. Moritsugu, and S. S. Farber. New York: Pergamon Press.

Billington, R. J., L. A. Washington, and E. J. Trickett. 1981. The research relationship in community research: An inside view from public school principals. *American Journal of Community Psychology* 4:461–79.

Bronfenbrenner, U. 1979. *The ecology of human development: Experiments by nature and design.* Cambridge: Harvard University Press.

Campbell, D. T., and J. C. Stanley. 1972. *Experimental and quasi-experimental designs for research.* Chicago: Rand McNally.

Caplan, N., and S. D. Nelson. 1973. On being useful: The nature and consequences of psychological research on social problems. *American Psychologist* 28: 199–211.

Cowen, E. L. 1973. Social and community interventions. *Annual Review of Psychology* 24:423–72.

Eron, L., and L. Walder. 1961. Test burning II. *American Psychologist* 16:237–44.

Iscoe, I. 1984. Social and community interventions. *Annual Review of Psychology* 35:333–60.

Kelly, J. G. 1966. Ecological constraints on mental health services. *American Psychologist* 21:535–39.

———. 1969. Naturalistic observations in contrasting social environments. In *Naturalistic viewpoints in psychological research,* edited by E. P. Willems and H. L. Raush. New York: Holt, Rinehart, and Winston.

———. 1970. Antidotes for arrogance: Training for community psychology. *American Psychologist* 25:524–31.

———. 1971. Qualities for the community psychologist. *American Psychologist* 26:897–903.

Kelly, J. G., and Associates. 1979. *Adolescent boys in high school: A psychological study of coping and adaptation.* Hillside, NJ: Lawrence Erlbaum Associates.

Langer, E. J., and J. Rodin. 1976. The effects of choice and enhanced personal responsibility for the aged: A field experiment in an institutional setting. *Journal of Personality and Social Psychology* 34:191–98.

Mann, P. A. 1977. *Community psychology: Concepts and applications.* New York: Free Press.

Moos, R. H. 1979. *Evaluating educational environments: A social ecological approach.* San Francisco: Jossey-Bass.

Munoz, R. F., L. S. Snowden, and J. G. Kelly. 1979. *Social and psychological research in community settings.* San Francisco: Jossey-Bass.

O'Neill, P., and E. J. Trickett. 1973. Ecological considerations in psychological testing. Paper presented at the Convention of the American Psychological Association. Montreal, Quebec, Canada.

———. 1983. *Community consultation.* San Francisco: Basic Books.

Pierce, W. D., E. J. Trickett, and R. H. Moos. 1971. Changing ward atmosphere through staff discussion of the perceived ward environment. *Archives of General Psychiatry* 26:35–41.

Price, R. H., R. F. Ketterer, B. C. Bader, and J. Monahan. 1980. *Prevention in community mental health: Research, policy, and practice.* Beverly Hills: Sage.

Ransen, D. L. 1981. Long-term effects of two interventions with the aged: An ecological analysis. *Journal of Applied Developmental Psychology* 2:13–27.

Sarason, S. B. 1981. *Psychology misdirected.* New York: Free Press.

Schneider, S. 1983. Some issues in training in health psychology. Invited paper for the National Working Conference on Education and Training in Health Psychology.

Schulz, R. 1976. The effects of control and predictability on the psychological and physical well-being of the institutionalized aged. *Journal of Personality and Social Psychology* 34:191–98.

Schwartz, G. E. 1984. Personal communication with author.

Trickett, E. J., J. G. Kelly, and D. M. Todd. 1972. The social environment of the high school: Guidelines for individual change and organizational development. In *Handbook of community mental health,* edited by S. E. Golann and C. Eisdorfer. New York: Appleton-Century-Crofts.

Trickett, E. J., J. G. Kelley, and T. A. Vincent. 1985. The spirit of ecological inquiry in community research. In *Knowledge building in community psychology,* edited by D. Klein and E. Susskind. New York: Praeger.

Vincent, T. A., and E. J. Trickett. 1983. Preventive interventions and the human context: Ecological approaches to environmental assessment and change. In *Preventive psychology: Theory, research, and practice,* edited by R. E. Felner, L. A. Jason, J. N. Mortisugu, and S. S. Farber. New York: Pergamon Press.

12

Health Psychology and Public Health

Ruth R. Faden

Health psychology and public health fit well together—in theory, in research, and in practice. In this brief paper, areas of mutual interest between the two fields are reviewed with an eye toward relatively untapped arenas where health psychology and public health can profitably interact.

What Is Public Health?

It is not easy to define public health. At least two strategies for sidestepping the problem come to mind. The first is to resort to the parable about the blind men and the elephant. The second is to paraphrase Roger Brown's classic description of social psychology and define public health more or less circuitously—public health becomes what public health professionals do.

Either way, we arrive at pretty much the same kind of description. Public health is a broad, almost boundless field of research and service embracing a wide array of scientific disciplines, health professions, political institutions, and social services. For example, all of the following can be viewed as the proper subject matter of public health: environmental health, disease prevention, health promotion, epidemiology, sanitation, health care organization, nutrition, injury control, food and water safety, health education, communicable disease control, health policy, health services administration, population policy, and biostatistics. What makes physicians, educators, administrators, engineers, and biostatisticians working in these diverse areas public health professionals is that their primary interest is the health of population groups rather than that of identifiable individuals. In contrast to clinically oriented health professionals whose primary focus is the individual patient, public health professionals "treat" the community, the aggregate unit. It is sometimes said that if you want to know where your true loyalties lie, ask yourself which most quickens your pulse—a decline in national lung cancer statistics or the fact that Ms. Smith has finally succeeded in quitting smoking. If your answer is the former, a career in public health may be worth considering.

Health Psychology and Public Health

Two observations concerning health psychology and public health are worth noting at the outset. First, there is tremendous overlap between public health and clinical health services. Interventions designed to prevent disease, particularly secondary and tertiary prevention strategies, are often targeted to clinical populations in health care facilities. As a result, much of what health psychologists do, particularly in the life-style and treatment adherence areas, may be described as public health psychology, even if it was not initially conceived as such. Secondly, because of the broad sweep of the field of public health, there is also tremendous overlap between it and other application areas covered elsewhere in this volume, for example, health policy and work in industrial, organizational, and community settings (see chaps. 10, 11 and 13).

Psychology has recently been formally recognized as basic to the training of public health professionals. The principal calling card of the public health professional is the Master of Public Health (MPH) degree. In 1983, the Association of Schools of Public Health (ASPH) officially increased its list of required areas for schools offering the MPH degree from four to five, adding the "behavioral sciences" to the existing core of epidemiology, biostatistics, health services administration, and environmental health. Insofar as we can safely assume that psychology is integral to the behavioral sciences, this represents a significant advance for health psychology and public health. Although this ASPH action is not likely to result in any immediate or dramatic changes in the faculty or curricula of schools of public health, it does represent official recognition of the role and importance of the behavioral sciences to public health.

LIFE-STYLES AND HEALTH BEHAVIOR

No where has this contribution been more widely recognized and accepted than in the life-style and health promotion areas. It is probably not necessary here to review the events that led to what is now popularly called the second revolution in public health—the shift from infectious disease to life-style and the environment as the major factors affecting health (Knowles 1977; LaLonde 1975). Thus far, psychology's major contribution to this area in public health has been in the development of interventions to modify life-style patterns and behavioral habits, most notably smoking behaviors, but also eating habits, exercise, injury control actions, etc. (e.g., Leventhal and Cleary 1980; McCaul et al. 1983; Dishman 1982; Ewart, Li, and Coates 1983; Sulzer-Azaroff and DeSantamaria 1980).

Although much of this work has been characterized by the individual, clinical approach that typifies psychology's varied paradigms of behavior change, several projects have employed theoretical models, research designs, and study samples of more direct interest and contribution to public health. For example, the Houston Project which uses mass media interventions to deter smoking in adolescents draws heavily on McGuire's pioneering work on an inoculation theory of persuasion and social influence (Evans et al. 1981). Schwalm and Slovic's (1982) report of the successful use of risk perception manipulations to improve the effectiveness of interventions designed to increase motorists' use of seat belts also falls under this category. Other projects and research programs could be cited, including two at the forefront of public health efforts to reduce life-style risk factors at the community level, the North Karelia Project (McAlister et al. 1982) and the Stanford Three and Five Community Studies (Farquar 1978).

Although health psychology has an obvious and important role in the development of effective behavior change interventions in public health, this does not exhaust health psychology's potential contribution to the life-style area. Health psychology also has an important role in the identification of new behavioral risks and compensatory factors, a scientific process of discovery that has thus far been dominated by an atheoretically oriented epidemiology. As Singer and Krantz (1982) have argued, psychology's focus on the mechanisms linking behavior and health should figure prominently in psychology's contribution to public health. Perhaps the best example of this to date has been psychological research on stress, particularly the relationship between the Type A behavior pattern and coronary heart disease (e.g., Dembroski et al. 1978; Matthews 1982). Recent work on social support, both as a mediator of stressors and as an independent factor, also holds considerable promise (e.g., Wallston et al. 1983).

Hazard Control

It is undesirable for health psychology's contribution to public health to be restricted to the identification and modification of personal life-style behaviors and habits. It is undesirable both because such a focus would fail to take full advantage of the range of interests and expertise within psychology of potential use to public health and because such a focus exacerbates, perhaps unwittingly, an important moral and political problem in public health policy, commonly referred to as the "blaming the victim" problem (Crawford 1977; Ryan 1971). The essence of this issue is that public health programs are morally unacceptable to the extent that they target interventions at the victims and not the causes of ill health and disease (Faden and Faden 1978). Again, smoking interventions are often used as the paradigmatic, but not the only, examples of such programs (Galanter 1977). Other examples include interventions in injury control (Barry 1975), alcoholism (Beauchamp 1975; Beauchamp 1976), and health services utilization (Hertz and Stamps 1977).

Health psychology must be sensitive to this debate. At very least, health psychology can contribute by identifying those areas where individually oriented behavior change strategies are likely to be unsuccessful and why this is so (Williams 1982). In addition, it must be remembered that the psychological principles of behavior change and social influence being explored for their usefulness in the modification of personal life-style habits could also be directed at modifying the attitudes and behaviors of public health officials, employers, and others who have power over both the factors that influence (if not control) many "personal health habits" as well as environmental health hazards.

The potential for health psychology in this area is enormous. Psychological research on risk perception and the evaluation of uncertain events has already had a significant impact on hazard management policy (Fischhoff et al. 1981). Consider also how the perspectives of environmental and organizational psychology could contribute to a better understanding of policies for controlling workplace hazards. Alternatively, consider how health psychologists with a developmental or cognitive orientation could contribute to an understanding of the effects of commercial marketing strategies designed to influence the eating habits of young children and the subsequent development of unhealthy eating patterns.

As this last example suggests, health psychology's contribution to this area is not limited to the development of interventions for the control of health hazards. There is also a central role for health psychology in the identification of new health hazards and in the explanation of the mechanisms of action of health hazards. The new field of behavioral toxicology, now recognized as an established component of the environmental health sciences (Weiss 1983; Fein et al. 1983), represents the most developed arena for psychology to contribute to the public health problem of hazard control. By focusing on the effects of environmental chemicals on how people feel and function, behavioral toxicology has helped expand the traditional public health conception of the nature and impact of health hazards. Also extremely important is research on noise and crowding in environmental psychology (e.g., Evans 1983; Baum, Deckel and Gatchel 1980; Irle 1975), although work in these areas has not been as firmly integrated with traditional public health approaches. Research on the effects of natural disasters (e.g., Quarantelli and Dynes 1972) and, more recently, nuclear power plant accidents (e.g., Collins, Baum, and Singer 1983; Baum, Fleming, and Singer 1982) represents yet another area of study in psychology that is extremely compatible with the public health interest in health hazard identification and control. Here again the focus is on the health threat or hazard as a behavioral stressor, a perspective that is becoming increasingly well accepted in public health.

ALLOCATION OF HEALTH CARE RESOURCES—HEALTH POLICY EVALUATION

It is arguably the case that the most important public health policy issue currently facing this nation is the allocation of health care resources, especially when this issue is coupled with related questions of health care cost containment. Thus far, analyses of alternative allocation policies have been dominated by economic, political, and to a lesser extent, legal and ethical concerns. Yet here, also, there is an important role for health psychology.

The question of how to allocate health-care resources is fundamentally a question of values and values trade-offs. However, there has been little attempt to study these values empirically as they are held by different segments of the public or the policy-making elite. There has been even less attempt to apply choice, moral development, or value theories to develop any systematic understanding of how decision problems involving health-related values are handled. Consider a somewhat artificial but not unrealistic situation in which there are not sufficient resources in the health care budget to publicly fund both heart transplantation for end stage coronary victims and improved living conditions for the institutionalized mentally infirm. What patterns or models of decision making and moral reasoning characterize how individuals approach this kind of hard choice? How do they frame the dilemma and how does their reasoning style affect their preferred policy? At a less complicated level, to what extent does the American public share the "health über alles" ethic that symbolizes much of the public health approach to allocation issues? What is the relationship between the public's perceived needs for preventive and curative services and their policy preferences? I could go on and on here with countless different examples. My point is simply that human judgment and value issues are at the core of the health care allocation policy problem and make ready subject matter for health psychology.

One area that has already received attention in health psychology is the measurement of health policy evaluation outcomes (Kaplan and Bush 1982). Almost all allocation policy analyses rely heavily on some kind of cost-benefit or cost-effectiveness assessment. A central problem for this methodology is how to define and conceptualize the benefits and outcomes that are to be maximized. Increasingly it is being recognized that life expectancy alone is an inadequate measure of health benefit. Quality of life is at least as important as years of life (e.g., Weinstein and Stason 1977). Also important are such "intangibles" as well-being, hope, and peace of mind. There is tremendous potential here for health psychology, as illustrated in a recent UCLA-Rand Corporation policy experiment on the effects of free health care on adult health (Brooks et al. 1983).

Still another area where health psychology can contribute to allocation policy is the assessment of new medical technologies. In traditional technology assessment, benefits are defined primarily in biomedical terms and costs primarily in economic terms. Yet the effects of new technologies are generally much broader than this medical-economics model suggests. Indeed, sometimes the social psychological consequences of offering or restricting a technology may be of central importance. This certainly has been our experience in psychosocial assessments of neonatal and prenatal genetic screening technologies (Faden et al. 1982).

Conclusion

Life-style, hazard control, and resource allocation are not the only issues in public health today, but they are arguably the most important. In taking the position that there is a broad role for health psychology in each of these areas, I am de facto also arguing that there is a major role for health psychology in public health generally and for public health in health psychology. Still, the future of health psychology and public health is as yet uncharted and many inter and intraprofessional issues have yet to be resolved. Chief among these is the extent to which the scientist/scientist-practitioner distinction, as it is emerging in health psychology (Stone 1983), fits with public health models of training and employment opportunity. Also unresolved is the relationship both in schools of public health and in public health agencies between health psychology, other behavioral and social sciences, and health education.

Although these issues pose important challenges to the development of public health psychology, the future is encouraging for this subfield of health psychology. The overwhelming overlap of interests shared by public health and health psychology is demonstrated in the 1984 issue of the *Annual Review of Public Health,* where one-third of the articles address central topics in health psychology (McNeil and Pauker 1984; Green 1984; Berkman 1984; Kasl 1984; Siegel 1984; Wingard 1984). In the face of this extraordinary degree of common ground and interest, it behooves both health psychology and public health to learn more about each other and to develop together effective models for professional training and interdisciplinary and interprofessional research and service.

REFERENCES

Barry, P. Z. 1975. Individual versus community orientation in prevention of injuries. *Preventive Medicine* 4:47–56.

Baum, A., A. W. Deckel, and R. J. Gatchel. 1980. Environmental stress and health: Is there a relationship? In *Social psychology of health and illness,* edited by G. S. Sanders and J. Suls, 279–306. Hillsdale, NJ: Lawrence Erlbaum Associates.

Baum, A., R. Fleming, and J. E. Singer. 1982. Stress at Three Mile Island: Applying psychological impact analyses. In *Applied social psychology annual: Volume III,* edited by L. Beckman. Beverly Hills: Sage.

Beauchamp, D. E. 1976. Alcoholism as blaming the alcoholic. *International Journal of Addiction* 11:41–52.

———. 1975. The alcohol alibi: Blaming alcoholics. *Society* 12:12–17.

Berkman, L. F. 1984. Assessing the physical effects of social networks and social supports. *Annual Review of Public Health* 5:413–32.

Brooks, R. H.; J. E. Ware, Jr.; W. H. Rogers; E. B. Keeler; A. R. Davies; C. A. Donald; G. A. Goldberg; K. N. Lohr; P. C. Masthay; and J. P. Newhouse. 1983. Does free care improve adults' health? *New England Journal of Medicine* 309: 1426–34.

Collins, D. L., A. Baum, and J. E. Singer. 1983. Coping with chronic stress at Three MIle Island: Psychological and biochemical evidence. *Health Psychology* 2: 149–66.

Crawford, R. 1977. You are dangerous to your health: The ideology and politics of victim blaming. *International Journal of Health Sciences* 7:663–80.

Dembroski, T. M., S. M. Weiss, J. L. Shields, S. G. Haynes, and M. Feinlieb, eds. 1978. *Coronary-prone behavior.* New York: Springer.

Dishman, R. K. 1982. Compliance / adherence in health-related exercise. *Health Psychology* 1:237–67.

Evans, G. W., ed. 1983. *Environmental stress.* Cambridge: Cambridge Univ. Press.

Evans, R., R. M. Rozelle, S. E. Maxwell, B. E. Raines, C. A. Dill, and T. J. Guthrie.

1981. Social modeling films to deter smoking in adolescents: Results of a three-year field investigation. *Journal of Applied Psychology* 66:399–414.

Ewart, C. K., V. C. Li, and T. J. Coates. 1983. Increasing physicians' antismoking by applying an inexpensive feedback technique. *Journal of Medical Education* 58:468–73.

Faden, R. R., A. J. Chwalow, N. A. Holtzman, and S. D. Horn. 1982. A survey to evaluate parental consent as public policy for neonatal screening. *American Journal of Public Health* 72:1347–51.

Faden, R. R., and A. I. Faden. 1978. The ethics of health education as public health policy. *Health Education Monographs* 6:180–97.

Farquhar, J. W. 1978. The community-based model of lifestyle intervention trials. *American Journal of Epidemiology* 108:103–11.

Fein, G. G., P. M. Schwartz, S. W. Jacobsen, and J. L. Jacobsen. 1983. Environmental toxins and behavioral development. *American Psychologist* 38:1188–97.

Fischoff, B., S. Lichtenstein, P. Slovic, S. L. Derby, and R. L. Keeney. 1981. *Acceptable risk.* Cambridge: Cambridge University Press.

Galanter, R. B. 1977. To the victim belong the flaws. *American Journal of Public Health* 67:1025–26.

Green, L. W. 1984. Modifying and developing health behavioral. *Annual Review of Public Health* 5:215–36.

Hertz, P., and P. L. Stamps. 1977. Appointment-keeping behavior reevaluated. *American Journal of Public Health* 67:1033–37.

Irle, M. 1975. Is aircraft noise harming people? In *Applying social psychology,* edited by M. Deutsch and H. A. Hornstein. New York: John Wiley and Sons.

Kaplan, R. M., and J. W. Bush. 1982. Health related quality of life measurement for evaluation research and policy analysis. *Health Psychology* 1:61–80.

Kasl, S. V. 1984. Stress and health. *Annual Review of Public Health* 5:319–42.

Knowles, J. H. 1977. The responsibility of the individual. In *Doing better and feeling worse,* edited by J. H. Knowles. New York: Norton.

LaLonde, M. 1975. *A new perspective on the health of canadians.* Ottawa: Information Canada.

Leventhal, H., and P. D. Cleary. 1980. The smoking problem: A review of the research and theory in behavioral risk reduction. *Psychological Bulletin* 88:370–405.

Matthews, K. A. 1982. Psychological perspectives on the Type A behavioral pattern. *Psychological Bulletin* 91:293–323.

McAlister, A., P. Puska, J. T. Salonen, J. Tuomilehto, and K. Koskela. 1982. Theory and action for health promotion: Illustrations from the North Karelia project. *American Journal of Public Health* 72:43–50.

McCaul, K. D., R. E. Glasgow, L. C. Schafer, and H. K. O'Neil. 1983. Commitment and the prevention of adolescent cigarette smoking. *Health Psychology* 2:353–65.

McNeil, B. J., and S. G. Pauker. 1984. Decision analyses for public health: Principles and illustrations. *Annual Review of Public Health* 5:135–61.

Quarantelli, E. L., and R. R. Dynes. 1972. When disaster strikes. *Psychology Today* 5(9):66–70.

Ryan, W. 1971. *Blaming the victim.* New York: Vintage Books.

Schwalm, N. D., and P. Slovic. 1982. *Development and test of a motivational approach and materials for increasing use of restraints.* Woodland Hills, CA: Perceptronics.

Siegel, J. M. 1984. Type A behavior: Epidemiologic foundations and public health implications. *Annual Review of Public Health* 5:343–67.

Singer, J. E., and D. S. Krantz. 1982. Perspectives on the interface between psychology and public health. *American Psychologist* 37:955–60.

Stone, G. C. 1983. Summary of recommendations: National working conference on education and training in health psychology. *Health Psychology* 2 (5):15–18.

Sulzer-Azaroff, B., and C. DeSantamaria. 1980. Industrial safety hazard reduction through performance feedback. *Journal of Applied Behavior Analyses* 13:287–95.

Wallston, B. S., S. W. Alagna, B. M. DeVellis, and R. F. DeVellis. 1983. Social support and physical health. *Health Psychology* 2:367–91.

Weinstein, M. C., and W. B. Stason. 1977. Foundations of cost-effectiveness analyses for health and medical practices. *New England Journal of Medicine* 296:716–21.

Weiss, B. 1983. Behavioral toxicology and environmental health science. *American Psychologist* 1174–87.

Williams, A. F. 1982. Passive and active measures for controlling disease and injury: The role of health psychologists. *Health Psychology* 1:399–410.

Wingard, D. L. 1984. The six differentials in morbidity, mortality and lifestyle. *Annual Review of Public Health* 5:433–58.

13

Health Psychology and Health Policy

Patrick H. DeLeon and Gary R. VandenBos

Health policy refers to the laws, regulations, guidelines, policies, priorities, and goals related to the delivery of health care; the conduct of health research; and the training of health professionals for local, state, national, and international governmental agencies, legislative bodies, foundations, associations, and other public and private groups. Health psychology is both influenced by health policy and can influence the formation of health policy. The participation of both practitioners and research psychologists in the development of public policy is an issue of increasing importance. (c.f., Bevan 1980, 1982a; Carpenter 1983; Fishman and Neigher 1982; Ginsberg, Kilburg, and Buklad 1983). Consequently, this chapter will focus on how health psychology can influence the development of health policy. Of primary concern is how our training institutions can assist the doctoral student in health psychology not only in appreciating the complexities inherent in developing health policy, but more importantly, by providing these future leaders of our profession with the necessary tools to actively participate in this all-important process. We would especially hope that in the foreseeable future graduate courses in health policy and the political process will be offered on a regular basis in every program.

Policy Development
POLICY FORMATION IS A POLITICAL PROCESS

This is true of both legislation and policy/program development within governmental agencies. By "political" we simply mean a situation in which two or more parties or individuals hold differing views and each attempts to assert their view in the establishment of goals, priorities, or procedures. Policy is developed within systems—be it a local public health department, a state legislature, or a federal agency. Getting legislation passed or establishing a new program initiative is, thus, a "systems problem" (Dörken 1983). It is important to understand the formal (as well as informal) process of policy formation with whatever organization one is attempting to influence. It is also important to be aware of all other groups who have an interest in the policy question under consideration: What do they want? How will they view our proposal? Is compromise possible? In the vast majority of policy debates health psychologists will not be the most powerful or central party involved in the discussions and resulting policy development. Therefore, an analysis of the "political" context will be important to having an impact on policy. In other words, effective policy efforts require knowledge of the "facts" about the context of the policy debate as well as facts about the health policy issue being debated. To make this more concrete, we might reflect on organized psychology's efforts to obtain hospital privileges. Today, services delivered in the hospital account for approximately half of all expenditures on personal health services. Dörken (1986) found in reviewing the fiscal year 1981 Department of Defense CHAMPUS mental health inpatient billings that only 3.1% of the procedures involved were outside of the scope of practice of a psychologist. Independent hospital practice is clearly an issue of major importance for health psychologists. Yet, merely "being right" is not sufficient. It took nearly a decade of intense effort by psychology and other nonphysician disciplines before the Joint Commission on Accreditation of Hospitals (JCAH) modified its medical staff membership standards to allow psychologists to have admitting privileges. And still, this is only when both the individual hospital and the local state legislature have authorized such practice. (Kilburg and Pallak, unpublished ms.; Tanney 1983; Zaro et al. 1982).

POLICY FORMATION IS AN EVOLUTIONARY PROCESS

Because policy is established in an ever changing system involving many interested parties who may hold widely differing views on "the problem" and acceptable solution, one rarely defines and achieves a desired policy initiative in a single year (or even in a couple of years). This is well illustrated by the ten-year process of modifying the federal conceptualization of quality health care from the more traditional concept of "medical treatment" to one that emphasizes behavioral health, thereby changing the national health priorities so as to make them more responsive to prevention and "wellness" efforts and, in particular, to health psychology activities (DeLeon and VandenBos 1983, 1984). The policy that is desired may very well need to serve as the long-term goal toward which one is working, moving toward it in a seemingly unorganized fashion of adding one piece or another as opportunity allows (Dörken 1977, 1981; Weick 1984).

INTERPERSONAL FACTORS AFFECT POLICY FORMATION

As educators we must assist the doctoral student in health psychology in appreciating that the interpersonal dimension of policy formation is often overlooked and undervalued. The most effective policy persons are generally seen as likeable, well-intended, reasonable people—despite the fact that one might disagree with them on specific matters in specific situations (Carpenter 1983). Health psychologists involved in policy development should have good interpersonal skills. They need to be emotionally secure, bright, and flexible. They need the ability to conceptualize a goal or outcome that they can work toward in a consistent manner while being flexible in making various diversions on the way to the end point. Needed interpersonal skills include the ability to negotiate a compromise by merging divergent views and come up with options acceptable to a wide range of parties. This latter skill may differ somewhat from research skills, which tend to take a more critical or even adversarial stance in relationship to the concerns, conceptualizations, and approaches of others. Teaching future health psychologists how to build a meaningful *interdisciplinary* consensus around the implementation of new scientific findings, such as using biofeedback to reduce high blood pressure, would be an important step forward by our educational institutions.

FACTS DO INFLUENCE THE DEVELOPMENT OF POLICY

Health psychologists may not always be fully satisfied with how their scientific research is utilized in the policy process (Parloff 1979), as their data may sometimes be overinterpreted or used after the fact to justify decisions. However, it is essential that the perspective and knowledge of health psychology be utilized in policy debate. Depending upon the issues involved, different types of data or different levels of specialized knowledge of health psychology may be required. For example, drafting a legislative bill dealing with a particular disease entity or health care treatment (such as renal dialysis) might well call for specialized, in-depth training related to that health care problem, whereas other health policy initiatives such as directing that a comprehensive range of behavioral health procedures be eligible for reimbursement might better be accomplished by someone with a broader expertise in health psychology, including perhaps additional knowledge in public health or health administration. The ability to access information and a range of experts in health psychology may, in many instances, be more important to the policymaker than any specific in-depth health psychology expertise per se.

Roles for Health Psychologists in the Policy Formation Process

As educators we should particularly assist the doctoral student in health psychology to appreciate that there are many positions and mechanisms through which health psychologists can contribute to the formation of health policy. Government is extensively involved in the health arena in the United States (Bevan 1982b). The federal government is centrally involved in the support of health research, health care delivery, and to a decreasing extent, the training of health professionals. State government is extensively involved in the support of health care delivery and the training of health professionals, and local government often has an important role in health care delivery.

Elected government officials—mayors, council members, governors, representatives, and senators—have significant influence over the basic laws that provide the core structure of health policy. However, to remain viable they must actively address a broad array of policy issues and thus they can only devote a small proportion of their energies to health policy. Relatively few elected officials are health professionals, and even fewer are health psychologists (DeLeon and VandenBos 1984). And those psychologists who have been successful in their bid for election have not necessarily been primarily concerned with health issues (Carpenter 1983).

Accordingly, professional staff members to elected officials are very important to the formation of health policy. These individuals frequently gather background information, identify critical issues, and outline possible policy options for the consideration of the elected official. It is usually the case, at all levels of government, that staff members are not health professionals and are personally quite unfamiliar with many issues of concern to health psychology. Moreover, in the U.S. Congress, there is a ninety percent turnover rate among personal professional staff members assigned to health issues every five years, and nearly seventy percent of these legislative assistants are holding their first post-college job (Grupenhoff 1982). Thus, it is important for health psychologists to routinely interact with elected officials and their staff so as to continue to shape their perspective on the societal contribution of behavioral health interventions. This must be a continuous process and one that could readily be incorporated into health psychology training programs (Forman and O'Malley 1984).

Health psychologists who are interested in actively participating in the formation of health policy will readily find professional staff positions to be roles in which their expertise and skills can be effectively utilized (DeLeon, Frohboese, and Meyers 1984). Undoubtedly, however, the interests and contributions of health psychologists would be more effectively addressed in policy deliberations if more psychologists choose to seek and accept professional staff positions at both the national and state level—thus resulting in a necessary "critical mass" of professional input. Realization of this potential led to the establishment of the APA Congressional Fellowship Program which provides psychologists with firsthand experience in the legislative process through a one-year full-time placement in the office of a congressperson. Other important policy fellowships include the White House and Robert Woods Johnson fellows.

Professional legislative staff positions represent potentially ideal jobs for health psychologists interested in mid-career or late-career changes. However, because psychology's involvement in health policy formulation is a relatively new development, it is crucial for the field that academic programs and future health psychologists begin to appreciate the very real contribution of those individual researchers and practitioners who decide to spend a period of time involved in legislative or policy development. And it is crucial, subsequently, that they be welcomed back into active academic careers. The medical profession understands the value of its members engaging in short periods of participation in public policy formation and encourages it. Psychology will not achieve its greatest policy impact until our educational institutions recognize this and make it more readily possible for university-based psychologists (particularly those at the assistant professor and associate professor levels) to enter government and later return to academic settings (DeLeon et al. 1985).

Appointed government policy positions and executive-level civil service positions are also important in policy development. There are a range of positions in government, at all levels, where the primary responsibility or work activity involves policy formation. Most of these positions are in the executive branch, although there are some in the legislative branch (such as with the Congressional Research Service or the Congress's Office of Technology Assessment) and in the judiciary branch (such as with the Federal Judicial Center or the Center for State Courts). Such positions range from major appointed posts (e.g., director of the National Institutes of Health) to staff assistant positions. Many executive branch positions involve dual responsibilities—participation in policy development as well as program management/policy implementation. The range of specific policy activities can, of course, be quite varied, but these positions can be thought of as "internal consultantships" and frequently involve proposing policy changes, reviewing and commenting on proposed policy changes, evaluating and describing the advantages and disadvantages of existing or proposed policy, and gathering and synthesizing available knowledge relevant to a given policy debate. The analytic, research, and conceptual skills of health psychologists, as well as their scientific knowledge in specific areas of health psychology, make them particularly well-qualified for such positions. Health psychology graduate students should strive to ensure that their own national student organization will begin to play a role similar to that of the American Medical Student Association in ensuring that policy positions become available for interested graduates.

At the present time, the majority of psychologists in governmental positions are mid-range executive-level administrators. Relatively few psychologists have been appointed to higher level policy positions (e.g., Institute director or above). Psychologists such as Richard Atkinson (former director of the National Science Foundation), Douglas Fenderson (former director of the National Institute of Handicapped Research), John Gardner (former Secretary of the Department of Health, Education, and Welfare), Carolyn Payton (former director of the Peace Corps), and Edward Zigler (former director of the Office of Child Development and the Children's Bureau) are notable exceptions. We are aware, however, of a number of instances where psychologists have been offered such high-level policy positions but unfortunately declined them. The difficulty in moving back and forth between university and government positions is one reason for the reluctance. This in turn influences which psychologists are seen as "qualified" for high-level appointed government positions. Because there is a critical shortage of psychologists in ranking administrative positions, psychologists are typically not considered for major federal appointments until they are extremely well known in their specialty area. This often means they are in their late fifties or early sixties and are involved in the projects that they see as "wrapping up" their careers. As a consequence, they are frequently "honored to be considered" and go through the nominations process, even though they are, in fact, quite reluctant to accept such an appointment (and decline them when offered). However, when they "reluctantly accept nomination," the strength of their credentials causes other younger colleagues (who are truly "willing to serve") to be eliminated from the list of possible candidates. The result is obvious— few psychologists are appointed to major government policy positions. As a further consequence, psychologists attempting to influence health policy continuously encounter policymakers who know little about psychology as a science or a profession (DeLeon, VandenBos, and Kraut 1984). It thus becomes continually necessary to educate them about behavioral perspectives and their relevance to the immediate issues at hand. This need has been evident, for example, in trying to convince those who set research funding priorities that "health psychology is considerably broader than merely mental health"; i.e., that its agendas should be considered by federal agencies other than the NIMH (VandenBos and Batchelor 1983).

External consultants play an important role in the policy development process and there are a variety of ways in which health psychologists can and do serve. The most frequent vehicle through which health psychologists contribute to policy development is through service on technical, scientific, and advisory boards. Examples of this type of activity include service on the Institute of Medicine panel studying health and behavior (Hamburg, Elliott, and Parron 1982), membership on the Department of Health and Human Services technical advisory panel on the development of goals for the promotion of health and prevention of disease, or service on a local health planning advisory panel considering the usefulness of developing a diabetics screening program for adolescents. Psychologists invited to serve, because of their expertise or personal interest, on such panels may have their primary employment in a wide range of settings which in themselves may also have an impact on health policy development—i.e., psychology departments, university-based or independent policy institutes (such as Rand or the Hastings Institute), professional associations (such as the APA), or other organizations (such as the Washington Business Group on Health).

The external consultant role may be more informal. For example, when a health psychologist has particular expertise in a given area and has, over time, expressed continuous interest in related policy issues, his or her own legislator may well enter into an in-depth discussion with the health psychologist about the evolving policy developments. Such informal consultation with an elected official does not have the same professional prestige value as serving on an advisory board of a major federal agency, but in the long run it may have a greater impact on the formation of national health policy. And, we would suggest that, given the gradual and evolutionary nature of health policy development, this would be a natural area in which university faculty and their health psychology graduate students could meaningfully contribute to the level of congressional understanding.

Our training institutions need to help tomorrow's health psychologists appreciate that they and their colleagues can significantly affect health policy through information dissemination and advocacy activities. For example, the APA Office of National Policy Studies and Divisions 12 (Clinical) and 38 (Health) engage in a concerted information dissemination project through a regular series of monthly policy dinners (DeLeon, O'Keefe, VandenBos, and Kraut 1982). Major federal policymakers are invited to an informal dinner with twenty to thirty psychologists to exchange information and perspectives on topics of mutual interest. Such dialogues educate policymakers about health psychology and educate psychologists about the problems, challenges, and issues facing a particular agency or congressional committee. At the Annual APA Conventions, Division 31 (State Associations) has held similar meetings for its leadership. The science seminars conducted by the Federation of Behavioral, Psychological, and Cognitive Sciences, the APA Board of Scientific Affairs, and the American Association for the Advancement of Science are also information dissemination efforts intended to inform and influence policy development in a collegial manner. Similar programs could be initiated at the state or local level, perhaps under the leadership of a graduate seminar or state psychological association. The subject matter may change, but the educational process would be the same.

Some health psychologists are actively involved in direct political advocacy efforts on behalf of specific legislation. This may be through such organizations as the American Psychological Association, various state psychological associations, or special task forces established by APA Divisions, and as individual congressional witness. While direct political advocacy activities are still viewed somewhat negatively by a few health psychologists, it is important that health psychologists testify before Congress, state commissions, and local government on specific legislation. Most educational institutions have their own legislative lobbyist (many on both the state and federal level) who could serve as an excellent additional vehicle for getting health psychology's message across.

The extent to which psychologists historically have not involved themselves in legislation by testifying may not be obvious. However, the data are compelling. Slightly over 155 public witnesses appeared in the various hearings before the Senate Appropriations Subcommittee on Labor, Health and Human Services, and Education in 1983. Two self-identified psychologists testified! Detailed checking of the witness lists reveals that two other psychologists did appear before the committee but did not identify themselves as psychologists. Is it surprising that legislative officials do not know what psychology is and the range of things psychologists do? Again, we feel that our educational institutions could, and should, take the lead not only in teaching future health psychologists how to present testimony, but even more importantly, in encouraging their faculty to serve as role models at the local level whenever possible (Hosticka, Hibbard, and Sundberg 1983; Kilburg and Ginsberg 1983; Portnoy et al. 1983).

Three Simple Activities for Individual Health Psychologists

There are a range of simple and quite concrete actions that health psychologists can take that will increase their impact on health policy at the national, state, and local level. These activities do not necessarily have to consume a lot of time. It is our hope that our nation's health psychology training programs will take the lead in educating their students as to the importance of periodically engaging in these efforts. The long-term effect of systematically sharing health psychology's message with the public at large, and especially with elected officials, will have demonstrable impact on the likelihood that health psychology's unique contributions will ultimately be recognized by those who set our nation's health and scientific priorities.

Maximize Individual Contact with Your Elected Official

The single most valuable political effort that those concerned with behavioral health can make is to develop, over time, a personal relationship with their own elected officials at various levels of government. Such relations should be built upon trust, respect, and mutual assistance. When urged to visit their elected officials during business or vacation trips to the nation's capitol, behavioral health professionals often reply, in good faith, that either they themselves are too busy or that they do not want to burden their senators or representatives with trivia. Instead, they want to wait until they have something "really important" to request and promise that they will follow through then. If taken at face value, their explanations might be reasonable. It is our judgment, however, that they are merely afraid they might look foolish if they call on their elected representatives for what is essentially a social visit (to drop off a reprint that "may be of interest to the congressperson"). We believe that visits and letters from behavioral health psychologists, before a crisis occurs, help prevent that crisis from occurring. By visiting they will sensitize the elected official to issues of concern to health psychologists long before it becomes too late to take effective action.

WRITE FOR A WIDER AUDIENCE THAN YOUR OWN PROFESSION

In addition to the scientific and professional writing that health psychologists do, it is critical that we inform the broader society about our work. It is our experience that there is no shortage of potential readership markets. One could write for the newsletter or journal of other professions, for one's local newspaper, or for national magazines geared toward the general public. If we hope to ultimately make the consumer responsible for his or her own health habits, we must provide the consumer with sufficient information to make informed decisions. Use of the print media is a cost-effective means of reaching the public. Although our present training models do not systematically encourage this type of knowledge proliferation, we are optimistic that as health psychologists become more involved in the overall health care system this will change (G. Kimble, personal communication, Public Information Committee meetings of the American Psychological Association 1983; Pallak 1984).

CULTIVATE THE MEDIA

If one takes the time to reflect on how we ourselves learn about developments in areas outside of our own professional expertise, such as foreign affairs, it is easy to see the significant role of the media—both electronic and print media. News anchorpersons and syndicated columnists play major roles in shaping our views (or, at the very least, influencing what we focus upon). The media, in a very real sense, creates the social/political agendas of our time—giving them importance and urgency. Most Americans do not really think about health care until they are ill. However, there is a clear public interest in remaining healthy. If the clinical interventions of behavioral health are nearly as effective as we expect, one must assume that the American public will respond enthusiastically, as long as behavioral health is presented in a credible and fashionable light by the media. It is important that health psychologists provide the media (both local and national) with the best of what we have to offer. This might be done, for example, by routinely sending short letters to the editors of local newspapers and the managers of local television stations which draw their attention to a recent health psychology publication (and enclosing a photocopy). Or, health psychology faculty could initiate interdepartmental programs with their colleagues in other parts of their university who are providing training for those students who will eventually become the media—for example, with schools of journalism. While national professional associations can handle information dissemination with national news agencies, only the efforts of individual health psychologists (or university departments or state psychological associations) can effectively reach local news sources. The communication should draw out potential implications and applications of the cited research, and individual psychologists should be willing to discuss the general area and specific topic with those in the media who follow up on the initial communication. It is important to stress that policymakers are *very* attentive to what is covered in the newspapers and on television (McCall, Gregory, and Murray 1984).

Summary

We have attempted to provide a broad overview of both the complexities inherent in being involved in formulating health policy and also the importance of psychology's educational institutions taking the lead in ensuring that our profession's future generations will actively accept this challenge. The political process is a fluid process; being involved is the most important ingredient. There are many roles that individual psychologists or psychological institutions can play. For the scientific and clinical knowledge base of health psychology to have its appropriate impact on our society, it is necessary that understanding the political process becomes an integral element of graduate education.

REFERENCES

Bevan, W. 1980. On getting in bed with a lion. *American Psychologist* 35:779–89.
———. 1982a. A sermon of sorts in three plus parts. *American Psychologist* 37: 1303–22.
———. 1982b. National policy and human welfare: A conversation with Stuart Eizenstat. *American Psychologist* 37:1128–35.
Carpenter, P. B. 1983. The personal insights of a legislator/psychologist. *American Psychologist* 38:1216–19.
DeLeon, P. H., R. S. Frohboese, and J. C. Meyers. 1984. Psychologists on Capitol Hill: A unique use of the skills of the scientist/practitioner. *Professional Psychology: Research and Practice* 15:697–705.
DeLeon, P. H., D. K. Kjervik, A. G. Kraut, and G. R. VandenBos. 1985. Psychology and nursing: A natural alliance. *American Psychologist* 40:1153–64.
DeLeon, P. H., A. M. O'Keefe, G. R. VandenBos, and A. G. Kraut. 1982. How to influence public policy: A blueprint for activism. *American Psychologist* 37: 476–85.
DeLeon, P. H., and G. R. VandenBos. 1983. The new federal health care frontiers: Cost containment and wellness. *Psychotherapy in Private Practice* 1:17–32.

————. 1984. Public health policy: Behavioral health. In *Behavioral health: A handbook of health enchancement and disease prevention,* edited by J. D. Matarazzo, S. M. Weiss, J. A. Herd, N. E. Miller, and S. M. Weiss. New York: Wiley and Sons.

DeLeon, P. H., G. R. VandenBos, and A. G. Kraut. 1984. Federal legislation recognizing psychology. *American Psychologist* 39:933–46.

Dörken, H. 1977. Avenues to legislative success. *American Psychologist* 32:738–45.

————. 1981. Coming of age legislatively: In twenty-one steps. *American Psychologist* 36:165–73.

————. 1983. Advocacy and the legislative process: Representation in a changing world. *American Psychologist* 38:1210–15.

————. 1986. The expanding role of clinical psychology in mental health services: The CHAMPUS experience. In *Professional psychology in transition,* edited by H. Dörken and Associates, 69–98. San Francisco: Jossey-Bass.

Fishman, D. B., and W. D. Neigher. 1982. American psychology in the eighties: Who will buy? *American Psychologist* 37:533–46.

Forman, S. G., and P. L. O'Malley. 1984. A legislative field experience for psychology graduate students. *Professional Psychology: Research and Practice* 15:324–32.

Ginsberg, M. R., R. R. Kilberg, and W. Buklad. 1983. State-level legislative and policy advocacy. *American Psychologist* 38:1206–9.

Grupenhoff, J. T. 1982. Turnover rates of members and staff who deal with medicine/health/biomedical research issues: Communication #1. Washington, D.C.: Science and Health Communication Group.

Hamburg, D. A., G. R. Elliott, and D. L. Parron, eds. 1982. *Health and behavior: Frontiers of research in the biobehavioral sciences.* Washington, D.C.: Institute of Medicine/National Academy Press.

Hosticka, C. J., M. Hibbard, and N. D. Sundberg. 1983. Improving psychologists' contributions to the policymaking process. *Professional Psychology: Research and Practice* 14:374–85.

Kilberg, R. R., and M. R. Ginsberg. 1983. Sunset and psychology: How we learned to love a crisis. *American Psychologist* 38:1227–31.

Kilberg, R. R., and M. P. Pallak. Unpublished manuscript. Psychology and medicine: Toward the understanding and management of complexity.

Kimble, G. 1983. Personal communication with author at Public Information Committee Meetings of the American Psychological Association.

McCall, R. B., T. G. Gregory, and J. P. Murray. 1984. Communicating developmental research results to the general public through television. *Developmental Psychology* 20:45–54.

Pallak, M. S. 1984. Report of the executive officer: 1983. *American Psychologist* 39:591–94.

Parloff, M. B. 1979. Can psychotherapy research guide the policymaker? A little knowledge may be a dangerous thing. *American Psychologist* 34:296–306.

Portnoy, S. M., S. J. Friedland, M. M. Norman, B. R. Calveric, E. J. Eisman, R. F. Zapf, and P. H. DeLeon. 1983. Effective state-level advocacy: A model for action. *American Psychologist* 38:1220–26.

Tanney, F. 1983. Hospital privileges for psychologists: A legislative model. *American Psychologist* 38:1232–37.

VandenBos, G. R., and W. F. Batchelor. 1983. Health personnel, service delivery, and national policy: A conversation with Tom Hatch. *American Psychologist* 38: 1360–65.

Weick, K. E. 1984. Small wins: Redefining the scale of social problems. *American Psychologist* 39:40–49.

Zaro, J. S., W. F. Batchelor, M. R. Ginsberg, and M. S. Pallak. 1982. Psychology and the JCAH: Reflections on a decade of struggle. *American Psychologist* 37: 1342–49.

Part Four

Professional Issues in Health Psychology

Editor: Cynthia Belar

Thus far we have discussed the emergence of health psychology, its knowledge base, and its application in a variety of settings from health care services to public policy. With the application of health psychology, issues of professional practice surface. In this part the authors delineate many of these issues, articulate concerns facing the field, and propose some guides for further professionalization in the field.

Health psychology will not escape, nor should it, issues of quality control in its application. Nelson Jones (chap. 14) outlines the current credentialling mechanisms in psychology for both individual psychologists and training institutions. In contrast to Matarazzo's view (chap. 4), Jones portrays the credentialling process as well established for a number of specialties and presently accessible to health psychology. On a cautionary note, he points out that conference guidelines for credentialling mechanisms exceed current practices in psychology as a whole and suggests that they will have to be brought into line.

Ethical standards are integral to professional practice. Charles Swencionis, Judy E. Hall, and Ruth Macklin (chap. 15) review the current "Ethical Principles of Psychologists," concluding that while the *principles* remain the same, different concerns may arise in health psychology which are related to specific setting and patient population issues. They propose a series of recommendations to facilitate the development and maintenance of ethical standards for health psychology.

Psychology's increasing concern with legal issues reflects changes in society as a whole. In health psychology, examination of these issues is just now getting underway. Robinsue Frohboese and Thomas Overcast provide the first analysis of the legal system's interactions with and impact on health psychology. Beginning with a general overview of the legal system, they subsequently delineate a variety of legal considerations, including regulations of practice, duties owed to others (e.g., reporting child abuse), professional standards, malpractice, practice management, and roles within the legal system for health psychologists.

This section closes with a chapter by David Altman and Jerry Cahn on employment options for health psychologists, without which, of course, there would be no concerns about professional practice. In a discussion directed particularly to students approaching graduation, they provide an overview of what they describe as the manifest and the latent health psychology job market, examining special issues that health psychologists will face and suggesting skills which may be helpful in making opportunities manifest.

14

Credentials for Health Psychologists

Nelson F. Jones

Throughout this volume references are made to psychology or to health psychology as professions. Peterson (1976) has made a cogent case for the broad field of professional psychology meeting the standards of a profession, but it is doubtful if health psychology as a specialty area of psychology could be so labeled convincingly. Peterson dealt with Flexner's (1915) criteria for evaluating a profession—criteria which are still consonant with current sociological thinking (Moore 1970). Criteria regarding the practical nature of the profession's objectives, the need for a professional society to monitor competence, and altruistic as well as self-serving motivations pose little problem for psychology. The state of the applicable knowledge base and the extent to which it can be taught were seen by Peterson to pose problems for some areas of psychology. Health psychology will need to demonstrate that it has met these latter criteria before claiming status as an independent profession.

The conference which gave rise to this book was, however, an effort to accomplish one of the functions of a profession, determination of standards for admission. The conference dealt with other issues such as the continuing need to enhance the body of knowledge basic to professional functioning and, in so doing, raised complications for the means by which the special qualifications of health psychologists are to be identified. Complicated identification, however, is not a new phenomenon for the broad profession of psychology, which has deliberately combined the roles of knowledge generation and service provision since its inception (Raimy 1950).

Quality control in the application of a body of knowledge for the protection of a consuming public not qualified to judge competence is a major concern of and rationale for professions. Maintenance of the knowledge base, a professional organization, training functions, and ethical standards are in service of protecting the public as well as maintaining the integrity of the profession. By the same token, professions survive by having active practitioners whose credentials are recognizable and meaningful, however much "surplus" meaning those credentials may carry. For psychology, this means identifying to the consumer the professional practitioners who provide services to the public in the most visible and persuasive fashion consonant with ethical standards, while simultaneously attending to the generation of new knowledge and to the setting of standards and training patterns. Imposing credentialing requirements which will protect the public but not hinder the other endeavors requires considerable sorting through of issues and goals.

In our short professional history we have made remarkable strides in these directions, although the process of adding a profession to an existing academic-scientific discipline has not always been universally welcomed by either the practitioners or the academicians. As the profession of psychology has grown, the complexity of credentialling issues has increased enormously. In 1949, when the training model which was to serve for twenty-five years was adopted at the APA-sponsored Boulder Conference (Raimy 1950), the decision that professional training be at the doctoral level seemed adequate. The Ph.D. was the only credential envisioned to be necessary for teaching, research, or clinical service by the educators of psychologists attending the conference.

However, clinical psychologists were already working in a broad array of settings, including independent private practice, and it had become apparent to these psychologists that the public interest would be better served by governmental regulation of practice than by relying only on academic requirements. With the passage of Connecticut's licensing law in 1945, the admission to practice was already beginning to pass from academic to governmental control, although it was 1977 before all states had statutory control of practice. Wisely, it now seems, the profession, serving as legislative consultants and lobbyists, pushed for generic laws, making psychology the core discipline to be regulated and leaving the designation of specialty areas to the profession. That licensing of activities rather than certification of the title psychologist eventually became the ideal for state legislation may not have been so wise, since many state boards of psychology have found enforcement of licensing laws to be difficult, if not impossible.

A third credentialling mechanism, the American Board of Professional Psychology (ABPP), was established in 1947 as an independent, nonstatutory agency to certify excellence in specialty areas within psychology. The three interlocking levels of credentialling became established much as they exist today. University training programs award the basic academic credential. The state regulates the practice of psychology through licensing, and the profession (via professional organizations) determines educational standards, makes recommendations regarding legislation, and establishes mechanisms for recognizing special competence.

The professional organizations referred to include APA, ABPP, and the Council for the National Register of Health Service Providers in Psychology. The Council for the National Register was established in 1975 to meet the growing need to identify those psychologists who were trained and experienced in rendering health services. While the Council for the National Register has not functioned as a credentialling organization itself, it has taken a leadership role in defining the educational and experience credentials which it verifies and lists for individual registrants.

Issues and Recommendations Regarding Entry-Level Credentials for Health Psychologists
SERVICE PROVISION VS. RESEARCH AND TEACHING

The 1983 National Working Conference on Education and Training in Health Psychology made recommendations which will affect all three sources of credentials described above (Stone 1983). The conferees attempted to differentiate professional service providers in the field from educators and researchers, although they strongly endorsed a single training model (the scientist-professional) for persons entering the service-provision area.

The profession has been on record for some ten years as endorsing a *practitioner* training model and a professional degree, the Doctor of Psychology (Psy.D.), as an appropriate basis for entering professional practice. At this point a number of accredited and recognized professional schools and departments of psychology offer the Psy.D., all states license Psy.D.'s for practice, and ABPP and the Council for the National Register recognize the degree. Thus, the Psy.D., as well as the more traditional Ph.D., is an entry-level credential for professional practice at this point. Most Psy.D. programs follow the practitioner rather than the scientist-professional training model.

While the conferees stopped short of recommending recognition of only the Ph.D. for entry into health psychology, they did recommend that doctoral-level training carry a strong component of research training because of what they perceived to be a lack of well-substantiated information in the field. Such a pattern continues support for psychology's (unique) scientist-professional training model but does little to clarify for the public the identity of the psychology practitioner or to separate academic from professional roles. While some existing Psy.D. programs can meet the recommended standards, as practitioner programs become more numerous and the health psychology area becomes more established, some reconsideration will have to be given to this recommendation. The professional training model will have to be recognized.

For those psychologists electing to enter the health field and to use the title health psychologist only as researchers or teachers, the doctoral degree was the primary credential recommended by the conferees, with a license and a postdoctoral training certificate for a research apprenticeship seen as desirable but not mandatory. For those rendering services to the public, even if those services are in the context of a research program, the recommended requirements change to include two years of postdoctoral training and a state license to practice as essential.

While this pattern would free teachers and researchers from the obligation to become licensed and would offer the public a measure of protection, it leaves unresolved the issue of appropriate role models in the course of training for professionally oriented students. APA accreditation standards have long recognized the problem of appropriate credentialed mentors for professionally oriented students in scientist-professional training programs, and it is an issue which will still need to be evaluated under these standards.

CREDENTIALS FOR PROGRAMS OR INSTITUTIONS

Programs preparing students for careers as service providers will need to attend carefully to several dimensions of general entry-level training for psychologists, the standards for which are becoming more consistent and more stringent. Some highly specialized doctoral programs will have to make changes in order to meet the standards for a doctoral degree in psychology set by the 1977 Conference on Education and Credentialling in Psychology (Wellner 1978). Those standards have been adopted by the Committee on Accreditation of APA, the American Association of State Psychology Boards, about two-thirds of the individual state licensing boards, and the American Board of Professional Psychology. They are also used by the Council for the National Register of Health Service Providers in Psychology as the basis for its system of designating programs in psychology. They will almost certainly form a large part of the standards of any program APA sets up in the future to designate doctoral programs in psychology. They will clearly influence any programs producing health psychologists. A detailed account of the need for these standards, the history of their development, and related issues can be found in *Education and Credentialing in Psychology* (Wellner 1978). The ten criteria developed by the 1977 conferees are:

1. Programs that are accredited by the American Psychological Association are recognized as meeting the definition of a professional psychology program. The criteria for accreditation serve as a model for professional psychology training OR all of the following criteria, 2 through 10.

2. Training in professional psychology is doctoral training offered in a regionally accredited institution of higher education.

3. The program, wherever it may be administratively housed, must be clearly identified and labeled as a psychology program. Such a program must specify in pertinent institutional catalogues and brochures its intent to educate and train professional psychologists.

4. The psychology program must stand as a recognizable, coherent, organizational entity within the institution.

5. There must be a clear authority and primary responsibility for the core and specialty areas whether or not the program cuts across administrative lines.

6. The program must be an integrated, organized sequence of study.

7. There must be an identifiable psychology faculty and a psychologist responsible for the program.

8. The program must have an identifiable body of students who are matriculated in that program for a degree.

9. The program must include supervised practicum, internship, field or laboratory training appropriate to the practice of psychology.

10. The curriculum shall encompass a minimum of three academic years of full-time graduate study. In addition to instruction in scientific and professional ethics and standards, research design and methodology, statistics and psychometrics, the core program shall require each student to demonstrate competence in each of the following substantive content areas. This typically will be met by including a minimum of three or more graduate semester hours (five or more graduate quarter hours) in each of these four substantive content areas:

    a) Biological bases of behavior: physiological psychology, comparative psychology, neuropsychology, sensation and perception, psychopharmacology;

    b) Cognitive-affective bases of behavior: learning, thinking motivation, emotion;

c) Social bases of behavior: social psychology, group processes, organizational and systems theory;

d) Individual differences: personality theory, human development, abnormal psychology.

In order to facilitate its processing of applicants for listing, the Council for the National Register has implemented a designation system for programs meeting these standards. While the 1983 edition of the designation list (Wellner 1983) includes some 780 programs, a sizable number of programs have not been accepted, even though they may have advertised themselves as offering degrees in psychology. A discipline-wide agreement on standards for programs in psychology, followed by a mechanism such as the Council for the National Register for determining whether the degree in fact represents a basic education in psychology, will be a necessity for evaluating health psychology programs.

Most programs in clinical and counseling psychology now require that a one-year internship be completed before the degree is granted. The 1983 conferees were very clear that both a predoctoral internship and a two-year postdoctoral fellowship were to be mandatory components of health psychology training for service provision.

Defining the minimum characteristics of an acceptable internship promises to be more complex than it might appear on the surface. Although APA has accredited internship programs for more than twenty years, there remain many nonaccredited internship programs in school, counseling, and clinical psychology. The addition of specialized health psychology internship programs promises to pose additional problems for evaluation.

Because of the existing numbers of nonaccredited internship programs, the Council for the National Register (1982) has promulgated for its own use a set of generic guidelines, consistent with those of the APA Committee on Accreditation and the Association of Psychology Internship Centers. They are as follow:

> Internships that are accredited by the American Psychological Association are recognized as meeting the definition, or all of the following criteria, 1 through 12.

1. An organized training program, in contrast to supervised experience or on-the-job training, is designed to provide the intern with a planned, programmed sequence of training experience. The primary focus and purpose is assuring breadth and quality of training.

2. The internship agency has a clearly designated staff psychologist who is

responsible for the integrity and quality of the training program and who is actively licensed/certified by the State Board of Examiners in Psychology.

3. The internship agency has two or more psychologists on the staff as supervisors, at least one of whom is actively licensed as a psychologist by the State Board of Examiners in Psychology.

4. Internship supervision was provided by a staff member of the internship agency or by an affiliate of that agency who carried clinical responsibility for the cases being supervised. At least half of the internship supervision was provided by one or more psychologists.

5. The internship provided training in a range of assessment and treatment activities conducted directly with patients seeking health services.

6. At least twenty-five percent of the trainee's time is in direct patient contact (minimum 375 hours).

7. The internship includes a minimum of two hours per week (regardless of whether the internship was completed in one year or two) of regularly scheduled, formal, face-to-face, individual supervision with the specific intent of dealing with health services rendered directly by the intern. There must also be at least two additional hours per week in learning activities such as: case conferences involving a case in which the intern is actively involved; seminars dealing with clinical issues; cotherapy with a staff person including discussion, group supervision, and additional individual supervision.

8. Training is post-clerkship, post-practicum and post-externship level.

9. The internship agency has a minimum of two interns at the internship level of training during the applicant's training period.

10. Trainee has title such as "intern," "resident," "fellow," or other designation of trainee status.

11. The internship agency has a written statement or brochure which describes the goals and content of the internship, states clear expectations for quantity and quality of trainee's work, and is made available to prospective interns.

12. The internship experience (minimum 1500 hours) is completed within twenty-four months.

The APA Committee on Accreditation, as psychology's accrediting agency, was asked to accredit postdoctoral training in health psychology as well by the 1983 conferees. Since all accreditation by APA is done on an invitational basis, there is a clear possibility that permanently nonaccredited programs will continue to exist at the postdoctoral level and be recognized by licensing boards for a variety of political reasons. Therefore, independent standards for designating both internship and postdoctoral training in the health psychology field will be needed. Designation could easily be accomplished through the same commission or interorganizational committee which designates doctoral programs as "in psychology," providing current efforts to establish such a group (APA 1983a) are effective. Including state licensing boards or the American Association of State Psychology Boards in the committee would allow them to recognize this level of designation as well as to set standards.

Thus, the apparently simple statement that entry-level credentials for the health-service provider in psychology should consist of a state license to practice based on a doctoral degree in psychology and a postdoctoral specialty fellowship isn't nearly so simple when the implementing mechanisms are considered.

Credentials Beyond the Entry Level

There presently exist two additional means of identifying the training, experience, and competence of practitioners in health-related areas of psychology.

The oldest is the ABPP diploma, which signifies that exceptional competence in one of the specialty areas of psychology has been demonstrated by examination. As indicated earlier, ABPP was established as an independent examining and certifying agency in 1947. By defining its mission as the certification of *exceptional competence,* however, ABPP both maintained a high-prestige level and rendered itself unsuitable as an agency to certify journeyman-level competence in the specialties. Indeed, ABPP has gone in the other direction, recently becoming an umbrella organization for several other specialty boards in addition to maintaining its own specialties in clinical, counseling, school, and industrial-organization psychology. At this time the ABPP diploma remains the most senior credential for practice in psychology, and it seems quite appropriate that a specialty examination in health psychology be proposed under its aegis to certify exceptional competence in this new area of practice. The designation of a specialty area in itself is an issue currently receiving a great deal of attention (APA 1983b). Recent developments are described in chapter 26 by Matarazzo.

The second mechanism is listing in the *National Register of Health Service Providers in Psychology.* Licensing laws in almost all states are generic. They cover educational and work-related practices as well as health-service provision. This posed a problem for patients seeking reimbursement from third-party carriers, for state and federal agencies in determining eligibility of individual psychologists to participate in funded programs, and for the political action groups within the profession who seek recognition of psychological services by third-party carriers. Due to the need for a mechanism to identify psychologists trained and experienced in rendering health services, in 1974 the APA Board of Directors requested ABPP to establish one. The result was the Council for the National Register of Health Service Providers in Psychology, now functioning as an independent organization and listing over 13,000 psychologists in its 1983 edition. The health services provided by registrants are most often mental health services and most registrants have been trained in clinical, counseling, or school psychology. It should be expected, however, that this vehicle for identification will be useful to the emerging specialty of health psychology as well. Criteria for listing in the *National Register of Health Service Providers in Psychology* are that the registrant have: (1) a current license or certificate from the State Board of Examiners in Psychology at the independent-practice level of psychology; (2) a doctoral degree in psychology from a regionally accredited educational institution; and (3) two years of supervised experience in health service in psychology, of which at least one year is in an organized health-service training program and one year is postdoctoral.

Thus, the health psychologist following the recommendation above, including the postdoctoral fellowship, will automatically meet the standards for listing and will probably find it a convenience to be listed in the *National Register*, whether or not he or she continues toward ABPP certification. There may be some confusion generated because the 1983 conferees recommended a two-year postdoctoral fellowship while the Council for the National Register has only required, to date, one year of such experience.

Continuing Education

To this point we have discussed the educational and regulatory patterns to be followed in becoming a fully credentialed health psychologist. That, however, is only the beginning. The 1983 conference did not make formal recommendations regarding continuing education, but it is obvious that health psychologists will need to keep themselves abreast of new developments in the field throughout their careers. The responsibility for making continuing education opportunities available, monitoring their quality and encouraging participation is one that APA has assumed to a substantial extent. Several states have passed laws or enacted board regulations requiring evidence of continuing education for continuation of licensing. Since the early 1970s, when attention was first focused on formal continuing education (Jones 1975), the concept has been challenged from many quarters. At least one state (Colorado), which enacted one of the earliest continuing education laws, has now repealed it as too cumbersome to administer. On the other hand, New York's Continuing Medical Education statute was recently upheld in court action (Johnson 1983), which will probably strengthen all such legislative efforts.

More workable than statutory requirements, continuing education provisions which are a contingency for continued membership in a specialty society are also less vulnerable to court challenges. Thus, it is quite within the scope of Division 38 of APA to set continuing education requirements for continued membership, and it is an issue which should be addressed at an early date. The Continuing Education Committee of APA has established mechanisms for recording and documenting whatever experience the Division may decide to require and such documentation could well become an essential part of the credentials of a health psychologist.

An issue which will need to be faced by the Division in setting continuing education requirements is whether they should apply to all Division members or only to service providers. Given the rapidly expanding knowledge base in the field and the pressures on researchers and academicians to become more and more specialized, it might be well to require everyone to update periodically rather than reserving the requirement for practitioners alone.

Summary

Dimensions along which the documentation of education, experience, and skills needed to be a health psychologist must be considered have all been well established as other specialty areas have developed. They consist of educational credentials of documented quality, statutorily required licensure or certification for service providers, and intraprofessional certification of competence and/or experience. Assuming that Division 38's efforts to have health psychology recognized as a specialty succeed (APA 1983b), the mechanisms exist for recognizing its practitioners, although the designation or accreditation of graduate programs, internships, postdoctoral training programs, and continuing education offerings will require ongoing monitoring for quality. Health psychology is perhaps the most rapidly growing segment of professional psychology. It is urgent that any system set up for identifying its practitioners be effective and hopefully durable. The number of changing elements in the pattern is large and special interests must somehow be accommodated. The opportunities presented by this field, however, make the process worth the trouble.

REFERENCES

American Psychological Association. 1983a. *Draft report of the task force on education and credentialing.* Washington, D.C.

————. 1983b. *Manual for the identification and continued recognition of proficiencies and new specialties in psychology,* second draft. Washington, D.C.

Council for the National Register of Health Service Providers in Psychology. 1982. *Register Report Number 16, May 1982.* Washington, D.C.

Flexner, A. 1915. Is social work a profession? In *Proceedings of the National Conference of Charities and Connections.* Baltimore, MD: Social Work.

Johnson, M. E. September 1983. *Continuing Medical Education Newsletter.* Chicago: AMA.

Jones, N. F. 1975. Continuing education: A new challenge for psychology. *American Psychologist* 30:842–47.

Moore, W. E. 1970. *The professions: Roles and rules.* New York: Russell Sage.

National Working Conference on Education and Training in Health Psychology, May 23–27, 1983. *Health Psychology* 2(5): 1–153, supplement section.

Peterson, D. 1976. Is psychology a profession? *American Psychologist* 31:576–81.

Raimy, V., ed. 1950. *Training in clinical psychology.* New York: Prentice-Hall.

Wellner, A. M., ed. 1978. *Education and credentialing in psychology.* Washington, D.C.: American Psychological Association.

————. 1983. *Designated doctoral programs in psychology.* Washington, D.C.: National Register of Health Service Providers in Psychology.

15

Ethical Concerns in Health Psychology

Charles Swencionis and Judy E. Hall

Ethical principles which apply for health psychologists are the same as ethical principles which apply to other psychologists. However, the settings, techniques, and populations of health psychologists dictate some specific concerns from those in more traditional areas. Since the Task Group in Ethical Concerns (Hall and Swencionis 1983) recommended that Division 38 should develop a casebook of critical incidents that have occurred or might occur in the health psychology setting, this paper illustrates how specific ethical principles apply to the health psychologist. This description is provided to show a difference in emphasis and not to argue that there are different principles which apply to the health psychologist.

"Ethical Principles of Psychologists" (APA 1981) describes these principles as falling within the following areas: (1) responsibility, (2) competence, (3) moral and legal standards, (4) public statements, (5) confidentiality, (6) welfare of the consumer, (7) professional relationships, (8) assessment techniques, (9) research with human participants, and (10) care and use of animals. We consider each of these principles in turn, identifying new or special considerations entailed by the settings in which health psychologists work. Principles 2–9 are illustrated with examples.

Much of the work being done in health psychology is in applied research. This is, of necessity, a combination of service delivery and research. Thus, most of the examples used in this article are derived from situations which have some service delivery component to them.

Principle 1   Responsibility

In providing services, psychologists maintain the highest standards of their profession. They accept responsibility for the consequences of their acts and

The authors thank Neal E. Miller, Michael J. Follick, Ruth Macklin, George Stone, and Cynthia Belar for their comments.

make every effort to ensure that their services are used appropriately (APA 1981).

The major difference between health psychology and other areas of psychology is that health psychology deals with physical health. More traditional areas of psychology are concerned with mental health, mental retardation, career decisions, marital problems, college students, organizations, children, and healthy people. Health psychology is concerned with these topics only insofar as they are related to and influence physical health. Thus, the health psychologist has an additional responsibility to those traditionally assumed: the responsibility for physical health. The physician has medical responsibility, and the individual has responsibility for him or herself, but the actions of the health psychologist have effects on the physical health of others. For those engaged in research removed from direct service delivery, for example in research on delivery systems, this is true only indirectly but must still be considered when making decisions concerning ethics.

Principle 2 Competence

The maintenance of high standards of competence is a responsibility shared by all psychologists in the interest of the public and the profession as a whole. Psychologists recognize the boundaries of their competence and the limitations of their technique. They only provide services and only use the techniques for which they are qualified by training and experience. In those areas in which recognized standards do not yet exist, psychologists take whatever precautions are necessary to protect the welfare of their clients. They maintain knowledge of current scientific and professional information related to the services they render (APA 1981).

The recommended training for a health psychologist involves predoctoral training in health psychology or a related area, but more importantly, also two years of postdoctoral training in health psychology (Stone 1983). The postdoctoral training should be specific and appropriate experience in service delivery if the trainee plans to be a health service provider, or in health research if the trainee plans to follow a research career. A trainee aiming toward an applied research career should pursue postdoctoral training combining both (Evans and Olbrisch 1983).

These recommendations come from a national training conference in health psychology held in 1983 (Stone 1983). The fully trained health psychologist needs to have as much experience with physically ill patients as the

health service provider psychologist has with mentally ill patients, but because of competing demands in the curriculum cannot be trained as thoroughly as those whose specialties are in dealing with psychopathology. The
internship in health psychology should be composed of assessment and intervention with physically ill patients and of experience with the effects of
physical illness on mental health as well as the reverse. The trainee in health
psychology must be taught to perform differential diagnoses and to recognize what the degree of psychopathology is and whether it requires referral
to a clinical or counseling psychologist, or in the case of a child, to a school
psychologist.

The difference in approach taken by health psychologists and more traditionally trained clinical psychologists is illustrated by the following case.
A 63-year-old, white, female was admitted to a hospital with a myocardial
infarction (MI). Despite direct, repeated information from physicians about
her condition, she insisted she was in the hospital for some digestive difficulty. As a member of a cardiac rehabilitation team, a health psychologist
saw her three times in the coronary care unit and after she had been transferred to the medical ward. She was monitored through her hospitalization
and as an outpatient by the nurse-practitioner member of the team. By the
third meeting as an inpatient, she allowed that, in addition to her digestive
problem, she also had, "You know, with the heart." This woman followed
recommendations regarding diet, exercise, risk factor reduction, and re-
sumption of normal activities well in the hospital and after discharge. Her
denial of the MI continued after discharge, but it did not need to be targeted
to be changed as a treatment goal. A more traditionally trained clinical psychologist might easily have made the error of attempting to change the denial as a treatment goal, or been untrained in dealing with the coronary care
unit (CCU), or been unable to deliver appropriate services in the context of
the team approach. A health psychologist with extensive experience with
cardiac patients was able to assess the denial as the patient's way of adap-
tively reducing anxiety, enabling her to proceed with risk factor reduction
and the return to normal life. This woman was far from psychotic and
seemed to have had no psychological disturbance prior to her MI. Her denial seemed to be purely a consequence of her MI.

A different treatment was required in the case of a 51-year-old, white male
admitted to the same hospital with an MI. The nurse-practitioner who
made the initial contact for the cardiac rehabilitation team noted that the
patient was depressed. A health psychologist saw the patient as an inpatient

and again after discharge. He was much more depressed than the usual post-MI patient. On the third outpatient visit, the patient appeared unshaven and admitted he was drinking a fifth of scotch per day and not taking his cardiac medications. Within several months before this man's MI his third wife had left him and his career had fallen apart. His first wife had attacked him with a knife. His second wife had become severely retarded and psychotic as a result of brain trauma; he was estranged from her and from the children of that marriage and felt considerable guilt related to this. Thus, the depression predated the MI, and the MI may have been partially a consequence of the depression, rather than the more typical course of depression being the usual consequence of an MI. The health psychologist attempted to have the patient admitted to the inpatient psychiatric unit for severe depression, but he refused. The patient was referred to a clinical psychologist for further outpatient care. In this case the extent of psychopathology was beyond that which could be treated within the competence of this health psychologist and the patient was referred.

The question of competence here is one of how much mental health the health psychologist should deal with and how much physical health the clinical, counseling, or school psychologist should deal with. Both types of specialists deal to some extent with both areas, but decisions on who should treat whom are properly decided on the basis of preponderance of physical versus mental problems in the patient, degree of psychopathology and proficiency in the particular techniques most appropriate to that patient. The depression that normally follows an MI might best be treated by a health psychologist with some training in interviewing, assessment, and some counseling, but the psychologist must certainly have extensive training in dealing with cardiac patients.

Such training allows the psychologist to compare the behavior, affect, and responses of the cardiac patient with those of many other cardiac patients. This background could enable the psychologist to assess the patient more quickly and effectively and to determine what about the patient's situation, treatment, and behavioral goals might most realistically be changed and how.

The issue of boundaries of competence becomes especially difficult in specialized interventions such as weight loss and smoking cessation. Health psychologists trained to perform applied research in such areas and with experience working with people would seem well-suited to such interventions. Such psychologists must, however, have experience providing service to people and experience in judging who should be referred, as well as specific competencies in specialized interventions.

Practically, it is impossible for all health psychologists to have these competencies, because education and training in health psychology is too new, and although psychologists have been trained in all the basic areas of psychology, the programs offering training specifically in health psychology have been available for only a few years. Most of the training has occurred on the job.

Many health psychologists today were trained as clinical psychologists. We do not mean to suggest that one cannot have both kinds of training and be competent in both areas. However, the competencies are different, and one need not be a clinical psychologist to be a health psychologist who provides service.

Principle 3   Moral and Legal Standards

Psychologists' moral and ethical standards of behavior are a personal matter to the same degree as they are for any other citizen, except as these may compromise the fulfillment of their professional responsibilities or reduce the public trust in psychology and psychologists. Regarding their own behavior, psychologists are sensitive to prevailing community standards and to the possible impact that conformity to or deviation from these standards may have upon the quality of their performance as psychologists. Psychologists are also aware of the possible impact of their public behavior upon the ability of colleagues to perform their professional duties (APA 1981).

Very relevant to health psychology is the question of cultural chauvinism. Prevailing community standards of what constitutes a healthy lifestyle varies enormously from subculture to subculture, although what constitutes a healthy lifestyle for an individual may be an objective, scientific matter. In the promotion of healthy behaviors, it is tempting to project an approach to health behaviors which is more appropriate to the subculture of the psychologist than to the patient. The health psychologist must be aware that his or her own notions of what is healthy for an upper-middle-class, well-educated American may not be appropriate for everyone. For example, an immigrant Italian-American aged 40 or above from an agricultural background is unlikely to take up jogging as an exercise regimen, regardless of how beneficial it might be. The health psychologist needs to be sensitive to cultural standards and propose regimens which would be more acceptable, such as a walk after dinner. A man on a high potassium diet who eats most meals at MacDonald's may be unwilling to change his diet so much as to cook green, leafy vegetables at home and eat fruit regularly, but he might easily be persuaded to replace some hamburgers with french fries.

Principle 4   Public Statements

Public statements, announcements of services, advertising, and promotional activities of psychologists serve the purpose of helping the public make informed judgments and choices. Psychologists represent accurately and objectively their professional qualifications, affiliations, and functions, as well as those of the institutions or organizations with which they or the statements may be associated. In public statements providing psychological information about the availability of psychological products, publications, and services, psychologists base their statements on scientifically acceptable psychological findings and techniques with full recognition of the limits and uncertainties of such evidence (APA 1981).

Health psychology, as a new and growing field, is especially sensitive to the pitfalls of false or misleading public statements. Health psychology has great potential for reducing risk factors, helping people acquire and maintain healthy behaviors and make optimal adjustments to chronic diseases, improving health, reducing health care costs, etc. However, we must be careful not to promise what we do not know we can deliver. Demonstration of the efficacy of health psychology in specific problems is a matter of painstaking and expensive research. Claims that we have effective treatments in areas where we should be saying we have promising approaches can alienate physicians and endanger support for the proper clinical trials or demonstration and education research.

Health psychologists have some ethical responsibility regarding what appear to be unwarranted claims by nonpsychologists. For example, the advertised claims by hypnotherapists to be able to end smoking in one session are without merit and should be criticized.

Principle 5   Confidentiality

Psychologists have a primary obligation to respect the confidentiality of information obtained from persons in the course of their work as psychologists. They reveal such information to others only with the consent of the person or the person's legal representative, except in those unusual circumstances in which not to do so would result in clear danger to the person or to others. Where appropriate, psychologists inform their clients of the legal limits of confidentiality (APA 1981).

The typical patient of a health psychologist has less of a confidential relationship than does a patient of an individual provider simply because of the setting and maintenance of records. In addition, the patient is most often seen by a team of providers, some of whom may not be able to guarantee privileged communication. All these issues must be explained to the patient. For example, a patient seen by a cardiac rehabilitation team, of which a psychologist is a member will typically have his or her case discussed in the group's meetings. The basic record for the patient may be the hospital chart which has wide access by staff.

The reader may wish to read chapter 7 on the issue of operating in multiprofessional situations and the issue of explicit or implicit conflict between members of a health team.

Principle 6   Welfare of the Consumer

Psychologists respect the integrity and protect the welfare of the people and groups with whom they work. When conflicts of interest arise between clients and psychologists' employing institutions, psychologists clarify the nature and direction of their loyalties and responsibilities and keep all parties informed of their commitments. Psychologists fully inform consumers as to the purpose and nature of an evaluative, treatment, educational, or training procedure, and they freely acknowledge that clients, students, or participants in research have freedom of choice with regard to participation (APA 1981).

Health psychologists are likely to be dealing with patients in precarious health who are at a greater risk of catastrophic events with irreversible consequences. It is the responsibility of the health psychologist to know what the special vulnerabilities are for his or her patients or research subjects and to see that they are adequately protected. "Such vulnerable people can sometimes be damaged by a behavioral situation that superficially appears to be bland. For example, one study has shown that patients in an intensive care unit for myocardial infarctions were five times as likely to suffer fatal fibrillations when grand rounds were in progress than at any other comparable period of time during the day" (Miller 1983).

This puts a responsibility on the health psychologst to know a great deal about the disease(s) he or she is working with and to maintain extensive communications with other relevant professionals: physician, nutritionist, nurse, etc. This is examined more closely in the next section.

Let us explore two particular examples. A cardiac patient who has had an MI and who has a high risk-factor profile (elevated serum cholesterol, cigarette smoking, hypertension, Type A behavior, obesity, and little exercise) needs information on the effects of risk factors and effective strategies to lower as many risk factors as possible. This is true whether or not the patient has been encountered in a service or a research situation. Alternatively, a person who has not had demonstrated cardiac disease, shows only one elevated risk factor, Type A behavior, and is in otherwise good health should not be unduly alarmed by warnings to lower the Type A behavior. Estimates of the prevalence of Type A behavior range up to 75 percent of the population, and the presence of one risk factor for cardiac disease may as much as double risk, but when two or more risk factors are present, their effect on risk is logarithmic, not additive. It may be commendable to reduce Type A behavior, or any other risk factor, but in isolation and without documented disease, there is not much relative risk. These two cases have been chosen to represent extremes, but usually the situations will not be so clear-cut. Here there is no substitute for the health psychologist having had extensive experience with the disease in question and having access to the other professionals involved in the person's care. The health psychologist needs to impress the patient with the gravity of the situation without causing anxiety in excess of the amount needed for change.

Special issues emerge in the ethics involved in invasive treatments. For example, cardiac catheterization is, in many instances, the only diagnostic procedure that can inform the cardiologist, internist, or surgeon of the proper treatment for the patient. It carries a low but real risk of fibrillation and death. Many patients are too afraid of the procedure to undergo it. Designing a program to reduce the patient's excessive fears, without minimizing the real risks, is a problem. It would be easy to produce a videotape modeling patients who have been through the procedure successfully and which would desensitize the patient to the procedure somewhat. However, it is difficult to produce a tape which accurately represents the risks for patients with different educational levels and degrees of understanding of biomedical models.

Special issues may arise in terms of protective welfare of the patient, especially where a different professional may have ultimate control, for example, a physician. If the psychologist and physician disagree as to the course of action which is best for a particular patient, the psychologist may have to clarify the nature and direction of his or her loyalties and responsibilities with the physician, patient, and any institution as well.

Principle 7   Professional Relationships

Psychologists act with due regard for the needs, special competencies, and obligations of their colleagues in psychology and other professions. They re-

spect the prerogatives and obligations of the institutions or organizations with which these other colleagues are associated (APA 1981).

Three issues are important here: adequate communications with physicians and other professionals involved in the patient's care; avoiding practicing medicine without a license; and conflicts with a profession having different ethical guidelines from psychology. Health psychology has enormous involvement with professionals in other disciplines. Issues and settings related to physical health lead to a different range of possibilities and problems from those encountered in other areas of specialization.

COMMUNICATION WITH OTHER PROFESSIONALS

Just as health psychologists are becoming increasingly important to health care, nutritionists, physical therapists, physicians, and other allied professionals each have their own areas of specialization and competence. It is impossible for the health psychologist to have all competencies, but it is essential to be aware of when each one should be called upon. The health psychologist can be very important in designing a nutritional program so as to maximize patient compliance, but the nutritionist is also essential to the design of such a program.

In some cases the collaboration can be so close that two or more professionals always see patients together, as in some diabetes teams. A more typical team may all be involved in patient's care and meet regularly to discuss progress. A psychologist in independent practice might consult with other professionals in the community as appropriate or call the physician responsible for the medical aspects of a patient's care. A psychologist helping a patient quit smoking might call the patient's physician to request that the physician prescribe nicotine chewing gum.

PRACTICING MEDICINE WITHOUT A LICENSE

Having the patient referred by a physician or having the physician perform a physical examination which rules out a physical cause for a problem is highly desirable. Is a psychologist practicing medicine when working with a patient suffering from a chronic illness, such as chronic back pain, and helping to rehabilitate the patient? Medical evaluation and referral avoids this problem, but without it the psychologist is in a gray area.

It is essential to have some collaboration with a physician when dealing with high-risk patients, or in cases where there is any doubt whether the patient is at high risk, whether in a research situation or in treatment. It is important that the physician is knowledgeable enough to decide that what the psychologist is doing is not medically contraindicated. The psychologist must make sure that any medical causes for his patients' or subjects' problems are adequately covered. For example, the health psychologist does not want to have been giving behavioral treatments for headache to someone who has a brain tumor that could have been surgically removed if caught in time. Clinical neuropsychological testing may be important here for diagnosis, and, in fact, the neurologist who does not make use of this may be guilty of malpractice.

The issue of functional versus organic etiology of illness is a potential source of problems. A psychologist who argues that there is a purely psychological cause to a particular set of symptoms may risk having that patient receive no further medical evaluation or treatment when, in fact, a condition such as undiagnosed cancer exists and needs appropriate care. Recurrent, or severe abdominal pain in a woman, for example, should always be examined by an obstetrician-gynecologist, because it could indicate any number of problems which even an internist might not be able to correctly diagnose. Such pains could be psychogenic, but this is a diagnosis of exclusion, even if the patient's psychological condition makes functional etiology likely.

The psychologist must be careful not to promise cure of a condition when self-control procedures are being employed to optimize maintenance of the condition, e.g., diabetes or headache. The patient must be helped to understand his or her responsibility in the treatment. For example, relaxation therapy for hypertension must be performed every day, like taking anti-hypertensive medication, in order to be effective. Performing relaxation for a period of time and then stopping because the hypertension is "cured" is dangerous unless the patient has external verification that the hypertension does not return.

The health psychologist ideally should work well and collaboratively with other professionals but also needs to be wary of the occasional medical chauvinist. Medicine was the first of the professions to organize, license, and legislate. Because of this, the definition of the practice of medicine in statute is so broad as to bear responsibility for all health care. Some physicians view the growth of health psychology and behavioral medicine enviously, and there have been legal attempts to ensure that biofeedback only be administered by physicians. Psychologists should work closely with physicians and other health professionals but not necessarily under their supervision. A further discussion of psychologists avoiding practicing medicine without a license is contained in Knapp and VandeCreek (1981).

CONFLICT WITH THE ETHICS OF OTHER PROFESSIONS

One problem with collaborating closely with other professionals is the difference in the codes of ethics. Psychologists need to be knowledgeable of the differences and aware of how to deal with them.

Principle 8   Assessment Techniques

In the development, publication, and utilization of psychological assessment techniques, psychologists make every effort to promote the welfare and best interests of the client. They guard against the misuse of assessment results. They respect the client's right to know the results, the interpretations made, and the bases for their conclusions and recommendations. Psychologists make every effort to maintain the security of tests and other assessment techniques within limits of legal mandates. They strive to ensure the appropriate use of assessment techniques by others (APA 1981).

Psychological assessment may be used to predict medical outcomes when there may be no relevant differential treatment, and/or treatment is controlled by others. For example, psychological tests may be used in predicting survival time, benefits from cosmetic surgery, or rehabilitation potential. In such cases, the decision of treatment is likely the physician's, and the psychologist is only a consultant.

Principle 9   Research with Human Participants

The decision to undertake research rests upon a considered judgment by the individual psychologist about how best to contribute to psychological science and human welfare. Having made the decision to conduct research, the psychologist considers alternative directions in which research energies and resources might be invested. On the basis of this consideration, the psychologist carries out the investigation with respect and concern for the dignity and welfare of the people who participate and with cognizance of federal and state regulations and professional standards governing the conduct of research with human participants (APA 1981).

A major difference from other psychological practices here has to do with the different implications of physical health findings for participants from the implications of mental health findings. If a patient-participant in a study is at high risk of a disease which is potentially life-threatening, and from which preventive measures can be taken, the responsibility is to inform the patient-participant. As in the example of the person with only one risk factor for heart disease in "Welfare of the Consumer" above, the psychologist also has the responsibility to present a balanced interpretation and not unduly alarm the participant.

The health psychologist also has some responsibility to moderate the stress levels of people he or she is involved in studying. Health psychology research is typically concerned with real and important situations to people, such as their health status. This is quite different from the "psychology of the college sophomore" where situations are more often simulated.

Principle 10   Care and Use of Animals

An investigator of animal behavior strives to advance understanding of basic behavioral principles and/or to contribute to the improvement of human health and welfare. In seeking these ends, the investigator ensures the welfare of animals and treats them humanely. Laws and regulations notwithstanding, an animal's immediate protection depends upon the scientist's own conscience (APA 1981).

The relevance of research results to human welfare may be more demonstrable in the case of health psychology than for other kinds of psychology. Cost / benefit analysis is relatively more advanced in health than in education, for example. How many rat lives equal one human life? Still, researchers must be cautious not to cause needless animal suffering. There may be questions which can only be answered through use of animal models, but this should be done to answer questions which cannot be answered in other ways.

Conclusions

Since health psychology is a new area and one which differs slightly from others within psychology, its practitioners, scientists, and educators have a responsibility to develop and maintain standards of ethics. This should involve at least the following steps: (1) the Division of Health Psychology of the American Psychological Association should develop a casebook of critical incidents that occur in health psychology; (2) the education and training of students in health psychology should involve information and knowledge in ethics as well as mock experience in peer review and in ethics committees; (3) standards should be established for intervening in situations involving possible unethical acts; (4) an ethics committee should be established within the Division of Health Psychology, with responsibility for review of ethics cases, development of educational materials, and dissemination of information about ethics in health psychology.

These and further recommendations for mechanisms for the development and maintaining of standards of ethics in health psychology are detailed in Hall (1983) and Hall and Swencionis (1983).

Summary

This chapter has focused on some of the features of health psychology which make it somewhat different from other areas of psychology. The principles which determine ethics in health psychology are the same as those which determine ethics for other areas of psychology, but the object of application, physical health, implies some differences from dealing with more traditional areas of concern of psychology.

REFERENCES

American Psychological Association. 1981. Ethical principles of psychologists. *American Psychologist* 36 (no. 6): 633–38.

Evans, Richard I., and Mary Ellen Olbrisch. 1983. Task Group on Applied Research. The Report of the National Working Conference on Education and Training in Health Psychology. In *Health Psychology* 2(5): 71–73, supplement section edited by George C. Stone.

Hall, Judy E. 1983. Ethics in the education and training of health psychologists. In *Sourcebook in Health Psychology*, edited by C. Belar and C. Swencionis for the National Working Conference on Education and Training in Health Psychology, Arden House, Harriman, New York, 23–27 May.

Hall, Judy E., and C. Swencionis. 1983. Task Group on Ethical Concerns. The Report of the National Working Conference on Education and Training in Health Psychology. In *Health Psychology* 2(5): 96–97, supplement section edited by George C. Stone.

Knapp, S., and L. VandeCreek. 1981. Behavioral medicine: Its malpractice risks for psychologists. *Professional Psychology* 12(6): 677–83.

Miller, Neal E. 1983. Some main themes and highlights of the conference. The Report of the National Working Conference on Education and Training in Health Psychology. In *Health Psychology* 2(5): 12, supplement edited by George C. Stone.

Stone, George C., ed. 1983. The Report of the National Working Conference on Education and Training in Health Psychology. *Health Psychology* 2(5): 1–153, supplement section.

16

An Overview of Health Psychology and the Law

Robinsue Frohboese and Thomas D. Overcast

The legal system is a critical factor affecting the nature and scope of activities in which health psychologists are engaged. Recognizing the legal system's pervasive influence on health psychology, conferees at the 1983 National Working Conference on Education and Training in Health Psychology recommended that instruction about legal issues be included at all levels of training of health psychologists (Task Force on Legal Issues 1983). Yet, despite the recognized importance of knowledge about the legal system's interaction with and impact on health psychology, no comprehensive analysis addressing these issues has been published to date. This chapter is a first effort to respond to the legal informational needs of health psychologists by presenting a broad overview of the legal system and relevant legal issues.

Overview of the Legal System

In order to understand how legal issues relate to and affect the activities of health psychologists, it is first important to understand how the legal system is structured and to have some knowledge of the elements of that system. For purposes of this chapter, the terms "law" and the "legal system" refer to statutes, administrative regulations and case law, and those branches of government that can generate them. Statutes are those pieces of law enacted by Congress and state legislatures. Administrative regulations are those rules promulgated by federal and state administrative agencies to interpret and implement their enabling statutes. Case law or common law consists of decisions about particular legal questions rendered by federal and state courts.

The courts serve as the ultimate legal authority on particular issues. Within both federal and state judicial systems there are trial courts, courts

The opinions stated herein reflect those of the authors and not necessarily those of the Department of Justice.

of appeal, and ultimately a supreme court. A host of complex rules dictates whether the contended issue is one that is appropriate for the federal or state court system. The precedential value of a case law decision may depend upon how widely accepted that decision is within the group of fifty states and among the various federal judicial districts. Thus, a decision rendered by a state court in Washington may not be followed in the state of Maryland. Similarly, a decision rendered by a federal court in San Francisco may not be followed by a federal court in Atlanta.

Given the complexity of the legal system and its dynamic nature, an answer to the question "what is the law of x?" or "is it legal to do y?" must always be accompanied by applicable qualifications. Even in situations where the Supreme Court of the United States has ruled definitively on a particular issue, the ruling oftentimes is limited to a very specific fact situation and therefore will only be binding upon precisely analagous circumstances.

Access to Legal Information

In order to function effectively in health psychology settings, pervaded as they are by legal influences, it is important for health psychologists to have both an understanding of legal information and some access to it. There are two primary means of access to needed legal information. The first is through a law library associated with a law school or perhaps with a city or county courthouse. Some rudimentary instruction in the use of the law library can be provided by law librarians and will permit health psychologists access to the most important sources of legal information, i.e., statutes, administrative regulations, case law, and law review articles. Although health psychologists should not rely on their own interpretations of these sources of information to make legal judgments, an understanding of the information they contain can heighten sensitivity to legal issues.

The second major avenue of access to legal information is through the services of an attorney who will be able to provide more definitive guidance and direction with regard to particular legal questions. Normally, however, the lawyer in general practice will only be minimally familiar with the scientific and/or professional interests that the health psychologist brings to the relationship. Thus, the lawyer will be able to perform his or her services more effectively to the extent that the health psychologist has a basic understanding of the legal system and legal issues and is able to frame a particular question narrowly.

Range of Legal Considerations

Given the complex myriad of state and federal case law, legislation and regulations that potentially bear upon the work of health psychologists and the range of activities in which health psychologists are engaged, it is impossible to delineate legal guidelines that are applicable to every health psychologist in every situation. Whether or not a legal issue is germane is always dependent on the specific and individual fact situations. Some of the relevant legal issues vary depending upon the state and setting (such as hospital, institution, university, or private practice) in which the health psychologist is engaged in activities. Other legal issues are dependent upon such factors as source of funding, nature of activities, and types of clients or subjects. The relevance of still other legal issues has yet to surface given the recent emergence of health psychology as a discipline and profession. Thus, the intent of this section is not to delineate all of the nuances of relevant law but rather to increase health psychologists' awareness, understanding, and appreciation of the laws bearing on their activities.

This section highlights the range of major legal considerations that could potentially impact upon the health psychologist depending upon the circumstances surrounding his or her activities. The breadth of material that could be covered prohibits delving into detail about the various topics outlined below. Where appropriate, sources have been cited that provide more detailed analyses. The reader is urged to consult all of the sources cited in each subsection for more information relevant to any particular topic.

Legal Standards of Professional Conduct
Duties Imposed by the Government

All professional activities carry the duty of acting in a legally appropriate and responsible fashion. Some of the duties of professional conduct are imposed by the government's legitimate interest in regulating the conduct of professionals. For example, the government has the right to set minimal competency standards for professional activities and to require licensing or certification prior to engaging in activities (Overcast, Sales, and Pollard 1982; Herbsleb, Sales, and Overcast 1985). Thus, the practice of psychology is regulated by law in every jurisdiction. Where it is providing funding for the activities, the government also has the right to impose standards and procedures regulating use of the money and to monitor activities to ensure compliance. In the case of the health psychologist researcher, this may mean that legal limitations are placed on the methods of experimentation and research design as well as the subject matter of research. For the health psychologist service provider, this may mean that limitations are placed on the mode of service delivery or the types of services that are permissible.

Duties Imposed by Professional Relationships

Professional standards. The duties of professional conduct are also determined and imposed by rights that clients and subjects have upon entering into a professional relationship with the health psychologist. When an individual holds himself or herself out to the public as a professional, the recipient of the professional activities has the right to expect that the professional possesses adequate training and skills to perform the responsibilities required by the professional activities and carries out those responsibilities according to the common practices and recognized standards of the profession. Where these standards are not met and injury is caused as a result of breach of the standards, the injured party has a right to bring legal action for malpractice based on the legal theory of negligence (Gable 1983).

These principles are applicable to the activities of the health psychologist. At this juncture, however, the specific standards to which health psychologists are held in their professional relationships with clients, subjects, and consumers are not readily identifiable because of the embryonic nature of health psychology as a profession. As the practices of health psychology become more widespread and better defined, the standards will become clearer and more firmly established (Overcast, Merrikin, and Evans 1985). Precisely what constitutes breach of the standards of professional conduct among health psychologists is, however, a question that can ultimately only be answered on a case-by-case basis (DeLeon and Borreliz 1978). It is an issue, for instance, in an $80 million lawsuit brought against two psychologist researchers by subjects involved in the researchers' efforts to study the effect of teaching alcoholics to drink in a "controlled fashion." The subjects claim that their conditions worsened significantly as a result of the psychologists' failure to meet minimal professional standards in carrying out the study ("Controlled Drinkers" 1983).

In order to prevail in an action for malpractice, an injury must occur as a result of the breach of professional standards. The nature of the harm that must be suffered to rise to the level of a recognizable injury is also an evolving area of the law. In a recent controversial case, a California Court of Appeals expanded the concept of injury to include the emotional distress suffered by parents when a psychologist misdiagnosed their son as having nonpsychotic brain syndrome in an attempt to ensure medical insurance reimbursement (Galante 1984). The Court of Appeals held that the parents' reaction to the diagnosis was foreseeable and the psychologist's actions therefore constituted negligent infliction of emotional distress.

Affirmative duties. In addition to the responsibility of meeting professional standards, the health psychologist may owe certain affirmative duties to clients and subjects prior to, during, and after service delivery and experimentation. To begin with, legal considerations may enter into the process of selecting clients or subjects. There are certain circumstances where the health psychologist may have a duty not to discriminate in client and subject selection. This is particularly true where the service or research may be classified as therapeutic rather than experimental and where potential clients or subjects fall within a legally protected group of persons, such as the disabled or elderly (Merrikin and Overcast 1985a). In these situations, constitutional considerations of procedural and substantive due process, equal protection, and federal and state statutes and regulations, such as the Age Discrimination Act and Section 504 of the Rehabilitation Act, may require that certain individuals not be overlooked in the selection process merely because of their status. The reverse is true, however, where the research or service may be classified as experimental rather than therapeutic. In these situations, care needs to be taken that individuals in a protected class (such as minors, incompetent adults, prisoners, institutionalized persons, disabled persons, or fetuses) are not targeted for experimentation merely because of their status (Levy 1983). This is particularly the case where the experimentation or service is considered to be intrusive or involves deprivation (Kassirer 1974; Martin 1975).

Whenever the activities of the health psychologist impact on the physical or mental functions of individuals, fundamental constitutional issues are involved (Merrikin and Overcast 1985b). All individuals have the right to privacy, personal autonomy, and self-determination, including the right to control their body and mind and to protect their body and mind from unwarranted invasions. These rights have been viewed as sacred by courts and have been construed broadly to encompass situations involving any type of behavior modification and therapy as well as physical intrusions (Wexler 1983). These rights are not violated, however, where the potential "intrusion" into body or mind is consensual. In most circumstances, therefore, health psychologists also have an affirmative duty to obtain informed consent from their clients or subjects prior to providing a service or conducting research. This normally entails ensuring that the client or subject has the capacity to consent, is provided with sufficient facts about the service or research to make an informed judgment about assent, is enabled to make the judgment free from any duress, and is advised of the right to terminate the service or research at any time desired (Herr, Arons, and Wallace 1983, chap. 3). Special protections and accommodations must be made if the client or subject is a minor, incompetent adult, mentally or developmentally disabled person, prisoner, or fetus to ensure that the elements of consent are met or, where necessary, substituted consent is legally provided (Turnbull 1977; Overcast, Sales, and Kesler 1983).

The duties owed to clients or subjects often also include those relating to information collection, management, confidentiality and disclosure. To begin with, the health psychologist may have legal obligations to ascertain certain types of information and to maintain various types of records. For example, federal and state laws and regulations as well as institutional policies may dictate the nature of records that must be kept prior to, during, and after service delivery or experimentation. The health psychologist may be legally obligated to keep such records or information confidential (Siegel 1979). This obligation, as that of informed consent, is premised on constitutional protections of privacy (Herr, Arons, and Wallace 1983, chap. 7). Record-keeping may also, however, raise legal issues of ownership and access. These legal considerations may impose upon the health psychologist an affirmative obligation to turn records over to the client or subject or to disclose information about diagnostic and testing results or research findings. Clients and subjects may also have rights to access information under federal or state Freedom of Information Acts (Morris, Sales, and Berman 1981). It is thus important for health psychologists to understand their obligations to protect information as well as the circumstances under which information can and must be divulged.

Finally, it is also possible that the nature of the relationship between the health psychologist and client or subject may require a referral of the client or subject to a physician or other health professional for health problems discovered during the course of providing services or conducting research. For example, the health psychologist conducting alcoholism or drug abuse treatment, smoking cessation, weight loss, or pain reduction programs may have a legal responsibility to refer the client to a physician for organic conditions of which the health psychologist is aware or suspects, or for medical complications that might stem from the program.

Duties Owed to Others

In addition to the legal duties owed to clients and subjects, the health psychologist may have legal responsibilities to other persons. At times these responsibilities can pose conflicts with those owed to the client or subject. This is particularly true in situations where ethical and legal responsibilities of maintaining confidentiality conflict with the duty to disclose to third parties records or information within the health psychologist's control and/or knowledge. Perhaps the best known and most troublesome example of this is the duty to warn others in situations where the client poses a threat to others (Brief of *Amici Curiae* 1986; Givelber, Bowers, and Blitch 1985). This legal responsibility, first established by the *Tarasoff* (1976) case that required a duty to warn identifiable victims, was recently expanded to include any forseeable victims by the California Appeals Court (*Hedlund v. Superior Court* 1983).

Equally troublesome in terms of weighing considerations of confidentiality are those state statutes that require the health psychologist to take initiatives to report information to authorities in cases of child abuse, spouse abuse, contagious diseases, and health hazards in industrial/organizational settings. Similarly, conflicts with confidentiality may arise from court-ordered searches, seizures, subpoenas of records, or requests for information within the control of the health psychologist (DeKraai and Sales 1982; DeKraai and Sales 1985). For example, a psychologist in Alaska was recently involved in a lengthy court battle because of his refusal to reveal confidential communications disclosed during court-compelled therapy with an alleged child abuser and his family. The case was finally resolved when the Alaska Court of Appeals decided that the state's psychotherapist-patient privilege protected the psychologist's duty not to disclose the communications (Brief for Amici Curiae 1983). Finally, conflicts with confidentiality may arise by virtue of the employment setting. For instance, the health psychologist operating a drug or alcohol rehabilitation program within a corporation by which he or she is employed may face conflicts as to whom primary responsibility is owed in the face of a corporate demand for confidential information.

Legal Considerations in Animal Experimentation

As illustrated by the much publicized case of psychologist Edward Taub (whose National Institutes of Health funding was revoked for failure to comply with NIH standards for animal use and care and against whom legal action was taken for alleged cruelty to animals), legal considerations are also critically important in the health psychologist's research with animal subjects (Chambers and Hines 1983). Most states have statutes prohibiting cruelty to animals and regulating their sale (although these statutes generally do not place legal restrictions on the use and treatment of animals during experimentation). The federal government has also placed legislative and regulatory restrictions on animal research in federally supported research institutions and facilities (U.S. Department of Health and Human Services 1985). For instance, the animal Welfare Act, which is currently the source of heated debates in the United States Congress (Griffin and Sechzer 1983), mandates stringent reporting requirements and compliance with Department of Agriculture standards designed to ensure humane treatment of certain warm-blooded research animals.

LEGAL CONTROL OF INSTRUMENTS AND DEVICES

Health psychologists who develop new and innovative research or treatment techniques may face legal considerations regarding copyrights and trademarks to protect ownership of their ideas, instruments, and products. Where the health psychologist is involved in the design, manufacturing, or marketing of a product, knowledge of the law related to products liability may also be important. The applicable legal doctrine generally requires that products be produced that are fit for their intended use, bear appropriate warnings about their use, be free from defects, and not result in unreasonable danger to potential users and others.

Additional care needs to be taken by health psychologists to ensure that it is legally permissible to use certain devices in their activities (Schwitzgebel 1977). For instance, the Food and Drug Administration has developed stringent regulations regarding medical devices, including review prior to their use in research and the necessity for physician consultation if they are used for treatment of a disease. Ironically, the Food and Drug Administration has classified "medical" as including such things as biofeedback devices, galvanic skin response measurement devices, conditioning devices that use an electrical stimulus, and even "enuresis treatment devices of the bed-and-blanket variety" (Schwitzgebel 1978, p. 481)—all of which were first conceived of by psychologists.

LEGAL LIMITATIONS ON TYPES OF ACTIVITIES

Health psychologists also face important legal considerations in deciding upon the nature of their activities. Great care needs to be taken, for example, that the activities do not constitute the practice of medicine without a license, which is a criminal offense in all states. Unfortunately, precisely what is encompassed under the rubric of practicing medicine is not always apparent. In addition to clear medical practices, such as performing surgery and prescribing medication, such practices as diagnosing diseases or encouraging a patient to withdraw from or refuse standard medical treatment could potentially be considered practicing medicine (Knapp and VandeCreek 1981).

As health psychologists continue to grow in number and expertise and gain important recognition, such as being given hospital staff privileges (Bersoff 1983) and being recognized as health providers in federal programs (Dorken 1979; DeLeon, VandenBos, and Kraut 1984), state insurance plans, and by private accreditation agencies, delineation of permissible activities will become clearer and could be expanded. The courts may also have a role to play in this regard. For example, in a case in which the American Psychological Association submitted an *amicus* brief, the United States Supreme Court has ruled that states cannot constitutionally preclude abortion counseling by nonphysicians (*City of Akron v. Akron Center for Reproductive Health, Inc.* 1983).

LEGAL ISSUES RELATING TO PRACTICE MANAGEMENT AND REIMBURSEMENT

An awareness of the legal issues relating to practice management can expand the health psychologist's professional opportunities and enhance his or her economic viability. For example, it is important for the health psychologist to be aware of the legal considerations involved in applying for and administering federal and state grants. In light of recent changes in the form and substance of the health care delivery system, particularly those relating to application of the antitrust laws to the health professions (Overcast, Sales, and Pollard 1982), it is also important to understand legal issues relating to alternatives to the traditional sole practitioner model of professional practice, such as: forming professional corporations (Overcast and Sales 1981); partnerships; multidisciplinary practices; health maintenance organizations; or other innovative forms of business organization.

An equally important and integral part of the health psychologist's professional opportunities and survival as a viable economic unit is an understanding of the reimbursement and financial incentive mechanisms that are tied to the health psychologist's services, such as: private insurance reimbursement, Medicare, state Medicaid plans, CHAMPUS (Civilian Health and Medical Program of the Uniform Services) programs, Veterans Administration programs, and tax deductions and tax disincentives for psychological services (DeLeon, VandenBos, and Kraut 1984).

Roles for Health Psychologists in the Legal System

Apart from the constraints that the legal system places on the activities of health psychologists, it offers many opportunities for their input and involvement. To begin with, health psychologists may conduct evaluations or assessments on behalf of the prosecution or defense for use in a civil or criminal case or an administrative proceeding. For example, a health psychologist may conduct an evaluation to determine whether a plaintiff in an automobile accident case is malingering. Similarly, the health psychologist could be involved in assessments for purposes of determining eligibility for federal or state benefits, such as vocational rehabilitation, social security disability insurance, or worker's compensation (Merrikin, Overcast, and Sales 1982; Sales, Overcast, and Merrikin 1983). Health psychologists may also prepare expert reports and/or serve as expert witnesses in court cases or at administrative hearings by providing expert opinions on contended issues (Motion for Leave to File Brief of *Amici Curiae* 1986). In addition, health psychologists may be involved in the legal system by providing services to a client pursuant to the order of a court or administrative tribunal. Finally, there are numerous opportunities for health psychologists to contribute their procedural and substantive knowledge to the important policy decisions that enter into the drafting of federal and state legislation, administrative regulations, plans and procedures (DeLeon, Frohboese, and Meyer 1984).

Conclusion

As health psychologists become better versed in legal issues and more aware of how the legal system affects their activities, they will be able to fulfill their responsibilities in a more effective and legally responsible fashion by being more sensitive to the legal rights of their clients, subjects, and consumers. In addition, they will be able to identify and avoid potential legal problems, thus protecting themselves from civil or criminal liability. Finally, health psychologists will be in a better position to expand their areas of involvement with the legal system and potentially have an impact on the future direction of the system as it pertains to their activities.

REFERENCES

Bersoff, D. 1983. Hospital privileges and the antitrust laws. *American Psychologist* 38: 1238–42.

Brief for Amici Curiae. 1983. *American Psychological Association and Alaska Psychological Association, State of Alaska v. R. H. and Mitchell H. Wetherhorn,* On a Petition for Review from the Superior Court of the Third Judicial District, October 17. Alaska Court of Appeals No. 7768.

Brief for Amici Curiae. 1986. American Psychological Association, Michigan Psychological Association and Michigan Psychiatric Society in Support of Defendant-Appellant. *Davis v. Yong-Oh Lihm.* Michigan Supreme Court No. 77726.

Chambers, K. T., and C. Hines. 1983. Recent developments concerning the use of animals in medical research. *The Journal of Legal Medicine* 4:109–29.

City of Akron v. Akron Center for Reproductive Health, Inc., 103 S.Ct. 2481 (1983).

"Controlled Drinkers" sue Sobells. 1983. *APA Monitor,* September, 3.

DeKraai, M. B., and B. D. Sales. 1982. Privileged communications of psychologists. *Professional Psychology* 13:372–88.

———. 1985. Confidential communications of psychotherapists. *Psychotherapy: Theory, Research and Practice* 21:293–318.

DeLeon, P. H., and M. Borreliz. 1978. Malpractice: Professional liability and the law. *Professional Psychology* 9:467–77.

DeLeon, P. H., R. Frohboese, and J. C. Meyers. 1984. The psychologist on Capitol Hill: A unique use of the skills of the scientist/practitioner. *Professional Psychology* 15:697–705.

DeLeon, P. H., G. R. VandenBos, and A. G. Kraut. 1984. Federal legislation recognizing psychology. *American Psychologist* 39:933–46.

Dorken, H. 1979. The forum. *Professional Psychology* 10:1–2.

Gable, K. 1983. Malpractice law. In *The professional psychologist's handbook,* edited by B. Sales. New York: Plenum.

Galante, N. A. 1984. Parents can sue for shock on child's misdiagnosis. *The National Law Journal* (August 13): 5, 19.

Givelber, D. J., W. J. Bowers, and C. L. Blitch. 1985. The Tarasoff controversy: A summary of findings from an empirical study of legal, ethical, and clinical issues. Washington, D.C.: United States Department of Health and Human Services, National Institute of Mental Health, Center for Studies of Antisocial and Violent Behavior.

Griffin, A., and J. A. Sechzer. 1983. Mandatory versus voluntary regulation of biomedical research. In *The role of animals in biomedical research* (vol. 406), edited by J. A. Sechzer, Annals of the New York Academy of Sciences. New York: The New York Academy of Sciences.

Hedlund v. Superior Court, 669 P.2d 41 (Cal. Sup. Ct. 1983).

Herbsleb, J., B. D. Sales, and T. D. Overcast. 1985. Challenging licensure and certification. *American Psychologist* 40:1165–78.

Herr, S. S., S. Arons, and R. E. Wallace. 1983. *Legal rights of mental health care.* Lexington, MA: Lexington Books.

Kassirer, L. B. 1974. Behavior modification for patients and prisoners: Constitutional ramifications of enforced therapy. *The Journal of Psychiatry and Law* 2:303–18.

Knapp, S., and L. VandeCreek. 1981. Behavioral medicine: Its malpractice risks for psychologists. *Professional Psychology* 37:517–25.

Levy, C. L. 1983. *The human body and the law: Legal and ethical considerations in human experimentation.* 2d ed. New York: Oceana Publications, Inc.

Martin, R. 1975. *Legal challenges to behavior modification.* Champaign, IL: Research Press.

Merrikin, K. J., and T. D. Overcast. 1985a. Patient selection for heart transplantation: When is a discriminating choice discrimination? *Journal of Health Politics, Policy, and Law* 10:7–32.

———. 1985b. Governmental regulation of heart transplantation and the right to privacy. *Journal of Contemporary Law* 11:481–514.

Merrikin, K. J., T. D. Overcast, and B. D. Sales. 1982. Worker's compensation law and the compensability of mental injuries. *Health Psychology* 1:373–87.

Morris, R., B. D. Sales, and J. Berman. 1981. Research and the freedom of information act. *American Psychologist* 36:819–26.

Motion for Leave to File Brief of Amici Curiae and Brief of American Psychological Association and North Carolina Psychological Association as *Amici Curiae* in Support of Appellant. 1986. *Horne v. Goodson Logging Co. & Self-Insured* N.C. App. Docket No. I-1608.

Overcast, T. D., K. J. Merrikin, and R. W. Evans. 1985. Malpractice issues in heart transplantation. *American Journal of Law and Medicine* 10:363–95.

Overcast, T. D., and B. D. Sales. 1981. Psychological and multidisciplinary corporations. *Professional Psychology* 12:749–60.

Overcast, T. D., B. D. Sales, and J. A. Kesler. 1983. Psychological evaluation of children at the request of noncustodial parents. *Psychotherapists in Private Practice* 1:65–74.

Overcast, T. D., B. D. Sales, and M. Pollard. 1982. Applying antitrust laws to the professions: Implications for psychology. *American Psychologist* 37:517–25.

Sales, B. D., T. D. Overcast, and K. J. Merrikin. 1983. Worker's compensation protection for assaults and batteries on mental health professionals. In *Assaults within psychiatric facilities,* edited by R. Lion and W. H. Reid. New York: Grune & Stratton.

Schwitzgebel, R. K. 1977. Federal regulation of psychological devices: An example of medical-political drift. In *Psychology in the legal process,* edited by B. D. Sales. New York: Spectrum.

———. 1978. Suggestions for the use of psychological devices in accord with legal and ethical standards. *Professional Psychology* 9:478–88.

Siegel, M. 1979. Privacy, ethics, and confidentiality. *Professional Psychology* 10:249–58.

Tarasoff v. Board of Regents of University of California, 118 Cal. Rptr. 129, 520 P.2d 533 (1974); Aff'd, 551 P.2d 334, 131 Cal. Rptr. 14 (1976).

Task Force on Legal Issues. 1983. The Report of the National Working Conference on Education and Training in Health Psychology. In *Health Psychology* 2(5): 98–102, supplement section edited by George C. Stone.

Turnbull, H. R., ed. 1977. *Consent handbook*. Washington, D.C.: American Association on Mental Deficiency.

United States Department of Health and Human Services. 1985. *National Institutes of Health guide for grants and contracts*. Volume 14, no. 8 (June 25). Special Edition. Laboratory Animal Welfare, 1–30.

Wexler, D. B. 1983. The structure of civil commitment: Patterns, pressures, and interactions in mental health legislation. *Law and Human Behavior* 7:1–18.

17

Employment Options for Health Psychologists

David G. Altman and Jerry Cahn

"Weeds spring up and thrive; but to get wheat, how much toil we must endure!"

(Midrash: Genesis Rabbah).

Introduction

Many students and professionals are intrigued by a career in health psychology. Before commiting to this career track, they should have a good sense of the job market and carefully consider what this commitment entails. What types of jobs and job settings now exist? What will exist in the future? What are the benefits and drawbacks of a career in health psychology? What skills and experiences are important? Will a career in health psychology provide personal and financial satisfaction? The purpose of this chapter is to provide an overview of the manifest and latent health psychology job market and to identify some of the issues a health psychologist-to-be should consider.

Today, the "health industry" is a major force in the American economy. In the past several decades, new health programs (e.g., Medicaid and Medicare) and new health providers (e.g., Health Maintenance Organizations, home health care) have come into existence and new technologies have been created to provide better care (e.g., the CAT Scan). Importantly, these forces and others (e.g., increased access to care, increased insurance coverage, and increased labor costs) have led health costs to skyrocket and outstrip even the double digit inflation of the 1970s. By 1983, almost $300 billion, or eleven percent of the U.S. Gross National Product was spent on health care. This escalation of costs in turn generated new forms of providers designed to reduce the costs of care (e.g., Preferred Provider Organizations, emergency care centers) and new government programs to control health costs (e.g., prospective reimbursement). In addition, major corporations (e.g., AT&T, Hewlett-Packard, and Aetna) that traditionally were not involved in the health care decision making of their employees have launched internal and cooperative programs to control health costs (Wolfson and Levin 1985).

As the "health industry" grows and takes new forms, the opportunities for professionals concerned with health issues also will grow. There are many professional groups, however, competing for the same jobs. They include public health administrators, medical sociologists, physicians, nurses, health educators, lawyers, hospital administrators, and psychologists. Health psychologists have the skills to function in a variety of settings (Altman and Cahn 1983) but having health psychology skills is not enough. Often, those obtaining employment are the ones who creatively define the job tasks and demonstrate that their skills and orientation can make a meaningful contribution. Belonging to a professional group which already has demonstrated its capacity to contribute makes this task easier. Since health psychologists are relative newcomers to the health field, many of the jobs they will find are not going to be advertised in job listings; rather they will be created. To be successful in the job market of the 1980s, health psychologists should have sound research and applied skills, a sense of adventure, an ability to accept uncertainty, and an educated understanding of the job market. Accordingly, this chapter focuses not only on what jobs now exist and could exist in the future but also on issues to consider in helping create the job market for health psychologists.

To put the current and future health psychology job market in perspective, it is useful to examine employment trends of psychologists. Unfortunately, at the time of this writing there are few data on the employment of health psychologists. As the field develops, data should become more readily available. As a result, gaining a perspective on employment options for health psychologists requires examining the job market for psychologists in general and extrapolating the data to health psychology.

Employment of Psychologists

As of 1981, there were 47,400 doctoral-level psychologists in the U.S. comprising 13.2 percent of the total population of doctoral scientists and engineers (National Research Council 1982). The social sciences are expected to grow more slowly than in the past due to the smaller pool of potential graduate enrollees (National Science Foundation 1979). There are data indicating that fewer psychologists will enter the job market in the future (Stapp and Fulcher 1983a). Along these lines, Stoup and Benjamin (1982) report that applications to psychology graduate programs have dropped from an average of 106 per program in 1973 to 85 per program in 1979.

As of 1981 (and excluding postdoctoral fellows, people unemployed, or people not reporting employment status), psychologists were employed in a variety of *settings* including educational institutions (50%), business/industry (24%), hospitals/clinics (14%), government (8%), and nonprofit organizations (4%) (National Research Council 1982). The primary *work activity* of these psychologists was consulting or professional service (38%), teaching (28%), management or administration (15%), research and development (14%), and other (5%). The 1975–80 graduates, compared to earlier cohorts, tend to be teaching less and consulting or providing professional services more (National Research Council 1982). Of the 1975–80 graduates, 2.5 percent were unemployed (with 1.4 percent seeking employment), 5 percent had postdoctoral appointments, 7 percent were employed part-time and 85 percent were employed full-time (National Research Council 1982).

Fulcher and Stapp (1982) report data on the status of 1981 doctoral recipients in psychology. They found that 79 percent were employed full-time, 8 percent employed part-time, 10 percent were postdoctoral fellows, and 1.5 percent were unemployed and seeking employment. The primary employment settings for these psychologists were academia (31%), hospitals or clinics (31%), business/government (17%), schools and other educational settings (8%), other human service settings (9%), and independent practice (4%).

A survey of APA members suggests that most members are employed full-time, consistent with findings from earlier surveys (Stapp and Fulcher 1983a). However, there have been changes in employment settings: since 1976, employment in university settings has declined, and employment in independent practice, government, business, and hospitals has increased. Interestingly, the percentage of *new* doctoral psychologists employed in university settings dropped from 33 percent in 1975 to 18 percent in 1980.

In terms of salaries, the median annual salary for the positions occupied by psychologists (National Research Council 1982) varied as follows: state or local government ($27,900); educational institutions ($29,000); hospitals or clinics ($30,100); nonprofit organizations ($30,500); and business/industry ($40,300). A survey of approximately 11,000 American Psychological Association members (Staff and Fulcher 1983b) indicates that the mean annual salary for psychology professors (based on the 1983 academic year) was $22,685 for assistant professors, $28,077 for associate professors, and $37,492 for full professors.

Employment of Health Psychologists

In recent years, greater numbers of APA members appear to be locating employment in health-related settings (Stapp and Fulcher 1983a). In 1979, Adler, Cohen, and Stone estimated the number of existing and potential positions in health psychology. At that time, they estimated that there were approximately 2,000 employed health psychologists. They predicted that over the next ten years, 2,400 new jobs in health psychology (or 200 per year) would appear. These data are conservative and do not reflect the current burgeoning interest in health psychology. Inevitably, this number could be much higher if the growth of direct service delivery positions and new employment settings were taken into account.

A survey of APA Division 38 members is useful in assessing what health psychologists are doing (Morrow, Carpenter, and Clayman 1983). Among the principal work settings for members are universities or colleges (28%), medical centers (25%), and private practice (20%). The professional activities of these psychologists, expressed in median percent time of involvement, included therapy (25%), research (15%), administration (10%), formal teaching (9%), and psychodiagnosis (9%).

Since June 1979, health psychology job announcements in the *APA Monitor* have been followed (Grzesiak 1984). In the period from July 1982 to June 1983, 330 health-related positions were advertised. Geographically, California and New York advertised the most positions. Hospitals/clinics, colleges/universities, and medical schools (in that order) were the most frequent employers of health psychologists. Of the jobs advertised during this period, 47 percent were clinical, 26 percent research, 1 percent administrative, and 26 percent a combination of the three types. These 330 jobs also were classified by position description area with the most frequent being neuropsychology/neuroscience (24%), health psychology (20%), behavioral medicine (16%), rehabilitation psychology (14%), and pediatric psychology (11%). Noticeably absent from this list are positions in the social, community, and health policy areas.

Job Qualifications for Health Psychologists

While health psychologists have been accepted in many university settings, the data illustrate that they have not been widely integrated into other job settings. Although other settings exist, the burden of obtaining employment in these settings typically rests on the shoulders of the health psychologist.

Obtaining positions in the full range of settings requires having the basic skills expected, being able to effectively communicate ones' capabilities, and having some experience demonstrating the application of these skills. At the National Working Conference on Education and Training in Health Psychology (Stone 1983), some of these basic skills were delineated as follows: posing questions and formulating hypotheses, use of various research methodologies, data analysis, written and oral communication skills, understanding the roles, values, and vocabularies of other health professionals, understanding the social-ecological context of the health system, and clinical or service delivery skills.

APPRENTICESHIPS

Depending on the particular job, additional skills are needed, as subsequent sections in this chapter illustrate. While some of these will be obtained in the classroom, many can only be obtained through an apprenticeship. The National Working Conference recognized that apprenticeships for health psychologists are essential to acquiring setting-specific skills and practical experiences not normally learned in the classroom (cf. Edwards and Holmgren 1979; Carroll, Werner, and Ashmore 1982; and chapter 24 in this volume). Indeed, health psychologists were encouraged to facilitate such opportunities for new students by offering internships whenever possible and by encouraging other professionals who could offer such positions to do so. Due to the newness of the discipline, students (and their faculty mentors) should expect to work just as hard on creating new apprenticeship positions as they will have to work on creating new job opportunities. Throughout the various health psychology employment settings, a number of excellent apprenticeship opportunities either now exist or could exist if students and faculty worked toward developing appropriate contacts.

In a survey of applied social psychology researchers and potential employers of applied psychologists about the skills needed to function as applied psychologists (Edwards and Holmgren 1979), the most important skills mentioned were the ability to communicate, interview, conduct impact evaluations, plan human resources, and utilize statistics. Obtaining relevant work experiences as well as a detailed knowledge of a specialized substantive area also were deemed critical. These findings suggest that to be successful, health psychologists interested in applied jobs must have knowledge of substantive and methodological issues and be proficient in written and oral communication.

OPPORTUNITIES IN ACADEMIA

Future employment opportunities for academic psychologists are somewhat discouraging. While health psychologists are marketable because of their ability to serve in medical, dental, and public health academic settings, there still is reason to be concerned about an undersupply of (or over-demand for) such positions. At this young stage in the development of health psychology, it is difficult to predict just how academic departments will accept health psychology. One hopes that the burgeoning academic intrigue with health psychology is more reflective of the sincere interest and dedication to the field than to what happens to be "in" or "faddish" at the time due to the availability of funds or to the glamour of conducting such research.

Regarding health psychologists in medical schools, Matarazzo, Carmody, and Gentry (1981) noted the large number of psychiatrists holding academic appointments in U.S. medical schools (2,336 in 1976). Similarly, Schneider (1980) noted the substantial rise in medical school and teaching hospital research positions from 1968 and 1978. In a survey of deans and psychologists in schools of public health, Matthews and Avis (1982) reported that psychologists accounted for just 5.7 percent of the full-time faculty. In some areas of health psychology, particularly those with a clinical orientation, academic jobs are relatively common (see Grzesiak 1984). Students pursuing academic careers are well advised to consider carefully the recommendations emerging from the National Working Conference on Education and Training in Health Psychology (1983).

Postdoctoral training for those pursuing academic careers is becoming more common. The National Working Conference recognized the importance of such training as did recent government bodies awarding training grants, grants which have shifted priorities from predoctoral support to postdoctoral support. While postdoctoral training for health psychologists has been encouraged (see chapters 25–27 in this volume), Zumeta (1983) presents an issue to consider in this regard. He compared the median income of Ph.D's with postdoctoral training in the basic medical sciences to Ph.D's without such training and found that the latter's income was higher and they were more likely to obtain tenured faculty appointments. Why? Several interpretations of these data are possible. For example, there is the possibility that the job market did not offer an adequate number of positions for both groups once the postdoctoral trainees were ready to enter the job market. Alternatively, the very best students might have been placed without postdoctoral training. While Zumeta did not study psychology postdoctoral training, the lesson is clear—the value of postdoctoral training is only as good as the skills obtained and the availability of employment positions. For some health psychology jobs, clearly not all, postdoctoral training may not be necessary.

Finally, there are two particularly illuminating articles on the academic job market (Darley and Zanna 1979; Heppner and Downing 1982). These authors discuss the details of the academic interviewing process and give suggestions for presenting oneself as a strong candidate.

OPPORTUNITIES WITH HEALTH CARE PROVIDERS

During the past decade, the problem of increasing access to health care has been eclipsed by questions of how to pay for the care. The number and variety of health care providers has proliferated, as evidenced by the increasing number of health maintenance organizations, preferred provider organizations, free-standing dental, optical, and urgent medical care centers, and corporate health programs. Furthermore, increased expectations about the quality of health care, the demand for sophisticated technology, and reimbursement systems that reward health care utilization have led to skyrocketing health costs. These events offer psychologists opportunities to contribute to the health care system.

Hospitals want to contain costs because insurance systems, especially Medicaid and Medicare, are limiting the degree to which they will reimburse certain procedures. Moreover, less profitable institutions are closing and being incorporated into chains of hospitals managed by professionals who use economies of scale and new technologies to reduce costs. Paralleling this trend among hospitals is one among nursing homes. In both cases, the pressures to provide high-quality services at lower costs are spawning new sets of service providers. Hospitals and physicians now compete with Health Maintenance Organizations, Preferred Provider Organizations, Emergency Care Centers, ambulatory care providers, and prevention-oriented providers. Alternatives to nursing homes also are being formed, including channeling programs, home health care programs, and community centers for the elderly.

These health service providers and programs clearly could benefit by collaboration with health psychologists because health psychologists understand basic principles of psychology as well as the unique demands associated with applying these principles to issues that arise in health settings. Health psychologists can contribute to planning, providing, and evaluating health services in various ways: (1) as providers of direct psychological services; (2) as administrators; and (3) as researchers and evaluators studying service delivery issues. Clearly, cost-containment and cost-effectiveness are issues of which health psychologists should be cognizant (Bugen 1983). Another area in which health psychologists can contribute is the use of simulation models to answer "what if" questions. In this regard, psychologists are uniquely skilled in predicting behavior and in developing sophisticated theoretical and quantitative causal models. As one example, psychologists could contribute to our understanding of the effects of raising insurance deductibles on health costs and on the health behaviors of consumers and health professionals.

The clinical and research/evaluation skills necessary to work as a health system provider are obtainable through health psychology coursework and apprenticeships. In contrast, the administrative skills (e.g., accounting, planning and management, cost-control) are not typically taught in psychology courses. Health psychologists with interests in administration might consider taking overview courses in organizational psychology, management, accounting, and marketing in order to gain an appreciation of how the key issues in these areas affect the activities of health care providers.

Opportunities with Government and Related Organizations

Both national and state governments are involved in the provision and regulation of health services. They reimburse health care (e.g., Medicare, Aid for Families with Dependent Children), regulate health service delivery and costs, formulate laws to regulate health behavior (e.g., drunk driving), operate health departments, and conduct demonstration programs. They also are responsible for regulating public health activities affecting the environment (e.g., the Clean Air Act).

To date, very few health psychologists have entered this employment arena, yet it offers an ideal setting for the application of psychological skills. Potential positions include working with legislative committees specializing in health issues (e.g., House and Senate subcommittees), executive agencies and administrative departments (e.g., Health Care Financing Administration, National Institutes of Health, National Institute of Mental Health, Environmental Protection Agency), government research organizations (e.g., Congressional Research Service, General Accounting Office and Office of Technology Assessment), special bodies empowered to help control health costs and quality (e.g., health systems review bodies, Professional Review Organizations), trade associations and lobbyists who provide government officials with information, and the military branches.

To stimulate interest in these settings, several organizations have created national fellowship programs to provide students with an opportunity to gain relevant experience. These programs include the following: Congressional Science Fellowship, Health and Human Service Fellowship, White House Fellowship, Judicial Fellowship, Robert Woods Johnson Fellowship, National Cancer Institute Office of Cancer Communications Internship, NIH Rotating Intern, and the Commissioned Officer Student Training and Extern Program of the Public Health Service. The best way to find out about these and other fellowship programs is through involvement in diverse professional associations. Most associations, for example, publish newsletters that advertise such positions.

To function effectively in these settings, it is important that the health psychologist be able to interpret research, evaluation, and policy findings, especially in regard to risk factor assessment, intervention, organizational/program development, and legal issues. Effective interpersonal and communication skills are essential.

Opportunities with Private Sector, Nonservice Providers

As health costs escalate and service providers practice in new ways, the number of private sector employers concerned with the health care system will increase. These employers are interested in why people choose particular health services and how behaviors concerning the use of health services can be altered to keep people healthier and reduce the total costs of health care.

Health insurance companies, constantly pressured by the demands of providers and consumers to reduce higher annual premiums, will seek assistance. They are increasingly being joined by industrial and commercial corporations who recognize that employee health benefit plans and occupational issues affect their bottom line. Indeed, these two groups are joining together to form business coalitions dedicated to addressing the health cost inflation issue. Think-tanks and consulting firms that work for the private sector or government also are looking for persons with expertise in health issues. Other firms that could benefit from the expertise of health psychologists include public relations, marketing, advertising, and survey research firms and health-related professional associations.

Employment in most of these organizations requires research, evaluation, management, and organizational skills. Likely roles for health psychologists in the private sector include research on and evaluation of programs or policies (e.g., does a program or policy really control health costs?) as well as administration of health programs. Since these settings employ professionals from multiple disciplines, health psychologists would be wise to have knowledge of organizational dynamics, consultation, risk factor assessment, health education, and cost-benefit analysis. Takooshian (1982) discusses opportunities for psychologists in nonacademic settings.

To date, few health psychologists have broken into the ranks of these firms. According to the survey of Division 38 members by Morrow, Carpenter, and Clayman (1983), less than 12 percent work for private industry. Accordingly, some of the most educational apprenticeship opportunities may only be available through mentors who are not psychologists. Therefore, a relationship should be formed between the health psychology community and these potential mentors in order to provide students interested in this employment setting with relevant training experiences. To be successful, these apprenticeships will require the joint supervision of faculty advisors and field mentors.

Health Psychology in Perspective

Health psychology is still in its infancy. As this chapter and others demonstrate, there are few limits to the issues a health psychologist with vision, dedication, and persistence can address. The newness of this discipline, however, will make entree into some employment arenas difficult. In the initial stages of the development of health psychology as a discipline, most jobs were located in universities and medical settings. While a potentially larger number of jobs can be found with private industry and government, few of these employers are disappointed when they cannot find a health psychologist to carry out their projects. Indeed, many do not even know what a health psychologist is. Therefore, health psychologists must be willing to break new ground and demonstrate that they have something useful to offer and of a quality that cannot be obtained from others. This necessitates utilizing research skills honed in graduate school to become experts on the job marketplace. A statement attributed to McGraw-Hill publications presents this argument cogently:

> I don't know who you are.
> I don't know your company.
> I don't know your company's product.
> I don't know what your company stands for.
> I don't know your company's customers.
> I don't know your company's record.
> I don't know your company's reputation.
> Now—what is it you wanted to sell me?

In a sense, the company health psychologists are working for is Health Psychology, Inc.; the products they sell are their health psychology skills.

Since there is stiff competition for positions, health psychologists must be creative in their strategy and convince potential employers of their value relative to what other professionals can offer. They must demonstrate their expertise and commitment to cost-effectiveness (cf. Fishman and Neigher 1982). In so doing, the next generation of health psychology students will have valuable role models as well as new employment options.

Participating in the activities of various professional organizations will help health psychologists learn about the job market. Professional associations of interest to health psychologsts, in addition to the American Psychological Association and its Division to Health Psychology, include the American Heart Association Council on Epidemiology, American Public Health Association, Association for Fitness in Business, American Orthopsychiatric Association, American Dental Association, Evaluation Research Society, and the Society of Behavioral Medicine, among others. Since many jobs are not formally advertised, it is important to find out about unpublicized openings through communication with appropriate gatekeepers in these organizations.

General Comments on Seeking Employment

A number of excellent sources exist on how to locate employment, write resumes and curriculum vitaes (there is a difference!), and behave in an interview. Limited space prevents a formal discussion of these sources but we highly recommend their perusal. A list of some of these sources follows the References section. In addition, articles by Huber (1982) and Takooshian (1982) are useful resources for graduate students and academicians seeking applied jobs.

Employment in Health Psychology: Looking Forward and Backward

The health field is going through major changes relating to the organization, delivery, and utilization of health services, the funding of services, environmental control and regulation, the prevention of disease and promotion of health, and the understanding of disease mechanisms. With exposure to other fields, health psychologists can make important contributions to the development, administration, and evaluation of health programs in many settings. Perhaps most important, they can obtain skills needed to formulate health policy.

The critical issue is whether health psychologists will be able to find job opportunities in appropriate and desirable settings. The responsibility for forging new pathways lies on the shoulders of the entire health psychology community. As stated in the report, "Health and Behavior: Frontiers of Research in the Biobehavioral Sciences" (Hamburg, Elliott, and Parron 1982):

> When young people have completed research training in health and behavioral sciences, they must be able to find acceptable career pathways, if their skills are not to be wasted. Relevant agencies and institutions must consider long-term career pathways through which the problems delineated in this report can be addressed effectively.
>
> (p. 23)

Current health psychologists, whether in academia or not, should be available at all times to counsel the new generation and help create jobs for them. The new generation should maintain close bonds with their already-established colleagues in order to facilitate the achievement of common goals. Only then will new employment options be created and capitalized upon for the good of all.

REFERENCES

Adler, N. E., F. Cohen, and G. C. Stone. 1979. Themes and professional prospects in health psychology. In *Health Psychology,* edited by G. C. Stone, F. Cohen, and N. E. Adler. San Francisco: Jossey-Bass.

Altman, D. G., and J. Cahn. 1983. The rest of the challenge: Position statement on employment opportunities. *Health Psychology* 2(5): 119–22, supplement section.

Bugen, L. 1983. The role of psychology in the Austin Regional Clinic/PRUCARE. *The HMO Psychologist* (Winter): 4.

Carroll, J. S., C. M. Werner, and R. D. Ashmore. 1982. Internships and practica in social psychology graduate training programs. *Personality and Social Psychology Bulletin* 8(2): 348–56.

Darley, J. M., and M. P. Zanna. 1979. On getting your first job in academic psychology. *Catalog of Selected Documents in Psychology* 9(3): 45. (m.s. #1916).

Edwards, J. D. and R. L. Holmgren. 1979. Some prerequisites for becoming a "really" applied, non-academic social psychologist. *Personality and Social Psychology Bulletin* 5(4): 516–23.

Fishman, D. B., and W. D. Neigher. 1982. American psychology in the eighties: Who will buy? *American Psychologist* 37(5): 533–46.

Fulcher, R. and J. Stapp. 1982. *Preliminary report: 1981 doctorate employment survey.* Washington, D.C.: American Psychological Association.

Grzesiak, R. C. 1984. Employment opportunities in health psychology: Four years of "Monitor" advertisements. *The Health Psychologist Newsletter* 6(1): 6–8.

Hamburg, D. A., G. R. Elliott, and D. L. Parron. 1982. *Health and behavior. Fron-*

tiers of research in the biobehavioral sciences. Washington, D.C.: National Academy Press.

Heppner, P. P., and N. E. Downing. 1982. Job interviewing for new psychologists: Riding the emotional rollercoaster. *Professional Psychology* 13(3): 334–41.

Huber, B. J. 1982. *Mastering the job market: Using graduate training in sociology for careers in applied settings.* Washington, D.C.: American Sociological Association.

Matarazzo, J. D., T. P. Carmody, and W. D. Gentry. 1981. Psychologists on the faculties of United States schools of medicine: Past, present and possible future. *Clinical Psychology Review* 1: 293–317.

Matthews, K. A., and N. E. Avis. 1982. Psychologists in Schools of Public Health. *American Psychologist* 37(8): 949–54.

Morrow, G. R., P. J. Carpenter, and D. A. Clayman. 1983. A national survey of health psychologists: Characteristics, training, and priorities. *The Health Psychologist Newsletter* 5 (2): 6–7.

National Research Council. 1982. *Science, engineering, and humanities doctorates in the United States: 1981 profile.* Washington, D.C.: National Academy Press.

National Science Foundation. 1979. *Projections of science and engineering doctorate supply and utilization, 1982 and 1987.* NSF 79–303.

Schneider, S. F. 1980. Positions of psychologists trained in research. *American Psychologist* 35(10): 861–66.

Stapp, J., and R. Fulcher. 1983a. The employment of APA members: 1982. *American Psychologist* 38(12): 1298–1320.

———. 1983b. *Salaries in psychology.* Washington, D.C.: American Psychological Association.

Stone, G. C., ed. 1983. National Working Conference on Education and Training in Health Psychology. In *Health Psychology* 2(5): supplement section.

Stoup, C. M., and L. T. Benjamin, Jr. 1982. Graduate study in psychology, 1970–1979. *American Psychologist* 37(11): 1186–1202.

Takooshian, H. 1982. Entering nonacademic social psychology. *Society for the Advancement of Social Psychology Newsletter* 8(5): 5–8.

Wolfson, J., and P. J. Levin. 1985. *Managing employee health benefits: A guide to cost control.* Homewood, IL: Dow Jones-Irwin.

Zumeta, W. 1983. A special news report on people and their jobs in offices, fields, and factories. *Wall Street Journal,* 19 July, p. 1.

References on the Jobmarket

Bestor, D. K. 1982. *Aside from teaching, what in the world can you do?* Seattle: University of Washington Press.

Billingsley, E. 1978. *Career planning and job hunting for today's student.* Santa Monica, CA: Goodyear Publishing Co.

Bolles, R. N. 1983. *What color is your parachute?* Berkeley, CA: Ten Speed Press.

Bostwick, B. E. 1982. *How to find the job you've always wanted.* 2d ed. New York: Wiley & Sons.

Dickhut, H. W. 1981. *The professional resume and job search guide.* Englewood Cliffs, NJ: Prentice-Hall.

Erdlen, J. D. 1976. *Job hunting guide.* Boston, MA: Herman Publishing.

Federal Yellow Book. Washington, D.C.: The National Press, most recent edition.

Feingold, S. H., and G. A. Hansard-Winkler. 1982. *900,000 plus jobs annually published: Sources of employment listings.* Fairfax, VA: Impact Publications.

Gale, B. 1979. *The national career directory: An occupational information handbook.* New York: Arco Publishing Co.

Greco, B. 1980. *How to get the job that's right for you.* Homewood, IL: Dow Jones-Irwin.

Irish, R. K. 1978. *Go hire yourself an employer.* New York: Anchor Books.

Jackson, T. 1978. *Guerilla tactics in the job market.* New York: Bantam Books.

Kocher, E. 1979. *International jobs—Where they are, how to get them.* Reading, MA: Addison-Wesley.

Lesko, M. 1983. *Information U.S.A.* New York: The Viking Press.

Meyer, M. C. and I. M. Berchtold. 1982. *Getting the job: How to interview successfully.* New York: Petrocelli Books.

Moore, C. G. 1978. *The career game.* New York: Ballantine Books.

Radin, R. J. 1983. *Full potential.* New York: McGraw-Hill.

Research Centers Directory. Detroit: Gale Research Co.

U.S. General Services Administration. 1983. *Consumer Information Catalog.* Pueblo, CO: Consumer Information Center.

Weinstein, R. V. 1983. *Jobs for the 21st century.* New York: Collier Books.

Part Five

Health Psychology and Segments of the Population

Editor: Judith Rodin

Research questions and treatment approaches within health psychology may differ as a function of the specific populations being considered. The authors of the next four chapters give examples of ways in which research that emanated from the study of a particular subject population relates to the knowledge base of health psychology and where gaps in our current level of information exist because of a lack of investigation, until recently, of the unique health issues relevant to each subpopulation. The chapters describe the opportunities for clarifying basic phenomena that can be realized in the study of these populations, the unique treatment needs of each population, and the implication of these needs for practice and application.

The issues relating to special populations are sufficiently unique to argue for subspecialties that confront these domains directly. Kurz, for example, argues that health assessment and treatment techniques must take into account the unique cognitive and motor capabilities of infants and young children and the family dynamics of the young child. Gatz and her collaborators argue the same point with regard to older adults. A full understanding of the life stage of a particular individual is needed to assess the role of stress in the etiology and duration of illness, the development of prevention strategies, and the types of diseases people get.

Sex and race, like age, are related to different types and patterns of illness and, quite notably, are associated with different responses from the health care system. It has been quite clear that men and women are treated differently by health professionals, a point well documented by Jansen. Similarly, blacks and other minority group members are often treated differently by the health care system than their white counterparts, both in terms of the quality of care and the types of treatment that are given. Biological as well as social aspects of intergroup differences need attention. Anderson and Jackson demonstrate the need for considering different interactions between risk factors and physiology in the case of blacks. Similarly complex patterns might be found in other racial subgroups and between the sexes if the possibility of their existence were adequately reflected in research designs. The possibilities of interactions among age, sex, and race, both in social and biological aspects of health processes, need to be kept in mind and investigated.

Jansen begins her chapter by considering the profound implications of being a woman patient in the health care system. She reviews data suggesting differential treatment and the consequences of this differential treatment for both physical and mental health. She considers, for example, how sexual biases may have contributed to the dramatic increase in the incidence of hysterectomy in the past decade. She notes that health psychologists, in their studies of patient-practitioner interactions have begun to detail how these interactions differ as a function of the sex of the patient. Jansen also considers the status of women as students and workers in the health care system, asking how training and colleagueship may vary as a function of sex. She considers the broad implications of the issues reviewed in her chapter for public policy and concludes with very clear recommendations for research and training issues that take the interface between the psychology of women and health psychology as a crucial domain of inquiry and attention.

Multiple reasons for focusing on health needs of racial and ethnic minorities are given by Anderson and Jackson in their chapter: members of such groups have higher incidence and prevalence rates for many diseases and illnesses; there is much evidence for differences in health and illness behavior; there are wide disparities in morbidity, mortality, and utilization rates among racial/ethnic groups. These authors elect to explore the many nuances of the ethnicity-health interface by exploring in-depth a specific problem—the excessive rate of essential hypertension in black Americans. In doing so they examine racial differences in the biological, behavioral, social/environmental, and applied dimensions of the problem. Their approach could well serve as a model for many other similar investigations.

Kurz begins his chapter on child health psychology by describing its domain and its relationship to other fields such as pediatric psychology and child clinical psychology. He describes the requisite skills for working with pediatric populations and specific important considerations essential for effective assessment and treatment of children. He then moves to an elegant analysis of the contribution of psychological factors in children's physical health and illness, using a common pediatric condition, asthma, to highlight the complexities involved. He discusses the selection of assessment techniques, the goals of psychological treatment of children in the pediatric health population, and the different approaches that have been taken to treatment. Brief coverage of the topics of prevention and pediatric health behavior reflects the great need for research and activity in this important area. Kurz concludes with a discussion of research on the effects of illness and medical procedures on children.

In common with other authors in this section, Gatz, Pearson, and Weicker open their chapter with an expression of concern that the intersection of health psychology with the psychology of their special population group, the aging, has received so little attention. Changing demographics are, however, forcing greater attention to this natural overlap in areas. They then discuss the physical, psychological, and social changes that occur with aging which must be understood in order to comprehend the etiology of good health and disease and must be taken into account for practice and treatment. The physical health of the aged population reflects both normal biological changes and the increased incidence of many diseases. Rates of decline vary among organ systems and from one individual to another. Of normal age-related psychological changes, cognitive function is most significant, highly variable among individuals, and essential to take into account in providing appropriate assessment and treatment. Gatz and her co-workers highlight important concepts from aging research that are relevant to health psychology. Most significant is the phenomenon of cohort (the generations in which the individual was born, grew up, and grew older), which impacts all of the variables relevant to health and illness. The phenomenon of increased interindividual variability with aging is also stressed. Finally, Gatz and her coauthors illustrate the collaborative potential that exists between health psychology and adult development and aging on such topics as attitudinal factors, health policy issues, preventive interventions, and service provision.

18

Women's Health Issues: An Emerging Priority for Health Psychology

Mary A. Jansen

In many ways, men's and women's health issues are similar; in many other ways health issues faced by men and women are very different. Yet, the reasons for these differences are not always clear. We know for instance that there is a higher incidence of depression diagnosed among women and that psychotropic drug use is higher among women than men. There are several possible explanations for these differences, ranging from an actual difference in depression rates for men and women, or differences in reporting between men and women, to differences in the way physicians perceive the symptoms men and women patients present or the ways they choose to treat these symptoms. Because we have not clearly identified all of the ways in which these differences may be accounted for, health differences between men and women should be acknowledged by health professionals and the factors which account for them identified. Many writers report, however, that these differences have led to a devaluing of women's health problems and differential treatment for women patients (Carmen, Russo, and Miller 1981; Marieskind 1980; Wallen, Waitzkin, and Stoeckle 1979). A review of the available literature reveals sharp distinctions between the ways in which men and women are perceived and treated in the health care setting. This literature will be examined in greater detail in following sections, and its implications for health care providers and for women as students in health care training will be noted.

The author is indebted to several individuals who provided assistance in the preparation of this chapter. These include Lois Beiner, Cheryl Brown Travis, Alexandra Todd, and Barbara Wallston. I am especially indebted to Nancy Felipe Russo who contributed valuable knowledge and expertise without hesitation and whose careful editing of previous drafts made publication of the final version possible.

Women as Patients in the Health Care System
IMPLICATIONS FOR MENTAL HEALTH

Before they receive any care at all from a physician, women patients may be faced with a bias not often readily apparent. Critics of physician training note that physicians have been systematically schooled in the belief that women are inferior, are less competent, present psychosomatic complaints, and are hysterical (Ehrenreich 1974; Greenhill 1965; Howell 1974; Novak 1970; Scott 1968; Walsh 1977; Wilson and Carrington 1979). Because physicians have been taught that women's illnesses are largely of emotional origin, they may believe that their complaints can be solved by prescribing a psychoactive drug (Ehrenreich 1974; Moore 1980). Additionally, beliefs of mental health providers affect the way they treat patients (Farina and Fisher 1982). When women are seen as anxious, depressed, and more helpless, dependent, and passive than men, there is a greater likelihood of treatment by psychoactive drugs. This belief can place women patients at a risk for receiving inappropriate health care and may well be a major reason for the well-documented overprescription of sedative drugs (Carmen, Russo, and Miller 1981; Moore 1980). We know that more women than men report depression and are treated by medication for depressive symptoms (Weissman and Klerman 1977). We also know that twice as many women use prescriptions for minor tranquilizers as men and fifty percent more women use prescriptions for barbituates than men (Wolcott 1979). Since the significant sex differences in drug use that are apparent when drugs are obtained by physician prescription disappear when one looks at drug use with illicitly obtained drugs (Carmen, Russo, and Miller 1981), it is likely that this difference in prescription drug use is attributable to sex-role stereotyping by physicians. It is not likely that this difference reflects more visits to physicians by women. In a study of all prescriptions written in Ontario in 1970–71 and 1973–74, Cooperstock (1978) reported higher prescription rates for women and went on to note that rates for physician visits were not different for men and women. Women accounted for fifty-four percent of the total physician visits, and most of these excess visits were made by younger women during their reproductive years.

Additionally, women report symptoms in greater detail than men, and since physicians tend to diagnose women's physical complaints as psychosomatic (Bernstein and Kane 1981) they may tend to assume that these complaints will be adequately treated by a psychoactive drug (Ehrenreich 1974; Howell 1974). One example is illustrative of this point. Until as recently as

1973, books, journal articles, and other scholarly presentations offered the view that nausea during pregnancy is the result of women's hysterical personality, immaturity, masochism, desire not to be pregnant, and other neurotic tendencies (Kasper 1980). This view was projected despite the fact that nausea during the early months of pregnancy is almost the sine qua non of being pregnant, occurring in seventy percent of all pregnancies (Jarnfelt 1982).

A further illustration of our limited knowledge in this area is apparent from recent research which has demonstrated an increase in the depression-related sex differential with increased family role obligations (Aneshensel, Frerichs, and Clark 1981) and which has shown that depression is mediated by social variables such as marriage and social contact (Cafferta, Kasper, and Bernstein 1983; Cleary and Mechanic 1983; Verbrugge 1982, 1983). Therefore to prescribe drugs for women for depression without realizing the impact of stereotyped social and family role expectations may be fruitless and inappropriate.

IMPLICATIONS FOR PHYSICAL HEALTH

Women's sexuality, reproduction, and responsibility for birth control have received much attention in the literature. It is frequently noted that despite the commonly available means of safe and effective birth control for males, invasive birth control methods such as the pill and IUD are prescribed uniformly to women when families seek information about birth control. This is so despite the potential for serious side effects including risk of stroke, unknown risks due to changes in hormonal balance and potential subsequent impact on the immunological system, possible risks of cancer, etc. (Seaman 1980; Seaman and Seaman 1977). Yet, the consequences of smoking while taking the pill are rarely communicated to women patients. The outcry over the potential risk of stroke to men who have had vasectomies and the decline in numbers of vasectomies performed stands in sharp contrast to the continued prescription without adequate warning of the potential risks from use of birth control devices for women (Ehrenreich 1974; Marieskind 1980).

Additionally, there is less questioning of costly health care expenditures for major surgery for women, such as hysterectomy, and more willingness on the part of insurers to pay for these costly procedures. This not only places the risks of these procedures on women, but in the case of hysterectomy, has reinforced the stereotypical notion that women have complete responsibility for birth control when a less costly and less risky procedure for men exists. Compared to a vasectomy operation, hysterectomy, which is a major surgical procedure, requires a hospital stay of several days, loss of productivity due to time for recovery at home, and considerable in-patient medical cost. The reluctance of the insurance industry, controlled to a large extent by the medical profession and which subsequently exerts great power on legislators (Starr 1982), to adopt vasectomy as the birth control method of choice may involve the fact that this procedure may increase the risk of stroke for men and the fact that physicians earn much more money for performing a hysterectomy than for performing the more minor male surgery, vasectomy.

Women's health experiences are distorted when phenomena unique to women (menstruation, pregnancy, menopause) are seen as sickness/disease experiences. This disease mentality contributes to the physician's justification for prescribing costly and invasive "curative" interventions such as hysterectomy, to eliminate the "diseased organ" (McBride and McBride 1981). The incidence of hysterectomy has risen dramatically; it is now the fourth most commonly performed surgery and, excluding biopsy, the most frequently performed procedure. Between 1968 and 1971 the number of hysterectomies performed by Los Angeles County at the University of Southern California Medical Center alone increased 293 percent. By 1979, 638,000 hysterectomies were performed in this country (U.S. Department of HHS 1982). The major reason for this astonishing escalation in hysterectomies is that this surgery was sold by the medical profession (particularly gynecologists who both recommend and perform the surgery for a typical fee of $2,000) as the sterilization and birth control method of choice. And gynecologists, ninety-seven percent of whom are males (Larned 1977), have promoted hysterectomy as everything from a convenient method for avoiding menstruation to the only logical way to avoid uterine cancer. Yet what hysterectomy advocates fail to tell patients is that the annual death rate for hysterectomy (a major surgery) is 1,000 of every 1 million women while the annual death rate for uterine cancer is 100 of every 1 million women and, of these, the National Cancer Society estimates that a majority could be avoided by routine (and inexpensive) pap smears (Larned 1977). In recognition of this overuse of hysterectomy, the American College of Obstetricians and Gynecologists recently adopted as policy a position stating that members should no longer perform hysterectomies for merely prophylactic reasons. In contrast to routine recommendations of hysterectomy, urologists have not historically recommended routine prostectomy despite the frequent occurrence of prostate cancer in men over fifty.

COMMUNICATION IN THE HEALTH CARE SETTING

Patient-practitioner interactions are also of relevance to psychologists. In a study of patient-practitioner verbal interactions, Wallen, Waitzkin, and Stoeckle (1979) demonstrated that male physicians respond differently to male patients versus female patients in their verbal interactions. Physicians tended to answer the male patient's technical questions more easily than they answered the female patient's technical questions. Women received lower-level, less technical explanations than male patients. This is not surprising in light of earlier research by McKinlay (1975) which showed that male physicians consistently underestimated female patients' level of comprehension of medical terms. In the 1979 study by Wallen, Waitzkin, and Stoeckle, the physicians were much more likely to match the level of technicality of questions asked by the male patients. Likewise, it has been observed by Korsch and Negrete (1972) that mothers who attempted to gain detailed information about their child's condition experienced communication difficulties with the child's physician.

Consistently, communication difficulties have been shown in studies using male physicians and female patients. Wallen and associates (1979) hypothesized that this may be because male physicians and female patients are operating on "different wave lengths" (p. 142). To date, communication difficulties have been demonstrated but not explained, and it may be that there is anxiety on the part of both physician and patient.

Additionally, physicians may attach less importance to the information seeking/providing component of the patient's verbalizations when that patient is a woman. The work of Alexandra Todd (1984) parallels the results obtained in the Wallen et al. (1979) study. In a study of the tape-recorded interactions between gynecologists and their patients, Todd found that the physicians consistently cut off the patients' questions, as if to say "You need not continue, I know exactly what you're going to say." Additionally, women are frequently patronized by male physicians if they do ask questions, are often treated as children (with whom they are often grouped, i.e., "women and children"), and told not to worry. Todd's work underscores the very traditional sex role stereotypes held by male physicians and displayed in the exhortations and advice that physicians in her study gave to their patients regarding sexual practices, family planning, reproductive decisions, and appropriate behaviors as wives and mothers. Further, physicians in this situation tended to exert power and control in communications with their patients.

When physician providers have been taught that the "core of the female personality is narcissism, masochism, and passivity" (Wilson and Carrington 1979), it is no wonder that they feel compelled to interact with women in demeaning, controlling ways. Thus, women may be left feeling powerless because the health care system which gives physicians the power to control life itself (Ehrenreich and English 1979) is a system which devalues women and their health problems. As a result, women are less likely to be involved as participants in their own health care or may encounter repeated frustration if they do assert their right to be informed and involved in health care decisions.

SOCIAL AND CULTURAL FACTORS

Sex role expectations are also of relevance because physicians' expectations about sex roles and illness have been shown to influence their perception of the seriousness of an illness and the resultant decision to hospitalize. Rosenfield (1982) studied individuals who were presented with symptomatology inconsistent with sex role expectation and found that men with neurotic or depressive symptomatology (feminine) were most likely to be seen as seriously ill and hospitalized. Women with symptomatology suggesting substance abuse (masculine) were more likely to be classified as seriously ill and hospitalized. Yet, women appear to be modeling the health risk behaviors of men with a resultant increase in alcohol and drug use, smoking, coronary risk (Type A) behaviors, etc. These problems are heavily influenced by behavioral factors, and health psychologists have a unique opportunity to significantly affect the health status of both men and women.

The Framingham study (Dawber 1980) points to a number of gender differences specifically related to heart disease. We know that women are advantaged with respect to mortality rates. Compared to men, women have roughly a fifty percent risk of cardiovascular disease at any level of combined risk factors (Moore 1980; National Center for Health Statistics 1978). This advantage of women is partially environmentally mediated, however. For example, wives of men who experienced cardiovascular disease have double the risk of those whose husbands do not have heart disease. Heart disease is more prevalent among those who occupy low-status jobs, have poor support systems, and who lack control over their lives and experience anxiety and depression related to this lack of control (Haynes and Feinleib 1980). Thus, executive women experience low-risk rates for heart disease compared to women who are employed in less competitive and less pressured positions.

THE ROLE OF PSYCHOLOGISTS IN HEALTH SETTINGS

Health psychologists can play a valuable role in assisting patients and physicians to look at ways in which their attitudes, values, and beliefs reflect stereotyped sex role expectations and influence behavior. The prejudicial attitudes of many physicians have very real consequences for women and their health. The quality of health care could be significantly enhanced if both physicians and women were taught to believe that women have a right and a responsibility to control their own health care. Women must be encouraged and trained to be assertive in their interactions with physicians and to press continually for adequate information so that they may make appropriate choices about their own health care. Likewise, physicians must be trained to respect their women and men patients and to pay serious attention to the questions and concerns raised by their patients. It is well known that treatment regimens are more likely to be followed when the patient feels understood, accepted, and respected by the physician (Kirscht and Rosenstock 1979; Francis, Korsch, and Morris 1969; Svarstad 1976). Psychologists in health settings can utilize their specialized knowledge of behavior to shape interactions between patient and provider so that the quality of patient care is enhanced.

Women as Students in the Health Care System

Doctoral level training is stressful for all students (Kutner and Brogan 1980) and women health psychology students may be at special risk for several reasons. Within the health care system, physicians form the pinnacle of the hierarchical power structure and eighty-eight percent of physicians are male (Leserman 1981; Lewis and Lewis 1977). In light of the probability of physician bias discussed earlier, students should recognize that this bias may be demonstrated in professor/student interactions. It has been noted that one common yet subtle form of bias is apparent when a physician professor hesitates to acknowledge a woman student's questions. One writer has pointed out that it may be that women's remarks are considered irrelevant or unimportant and this more subtle discrimination occurs frequently. Often a woman student's very cogent, enlightened statements are given little credence or paid little attention. These unacknowledged comments can be restated by a male student and taken more seriously (Howell 1974). An additional assumption that women students in the health care system may face is that they are students of nursing, medical technology, or some other nondoctoral-level profession. Women students in health psychology training programs must be aware that the value of their profession and indeed their worth as individuals may be called into question. Feelings of anxiety, depression, frustration, irritation, and resultant lack of self-esteem and self-worth may occur and may contribute to early burnout among women health psychologists. For these reasons women students in health psychology training programs should become aware of support systems which can provide objective, unbiased assistance and should establish liaisons with other women professionals with whom they can develop mutually supportive relationships.

Women as Colleagues

Health psychologists function as providers of mental health services and as consultants to other health care professionals about a variety of behaviorally related issues. Women health psychologists serve as role models for students and colleagues and can help shape the attitudes and behavior of students, patients, and other health professionals with whom they have contact.

As noted earlier, the status differential which exists in interactions outside the health care system also exists when one examines professional health disciplines. Most physicians are male; many nonphysician health providers are female. Physicians have power; nonphysicians are lower on the status hierarchy and have less power. This is apparent in rates of pay, parking privileges at health care facilities ("doctors' parking"), hospital staff privileges for physicians versus refusal to grant hospital privileges to nonphysician providers, and physician authority for determining the most appropriate treatment for patients. Female health psychologists interacting with male physicians should be aware that their credibility as professionals may be questioned first because they are nonphysicians and secondly because they are women. Women health psychologists need to develop ways to support each other and to form networks of support across health disciplines. Health psychologists may be more sensitive to the need for, and implications of, research surrounding women's issues. Therefore, we have a professional responsibility to enlighten other colleagues who may not as readily see these relationships.

Implications for Public Policy

The issues and questions raised above also have implications for public policy. A fundamental goal for women in national health policy must be to shift the concept of women's health care as primarily related to reproduction and therefore under the domain of obstetricians and gynecologists. We need to recognize that most of women's health needs are similar to the health needs of men and require a wide range of providers along with equalized allocation of research dollars (Marieskind 1980).

Although policymakers are sensitive to the needs and requests of their constituents, most policymakers are male and most have not paid enough attention to policies which ultimately affect women and their health. Many diseases which strike women with higher frequency have been underfunded such as lupus and muscular dystrophy. Women at all ages are dying of breast cancer with increasing frequency. Two years ago one woman in thirteen was likely to develop the disease—now one woman in eleven has a likelihood of developing breast cancer. It is the primary cause of death for middle-aged women and by far the leading cancer killer of women (National Center for Health Statistics 1982). Despite the increased incidence of this disease and the very great toll it takes on women's lives, only 4.1 percent of the nation's annual research dollars are allocated for research on breast cancer (Clark 1982). At the same time, however, heart disease and respiratory illness which are major causes of death among men receive a large share of the nation's research dollars. Likewise, breast examinations for women are rare during the course of routine office visits. Yet, physicians listen to the heart and lungs of every patient who reports for a routine office visit. While a part of this difference may be accounted for by embarrassment, it is likely that physicians attach a higher priority to early detection of heart and lung disease, and a lower priority to early detection of breast disease.

Differences in funding priorities are also revealed if one compares the number of studies dealing with female fertility versus the number of studies dealing with male fertility. Between 1973 and 1978 the ratio ranged from 1:1 to 1:4 (Clark 1982). In 1978 six million dollars were spent for the development of female contraceptive methods as opposed to less than one million dollars for male contraceptive development. Yet, when one looks at the amount spent for evaluating the safety and efficacy of female versus male contraceptives a very different picture emerges. In 1978 four and one half million dollars were spent on evaluating female contraceptives as opposed to slightly over two million dollars for male contraceptive evaluation studies (Women and Health Roundtable 1979). Though this trend has moderated somewhat, the pattern remained consistent between 1978 and 1982 (U.S. Dept. of HHS 1983). The message from our nation's policymakers seems clear: Women should bear the major responsibility for birth control and, as a nation, we are willing to develop birth control measures to help them do so. Moreover, a small amount of research dollars have been allocated for development of male birth control measures. However, as a nation, we are not willing to allocate a large amount of money to evaluate the safety and efficacy of birth control methods for women but do in fact place a high priority on evaluation of safety and efficacy of birth control measures for males. So high in fact that in 1978 two and a half times as much was spent evaluating the safety and efficacy of birth control methods for males as was spent developing these methods for males, while three fourths as much was spent evaluating the safety and efficacy of birth control methods for women as was spent developing these methods.

We must develop a national health policy which insures that adequate development and testing of new drugs and procedures will be carried out before they are approved for use. Recent examples which illustrate the ineffectiveness and danger of current policy include the prescription of DES, estrogen replacement therapy, the contraceptive pill, IUDs, and use of mammography, all approved for use without adequate knowledge of the effects and implications for female users. The risks to women of hysterectomy and the birth control pill have been well documented (Ehrenreich 1974; Larned 1977) and the dangerous implications of use of the procedures and devices mentioned above are just now coming to light after years of use by women (Marieskind 1980).

Women also have greater need for health care under publicly funded medical programs such as Medicare and Medicaid than men. Larger numbers of women fall below the poverty level than men and more women than men live beyond age 65. These factors lead to a greater need for health services by poor and elderly women who qualify for these public programs. Yet Medicare and Medicaid provide only limited access to much needed physical and mental health services for the elderly and disabled poor of our country. National health policy reforms must ensure more equitable access to health and mental health care for the elderly and poor under these public programs, many of whom are women.

Finally, professional health psychologists must be strong advocates for changes to health care policies and practices that directly discriminate against psychologists as health care providers and indirectly discriminate against patients, many of whom are female. Professional women health psychologists must also work toward increased recognition of women as professional health care providers and as professionals with equal status to male physicians. All health psychologists face both a challenge and an opportunity to assist our nation's health care system to move in less discriminatory, more equalitarian directions for the benefit of those who work within the system and for those served by it.

Research Issues and Recommendations

Recent research has revealed differences between men and women in mortality rates. It is likely that several factors account for this. Certainly, women seem to be hardier than men and at all age levels have lower mortality rates. The reasons for this are as yet unclear and need further study. Environmental factors play a part, yet the relationship of these factors to mortality rates is unclear. For instance, unmarried men are at greater risk than are married men, yet unmarried women and those women who are married face essentially the same risk. Further, availability of social contact seems unimportant for men who demonstrate similar mortality rates regardless of the number of social interactions. Women, however, are at much greater risk when they are without social contacts than when they participate in social interactions (Aneshensel, Frerichs, and Clark 1981; Gove, Hughes, and Syle 1983). These effects are mediated by age and impact on internal versus external causes of mortality. The interactions are unclear, however, and one reason for this lack of clarity is that good epidemiological studies which tease out these relationships are lacking. Clearly, health research must begin to focus on a variety of psychological and behavioral variables and must include age and gender as factors.

Minority women are at particular risk when one considers the effects of stress from economic deprivation and this relationship needs further study. Additionally, the demeaning and demoralizing effect of physician-patient interaction and status inequity are further compounded when the patient or student is a minority woman. We need to study the effects of subculture specific behaviors on the health care system. For instance, practices and behaviors specific to one ethnic group may impact on the patient-physician relationship and may determine whether or not treatment regimens are followed by ethnic women. Health practices, behaviors, and attitudes specific to ethnicity and subculture must be considered in all aspects of research.

Research paradigms need to look at the dynamics which influence men and women in their health-risk behaviors. For instance, despite the fact that men continue to smoke, they have been more responsive to campaigns which have encouraged them to quit smoking. Women, on the other hand, have been less responsive and this points to the fact that there are most likely different factors which reinforce smoking behavior in men and women. Since deaths from respiratory disease are increasing as a major cause of death among women, it is critical that researchers turn their attention to the variables which encourage women to continue smoking. Additional health risks for women include the increased stressors of work and family which dual-career women experience, the low prestige of the homemaker role, and the potential for women to experience stressful life events over which they have little control. It appears that multiple roles as spouse and mother may be adaptive for a woman's health but as family role expectations become greater, and potentially overwhelming, this edge is likely lost (Cleary and Mechanic 1983; Verbrugge 1982; 1983). A need exists to address questions related to the notion that power, control over, and general predictability of one's life will have a positive influence on a woman's health (Antonovsky 1979; Strickland 1978). For instance, we have only begun to touch on the relationships to mental health of marital commitment, employment, presence versus absence of children, responsibility for primary care of children, and a host of other psychological and behavioral factors. Additionally, we can not say with certainty that the same environmental stressors will produce the same effects on men and women. It is clear that psychological and social variables must be explored much more fully before we can know the effects of these variables on the differential health of men and women. As noted earlier, the higher prevalence of depression among women (Weissman and Klerman 1977; Brown and Harris 1978; Aneshensel, Frerichs, and Clark 1981) must be reviewed in light of the various factors which impact on development of depression and the factors which impact on symptom presentation. We need studies which will tease out those complex interactions so that interventions aimed at preventing illness and disability in both sexes can be appropriately designed. Finally, investigations into the ways in which women as students in the health care system are differentially evaluated from their male counterparts are needed. In order to heighten awareness of current practitioners and trainers, selection methods for postdoctoral residency training programs should also be studied.

Training Issues and Recommendations

Training in health psychology must include emphasis on heightening the awareness of future health psychologists concerning the issues that confront women throughout the health care system. It is important that pre- and postdoctoral training programs in health psychology incorporate a course which embodies the most current research findings in this area. Textbooks used at both levels of training should also be written so that traditional sex role stereotypes which pervade medical education and the health care system are eliminated.

The training system itself must also be flexible enough to incorporate students with special needs. In our society, women are generally responsible for the care of children. This presents several problems for a woman who wishes to attend graduate school. Rigid curriculum expectations and course schedules prohibit women with child care responsibilities from attending courses, practicum and internship experiences, lab experiences, etc., which are not designed so that special needs can be accommodated. Some remedies for this problem include: competency-based approaches to instruction which provide research, skill training, and self-instruction as alternatives and variable schedules which allow women who are responsible for child care to complete the requirements for course work at times other than the scheduled time. Questions surrounding access to appropriate research and training opportunities, facilities, mentors, as well as equal access to personal convenience and necessity items such as locker rooms in medical facilities for storing belongings, sleeping quarters for students on emergency call, and access to stress relieving recreational facilities, need to be investigated. It must also be realized that many women are economically disadvantaged [women still earn 59 cents for every $1.00 that men earn among full-time, year-round workers (Women's Bureau 1983)] and costs for tuition, housing, and related expenses may be especially burdensome for women.

Training experiences in clinical and research settings should include an emphasis on research pertaining to the particular health problems of women and minorities, such as research paradigms which recognize the complexity of factors influencing the health status of both men and women. Jansen and Wellons (1983) point to the diversity of training experiences which are necessary if health psychology is to maintain the consistent and focused emphasis on women's issues that is needed over the next several years.

Summary

Psychologists in health settings must be aware of the differential implications of the health care system for men and women. In women's interactions as patients, students, and as colleagues, a status differential exists and women are often devalued and treated as if they are inferior to their male counterparts. This differential impact extends to funding for research priorities and national health care policies.

Health psychologists have a unique opportunity to influence the future direction of our health care system. As behavioral scientists, psychologists can provide information, serve as appropriate role models, and directly and indirectly shape the attitudes and behavior of patients and providers in the health care system. This unique opportunity offers both a challenge and a promise and is one to which health psychologists must pay serious attention over the next decade.

References

Aneshensel, C. S., R. R. Frerichs, and V. A. Clark. 1981. Family roles and sex differences in depression. *Journal of Health and Social Behavior* 22:379–93.

Atonovsky, A. 1979. *Health, stress, and coping.* San Francisco: Jossey-Bass.

Bernstein, B., and R. Kane. 1981. Physicians' attitudes toward female patients. *Medical Care* 19:600–608.

Brown, G. W., and T. Harris. 1978. *Social origins of depression: A study of psychiatric disorders in women.* New York: Free Press.

Cafferta, G. L., J. Kasper, and A. Bernstein. 1983. Family roles, structure and stressors in relation to sex differences in obtaining psychotropic drugs. *Journal of Health and Social Behavior* 24:132–43.

Carmen, E., N. F. Russo, and J. B. Miller. 1981. Inequity and women's mental health: An overview. *American Journal of Psychiatry* 138(10): 1319–30.

Clark, A. H. 1982. Letter to the editor, *Women and Health* 7(1): 87–88.

Cleary, P. D., and D. Mechanic. 1983. Sex differences in psychological distress among married people. *Journal of Health and Social Behavior* 24:111–21.

Cooperstock, R. 1978. Sex differences in psychotropic drug use. *Social Science Medicine* 12B:179–86.

Dawber, T. R. 1980. *The Framingham study.* Cambridge, MA: Harvard University Press.

Ehrenreich, B. 1974. Gender and objectivity in medicine. *International Journal of Health Services,* 4 (4): 617–23.

Ehrenreich, B., and D. English. 1973. *Complaints and disorders.* Old Westbury, NY: The Feminist Press.

Farina, A., and T. D. Fisher. 1982. Beliefs about mental disorders: Findings and implications. In *Integrations of clinical and social psychology,* edited by G. Weary and H. F. Mirels. New York: Oxford University Press.

Francis, V., B. M. Korsch, and M. Morris. 1969. Gaps in doctor-patient communication—Patients' responses to medical advice. *New England Journal of Medicine* 280:535–40.

Gove, W., M. Hughes, and C. B. Syle. 1983. Does marriage have positive effects on the psychological well-being of the individual? *Journal of Health and Social Behavior* 24:123–31.

Greenhill, J. P. 1965. *Office gynecology.* Chicago: Year Book Medical Publishers, Inc.

Haynes, S. G., and M. Feinleib. 1980. Women, work, and coronary heart disease: Prospective findings from the Framingham Heart Study. *American Journal of Public Health* 70(2):133–41.

Howell, M. 1974. What medical schools teach about women. *The New England Journal of Medicine* 291(6):304–7.

Jansen, M., and R. Wellons. 1983. Task group on women and ethnic minorities. *Health Psychology,* 2(5):103–6.

Jarnfelt, A. 1982. Paper presented at the World Congress of Gynecology and Obstetrics. *Women and Health Roundtable Report,* section VI, p. 10.

Kasper, A. S. 1980. Nausea of pregnancy: A historical medical prejudice. *Women and Health* 5(1):35–43.

Kirscht, J. P., and I. M. Rosenstock. 1979. Patients' problems in following recommendations of health experts. In *Health psychology,* edited by G. C. Stone, F. Cohen, and N. E. Adler. San Francisco: Jossey-Bass.

Korsch, B. M., and V. F. Negrete. 1972. Doctor-patient communication. *Scientific American* 227(2):66–74.

Kutner, N. G., and D. R. Brogan. 1980. Persistent sources of sex-role related stress among women medical students. *International Journal of Women's Studies* 3(1):19–27.

Larned, D. 1977. The epidemic in unnecessary hysterectomy. In *Seizing our bodies,* edited by C. Dreifus. New York: Vintage Books.

Leserman, J. 1981. *Men and women in medical school.* New York: Praeger.

Lewis, C. E., and M. A. Lewis. 1977. The potential impact of sexual equality on health. *New England Journal of Medicine* 297:863–69.

McBride, A. B., and W. L. McBride. 1981. Theoretical underpinnings for women's health. *Women and Health* 6(1/2):37–49.

McKinlay, J. B. 1975. Who is really ignorant? *Journal of Health and Social Behavior* 16(1):3–11.

Marieskind, H. I. 1980. *Women in the health system.* St. Louis: C. V. Mosby Co.

Moore, E. C. 1980. Women and health, United States, 1980. *Public Health Reports,* a supplement to the September-October issue 1–84. Washington, D.C.

National Center for Health Statistics. 1978. *Chartbook for the conference on the decline in coronary heart disease.* Hyattsville, MD.

———. 1982. *Health, United States.* DHHS Publication no. (PHS) 83–1232. Washington, D.C.: U.S. Government Printing Office.

Novak, E. R. 1970. *Novak's textbook of gynecology.* Baltimore: Williams & Wilkins Co.

Rosenfield, S. 1982. Sex roles and societal reactions to mental illness: The labeling of "deviant" deviance. *Journal of Health and Social Behavior* 23(1):18–24.

Scott, C. R. 1968. *The world of a gynecologist.* London: Oliver & Boyd.

Seaman, B. 1980. *The doctors' case against the pill.* 2d ed. New York: Doubleday.

Seaman, B., and G. Seaman. 1977. *Women and the crisis in sex hormones.* New York: Rawson.

Starr, P. 1982. *The Social Transformation of American Medicine.* New York: Basic Books.

Strickland, B. R. 1978. Internal-external expectancies and health-related behaviors. *Journal of Consulting and Clinical Psychology* 46:1192–1211.

Svarstad, B. 1976. Physician-patient communication and patient conformity with medical advice. In *The growth of bureaucratic medicine,* edited by D. Mechanic. New York: Wiley.

Todd, A. D. 1984. The prescription of contraception: Negotiations between doctors and patients. *Discourse Processes* 7:2.

U.S. Department of Health and Human Services. 1982. *Detailed diagnosis and surgical procedures for patients discharged from short stay hospitals.* DHHS Publication no. (PHS) 82–12741. Washington, D.C.: U.S. Government Printing Office.

———. 1983. *Inventory and analysis of federal population research.* DHHS Publication no. (NIH) 83–133. Washington, D.C.: U.S. Government Printing Office.

Verbrugge, L. M. 1982. Women's social roles and health. In *Women: A developmental perspective,* edited by P. W. Bergman and E. R. Ramey. U.S. Department of Health and Human Services, Public Health Service NIH Publication no. 82–2298.

———. 1983. Multiple roles and physical health of women and men. *Journal of Health and Social Behavior* 24(1):16–30.

Wallen, J., H. Waitzkin, and J. Stoeckle. 1979. Physician stereotypes about female health and illness: A study of patients' sex and informative process during medical interviews. *Women and Health* 4(2):135–46.

Walsh, M. R. 1977. *Doctors wanted, No women need apply: Sexual barriers in the medical profession, 1835–1975.* New Haven: Yale University Press.

Weissman, M., and G. Klerman. 1977. Sex differences in the epidemiology of depression. *Archives of General Psychiatry* 34:98–111.

Wilson, J. R., and E. R. Carrington. 1979. *Obstetrics and gynecology.* 6th ed. St. Louis: C. V. Mosby Company.

Wolcott, I. 1979. Women and psychoactive drug use. *Women and Health* 4(2):199–202.

Women and Health Roundtable. 1979. Federally sponsored contraception research and evaluation projects. *Roundtable Report* 3:2, 3.

Women's Bureau. 1983. *Twenty facts about women workers.* U.S. Dept. of Labor. Washington, D.C.: U.S. Government Printing Office.

19

Race, Ethnicity, and Health Psychology: The Example of Essential Hypertension

Norman B. Anderson and James S. Jackson

The field of behavioral medicine, particularly health psychology, has grown phenomenally in a relatively brief period (Krantz, Grunberg, and Baum 1985; Matarazzo 1980; Miller 1983). Work within health psychology on factors affecting physical health and illness include stress, psychoneuro-immunology, cardiovascular disorders, health damaging behaviors, compliance, and primary prevention. Very little of this extensive literature, however, has focused on racial and ethnic minorities. This lack of attention is problematic for at least two reasons. First, members of racial and ethnic groups within this society have higher incidence and prevalence rates for a large number of diseases and physical illnesses (Jackson 1981; Harwood 1981; Hamburg, Elliott, and Parron 1982; National Center for Health Statistics 1984; U.S. Department of Health and Human Services 1985). Second, a great deal of research points to the existence of sociocultural and socioeconomic differences in behavior and reactions to illness, both among and within racial and ethnic groups, that have implications for physical health and illness (Harwood 1981; Hamburg, Elliott, and Parron 1982). These two considerations suggest that health psychology models should be sensitive to the variation between and within racial and ethnic groups. Before such general models can be developed, however, understanding is needed of the factors related to physical health, health behaviors, and biological processes within the major racial and ethnic groups (Harwood 1981).

The population growth of racial and ethnic groups in the United States over the last fifteen years has been significant (U.S. Department of Health and Human Services 1980; American Public Health Association 1982). The major groups (blacks, Asian Americans, Hispanic, and Native Americans) now constitute approximately 23.1 percent of the U.S. population. In some regions of the country, racial and ethnic minorities represent a larger proportion of the population than white Americans. Much of this growth is due to the influx of immigrants, as well as greater fertility in some groups. The most recent Census information (National Center for Health Statistics 1984) indicates that blacks in 1980 represented 11.7 percent, Hispanics 6.4 percent, Asians 1.5 percent, and Native Americans approximately 0.6 percent of the total U.S. population. For all racial and ethnic groups, recent statistics show wide disparities, in comparison to whites, in morbidity, mortality, and health care utilization (American Public Health Association 1982; National Center for Health Statistics 1984; U.S. Department of Health and Human Services 1980).

Clearly, some of the racial and ethnic disparities in physical health, physical illness, and service utilization can be attributed to significant deficits in socioeconomic status among many minority group members (U.S. Department of Health and Human Services 1980; Hamburg, Elliott, and Parron 1982). Thus, while many of the racial and ethnic differences in health behavior (Baquet 1985), in attitudes and barriers to health care utilization (Woolander et al. 1985), and reactions to illness (Wolinsky 1982) may decrease as the socioeconomic status of disadvantaged minorities improves, many differences may remain (Anderson, Kravitis, and Anderson 1975). This would suggest the need for greater attention to sociocultural factors above and beyond socioeconomic status, as well as to the interface between the individual and the health care system (Stone 1982).

In discussing health psychology issues for minority groups, a difficulty immediately encountered is that not only is there considerable variation across racial and ethnic groups, but also within ethnic groups. This variation can take the form of observed differences in the prevalence rates of certain illnesses (Bullough and Bullough 1972; Shiloh and Selavan 1973), as well as in health beliefs and health behaviors within and across groups (Adair and Deuschle 1970; Anderson et al. 1975; Weaver 1970). Given this heterogeneity, one must caution against drawing general conclusions concerning the needs or issues relevant to "minority groups" without being sensitive to the often large intragroup variability. Yet, it is beyond the scope of this chapter to address comprehensively the health psychology issues for each ethnic group, as well as the complex intragroup differences in attitudes and behavior related to health. Therefore, we have chosen to illustrate the potential role and value of health psychology in the health status of racial and ethnic minorities by focusing on a health problem of particular importance to black Americans, essential hypertension.

The choice of hypertension as an illustrative example implies neither that it is the only health problem facing blacks, nor that it is necessarily the most significant health problem in other racial and ethnic minorities. However, a detailed examination of essential hypertension in blacks, as a way of illuminating the potential role of health psychology in blacks and other racial and ethnic groups, is attractive for several reasons.

First of all, essential hypertension is a common problem in the general population, affecting 18 percent of adults between the ages of 25 and 74 (Roberts and Rowland 1981). Yet, blacks are roughly twice as prone to develop hypertension as whites. The hypertension rate is roughly 18.1 per 100 for white males ages 25 to 74, as compared to a rate of 35.3 per 100 for black males of the same ages. Similarly, the rate for white females between the ages of 25 and 74 is 14.8 per 100 compared to 29.7 per 100 for black females (Roberts and Rowland 1981). Moreover, blacks with hypertension between the ages of 33 and 54 are six to ten times more likely than whites to suffer from the hypertensive vascular diseases (National Center for Health Statistics 1984), a rate far out of proportion to the approximate two times excess of hypertension in blacks (Gillum 1979). Thus, it is not surprising that hypertension is frequently considered the number one health problem among blacks today (Saunders and Williams 1975).

Another reason essential hypertension is a particularly useful example is that health psychologists have already made significant contributions to the research on and treatment of essential hypertension. Psychologists have been instrumental in proposing and studying the mechanisms by which behavior might contribute to hypertension development (Obrist 1981), as well as identifying and evaluating nonpharmacologic treatment approaches (Surwit, Williams, and Shapiro 1982). Despite this involvement by health psychologists, very little scientific and applied attention has been directed toward hypertension in black populations. As illustrated in this chapter, there may be important racial differences in the dimensions of hypertension at four different levels of analysis: biological, psychological, social/environmental, and applied. These considerations suggest the need for new models and hypotheses concerning the etiology, maintenance, and treatment of hypertension in blacks and in the general population.

Using essential hypertension as an example is also attractive because clinical health psychologists employed in medical centers which serve large numbers of blacks will likely encounter this disorder in their patients. It is thus imperative that health psychologists have an understanding of the features of the disorder as exhibited by black patients, as well as the associated treatment implications.

Finally, essential hypertension in blacks serves as an instructive example since many of the important components of hypertension (i.e., biological, psychological, and social/environmental) are also important aspects of other disorders across all racial and ethnic minority groups. For example, many forms of cancer are more prevalent in certain ethnic groups than in others (Young, Ries, and Pollack 1984). Additionally, there are considerable ethnic and racial differences in cancer mortality, even with similar cancer sites (Baquet 1985). Adequate explanations for these discrepancies will no doubt require consideration of biological as well as behavioral and social/environmental factors.

The next section provides an overview of essential hypertension in blacks, concentrating on the components of the problem which are particularly important from a health psychology perspective. Four areas will be discussed: biological issues, behavioral and psychological issues, social and environmental factors, and applied issues. Within each area, a brief review of the current state of knowledge related to hypertension in blacks will be presented, along with recommendations for health psychology research to help clarify unresolved issues. It should be emphasized that this partitioning of the various aspects of hypertension is solely for organizational purposes. The status of any one of the components of the disorder is partially determined by its interaction with the others. Thus, each area is viewed both as influencing and being influenced by the other areas.

Essential Hypertension in Blacks: Health Psychology Issues
BIOLOGICAL ISSUES

Essential hypertension is a disorder of unknown origin. However, it is generally agreed that the onset of sustained high blood pressure could involve any number of pathophysiological mechanisms (Page 1960). Studies on the pathophysiological basis of hypertension in blacks have centered primarily on two factors which are generally believed to be critical to blood pressure regulation and hypertension development: the autonomic nervous system, particularly the sympathetic branch, and sodium regulatory mechanisms operating through the kidney. Biobehavioral researchers, however, have heretofore concentrated their attention on the sympathetic nervous system. Therefore, we will center our discussion on this system. Most studies on sympathetic involvement in black hypertension have been designed to compare black and white hypertensives and/or normotensives on activity within this system.

Sympathetic Nervous System (SNS) Activity

The role of the SNS in essential hypertension has been evaluated primarily through the measurement of plasma norepinephrine (NE) which is released via sympathetic nerve endings and from the adrenal medulla (Guyton 1981). Norepinephrine acts to raise blood pressure by causing blood vessels to constrict, producing greater resistance against the circulation, and hence, elevating blood pressure. Plasma norepinephrine has been found to be elevated in many patients with essential hypertension (Goldstein 1981) and is believed to play a key etiological role in hypertension development in certain subgroups of patients (de Champlain, Cousineau, and Lapointe 1980).

In order to determine whether heightened NE levels are important in racial differences in hypertension, a number of studies have examined plasma NE levels in groups of black and white hypertensives and normotensives (Jones, Hamilton, and Reid 1978; Rowlands et al. 1982; Sever et al. 1979). These studies have generally not provided evidence of higher resting sympathetic nervous system activity in blacks. Using factory workers, Sever et al. (1979) found no black/white differences in NE activity, although NE increased with age in both groups. Rowlands et al. (1982) examined resting NE levels in sixteen untreated blacks with mild to moderate hypertension and sixteen white hypertensives matched on age, sex, casual blood pressure, and socioeconomic status. Again, no differences were found between racial groups. In light of the consistent failure to demonstrate higher levels among blacks, it has been suggested that sympathetic overactivity as measured by resting NE is not a feature of hypertension in blacks and probably is not a contributor to the racial differences in morbidity rates.

Another index of SNS functioning, plasma renin, has also been examined in relation to hypertension in blacks. Renin is released by the kidneys in response to SNS activity, as well as to numerous other factors (Vick 1984). Once released, renin aids in the production of angiotensin II, a powerful vasoconstrictor, which in turn increases arterial pressure. Renin has been implicated as a contributor to elevated blood pressure and hypertension (Brunner, Sealey, and Laragh 1973). Studies have consistently shown racial differences in plasma renin activity but not in the expected direction. Blacks with hypertension, more frequently than whites, exhibit *low plasma renin* levels. It has been noted that roughly 36 to 62 percent of black hypertensives have relatively suppressed renin levels as compared to 19 to 55 percent of white hypertensives (Gillum 1979; Wisenbaugh et al. 1972). In sum, the plasma renin studies suggest that certain aspects of the SNS may be inhibited rather than overexcited in blacks.

Although most of the studies reviewed above have come from biomedical research, biobehavioral scientists have also been active in the theorizing and research on the biological mechanisms involved in hypertension. The focus, however, has been on the influence of behavior and environmental stressors on transient increases in SNS activity. The importance of these transient situational changes in SNS activity grew out of animal research by James Henry and others which demonstrated that factors such as territorial conflict, crowding, and other psychosocial stressors produced sustained high blood pressure (Henry and Cassel 1969). This sustained high blood pressure has been shown to be preceded by transient activation of the "defense alarm" or "fight-flight" pattern of beta-adrenergically mediated sympathetic outflow. Stimulation of the beta-adrenergic branch of the SNS produces increases in heart rate, blood pressure, catecholamine and renin release, and muscle vasodilation. It has been hypothesized that repeated elicitation of this response, when incongruent with metabolic needs, might ultimately lead to sustained high blood pressure (Charvat, Dell, and Folkow 1964; Obrist 1981).

In human studies, there have been repeated demonstrations that heightened SNS reactivity to behavioral challenges is present among hypertensives compared to normotensives (Brod et al. 1959; Hollenberg, Williams, and Adams 1981; Fredrikson et al. 1985). Further, there is evidence indicating that exaggerated SNS mediated cardiovascular responses to behavioral challenges (e.g., mental arithmetic, shock avoidance reaction time) precedes the onset of hypertension in persons with a genetic predisposition to the disorder (Hastrup, Light, and Obrist 1982; Jorgensen and Houston 1981; Manuck and Proietti 1982). Most of these experiments have shown that young white males or females with a parental history of hypertension exhibit heightened blood pressure or heart rate responses compared to those subjects who have no family history. There is some evidence from the previously cited psychophysiological studies that beta-adrenergically mediated cardiovascular reactivity to behavioral stressors may be important in hypertension development in whites. Published reports, however, were not found which examined this association in blacks.

Several recently completed studies suggest the presence of racial differences in patterns of SNS reactivity to stressors. Fredrikson (forthcoming) examined SNS reactivity during an aversive reaction time task in three groups of black and white subjects: established hypertensives, borderline hypertensives, and normotensive controls. Fredrikson found that while resting cardiovascular activity was similar in black and white hypertensives and controls, heart rate and systolic blood pressure increased less in black patients and controls compared to whites. However, muscle vascular resistance increased more in the black subjects, suggesting enhanced vasoconstriction. Similarly, Anderson, Muranaku, Williams, and Lane (1986) explored potential racial differences in vasoconstrictive responses in black and white normotensives. Measures of blood pressure, heart rate, forearm blood flow, and forearm vascular resistance were taken during a resting baseline and while subjects had an ice pack placed on their foreheads. This maneuver has been shown to elicit a profound peripheral vasoconstriction (Abboud and Eckstein 1966). In response to the cold stimulus, black subjects exhibited significantly greater systolic, diastolic, and forearm vascular resistance increases than white subjects. No racial differences were observed on heart rate, suggesting perhaps greater vascular as opposed to cardiac sensitivity in blacks. Finally, Anderson, Williams, Lane, and Houseworth (1985), studied cardiovascular reactivity to a mental arithmetic task in a group of young normotensive black women divided on family history of hypertension. Unlike the findings with white subjects, females with a family history of hypertension exhibited significantly lower cardiovascular responses than their counterparts who did not have a family history of the disorder. In light of these preliminary findings, it seems necessary to determine whether in fact the relationships between behavioral stressors and the SNS observed in whites is the same in blacks and to speculate as to the relevance of these potential differences to essential hypertension development.

Other Biological Factors

Space limitations do not allow for a detailed overview of the abundance of other physiological factors which have been explored in blacks that may be related to hypertension development. However, some mention of one of these factors, sodium retention, is warranted since striking racial differences have been noted on this variable, and it may be affected by behavioral psychosocial factors. Sodium and water regulation by the kidneys is felt to be crucial to maintaining appropriate blood volume. Yet, inhibited excretion of sodium results in volume expansion and augmented blood pressure (Vick 1984). Luft, Grim, and associates at Indiana University have conducted a series of studies on sodium homeostasis in blacks (for review see Luft, Grim, and Weinberger 1985). Using protocols involving the administration of fixed amounts of sodium (sodium load) to normotensive subjects, these researchers found several racial differences in the effects of this procedure. Following sodium loading black subjects have been shown to excrete less sodium in urine and exhibit greater blood pressure increases than their white counterparts (Luft et al. 1977; Luft et al. 1985). Although genetic explanations have been proposed (Helmer 1967), the results from salt loading studies are potentially relevant for health psychologists working in the hypertension field. For example, Light, Koepke, Obrist, and Willis (1982) found that behavioral stressors can actually inhibit sodium excretion in white subjects who have a family history of hypertension. One might speculate as to the role of environmental and behavioral stressors in the enhanced sodium retention in blacks. For example, environmental stressors might be particularly hazardous among blacks, since they seem to already possess exaggerated sodium retention mechanisms.

In summary, the literature on biological factors in hypertension and blood pressure control appear to support the notion of important racial differences in certain pathophysiological characteristics of the disorder. These differences have been found primarily in plasma renin activity and response to sodium administration. Preliminary results from psychophysiological studies on cardiovascular responses to behavioral stress indicate the possibility of important racial differences in patterns of cardiovascular adjustment. Health psychologists conducting basic research on hypertension could contribute to our knowledge and understanding of mechanisms involved in black hypertension. Stress reactivity paradigms could be used to examine simultaneously several potentially important factors: environmental (e.g., various types of stressors), genetic (e.g., family history of hypertension), and biological (SNS reactivity, sodium excretion). Research designs should be used which not only explore potential differences between black and whites, but which also examine variation within black populations. This would permit an identification of those black individuals who may be most prone to develop hypertension.

BEHAVIORAL AND PSYCHOLOGICAL ISSUES

Research on the role of behavioral and personality factors and essential hypertension has had a long history. Alexander (1939) hypothesized that hypertensive patients were characterized by an inability to express anger, often labeled as suppressed hostility. The suppressed hostility hypothesis has been a consistent theme over the years in personality research related to hypertension. The results, however, have been far from conclusive. Most of the studies on personality factors in hypertension have been conducted using predominantly white samples; only a few have examined behavioral and personality factors among black hypertensives.

The most significant work related to the idea that suppressed hostility may be involved in hypertension among blacks comes from the epidemiologic studies conducted in Detroit by Harburg and associates (Harburg et al. 1973; Harburg, Blakelock, and Roeper 1979). These studies were based on community samples of black and white subjects residing in either high or low socioecological stress areas. (The socioecological stress concept will be discussed in the next section.) In the initial study (Harburg et al. 1973), suppressed hostility was determined by the subjects' responses to two hypothetical situations: being verbally attacked by a police officer unjustifiably and experiencing housing discrimination. For both black and white males residing in high-stress residential areas, a tendency to not express anger when provoked (anger-in) was associated with higher mean diastolic pressures and a greater prevalence of documented hypertension compared to subjects who reported an anger-out coping style. A similar study by Gentry, Chesney, Gary, Hall, and Harburg (1982) suggested that the "anger-in" or suppressed hostility hypothesis may also be relevant with black and white females. All the findings, however, have not been supportive of a simple "anger-in" high blood pressure relationship. Johnson and Broman (1985) found in a national sample of black adults that anger expression was associated complexly to increased health problems. Blacks who were unemployed, single, and possessed less than a high school education were particularly at risk if anger was expressed outwardly at high levels during periods of emotional distress.

Recently, Sherman James hypothesized that a stress coping style labeled "John Henryism" may be a key behavioral factor in hypertension development, particularly among blacks (see James 1984b for review). This active coping style was named after the legendary black American folk hero, John Henry, who epitomized hard work and determination against overwhelming odds. James speculated that individual blacks who exhibit this type of determination but who also have few resources to help them succeed (i.e., low levels of formal education) might be at greatest risk for hypertension development. This hypothesis was tested in an epidemiologic study in rural North Carolina using black males (James, Hartnett, and Kalsbeek 1983). It was found that men who scored below the median on formal education (less than or equal to eleven years) but above the sample median on John Henryism had the highest mean blood pressure levels.

In summary, the research on behavioral and psychological factors and hypertension among blacks has identified two potential contributors: suppressed hostility/anger-in and John Henryism. Although several published studies have supported a relationship between suppressed hostility and resting blood pressure in hypertension among blacks, more research is needed to clarify the nature of this relationship. Prospective epidemiological studies may help to determine whether in fact suppressed hostility is a risk factor for the subsequent development of hypertension. It would also be useful to clarify some of the biological mechanisms whereby suppressed hostility or anger-in leads to elevated blood pressure levels among blacks. Field studies could examine 24-hour blood pressure and neuroendocrine reactivity, as well as 24-hour sodium excretion among blacks reporting anger-in vs. anger-out coping styles.

Understanding these underlying biological mechanisms is important. As reviewed in the previous section, the development of hypertension may involve different biological mechanisms in blacks as compared to whites. Differences in biological mechanisms suggest that the relationship between personality factors and pathophysiologic mechanisms may be different as well. For example, data from white hypertensives indicate that those individuals with high renin essential hypertension are more often characterized by an anger-in coping style compared to individuals with low renin hypertension (Esler et al. 1977). Yet, black hypertensives tend to have *low renin* hypertension, which apparently is not associated with anger-in among whites. Finally, the John Henryism concept shows early promise as a possible behavioral risk factor for hypertension development.

SOCIAL AND ENVIRONMENTAL ISSUES

Numerous sociocultural and environmental factors have been examined in relation to hypertension in blacks, such as socioeconomic status (SES), stressful living conditions, and career mobility (Myers 1984; Michaels 1983; James 1984a; Kasl 1984). The sociocultural factor that has received the most attention is SES, as measured by income, occupation, or education (James 1984b, 1984c; Kasl 1984; McDonald 1984). Consistent with the general health literature, the major research focus has been on whether SES, as measured by income or education, can explain race differences in hypertension prevalence. Studies have generally found that although the discrepancy between blacks and whites in the prevalence of hypertension is reduced when income and education are similar, the differences are not totally eliminated (Hypertension Detection and Follow-Up Program 1977).

Harburg (1978) conducted some of the more notable research on environmental factors by demonstrating that high-stress geographical areas are related to elevated blood pressure in blacks. High-stress neighborhoods in Detroit were defined as those which were low in SES (low income, high unemployment) and high in social instability (SIS) (high crime rate, high divorce rate, etc.). Low stress areas were defined as high SES and low SIS. In a series of studies, Harburg and his co-workers found that black males residing in high-stress areas had significantly higher age- and weight-adjusted blood pressures than those living in low-stress areas (Harburg et al. 1973). This relationship was not found for white males. The highest blood pressures were found in those black males in high-stress areas who also exhibited an anger-in coping style (Gentry et al. 1982).

Another major area of investigation in the biobehavioral sciences in recent years has been the function of social networks and social support in alleviating the effects of stress, promoting health behavior, and enhancing health outcomes (Berkman 1985; Hamburg et al. 1982). While there has been a plethora of research devoted to examining this issue (Baum, Singer, and Taylor 1984), little of this research has been devoted to racial and ethnic minority groups. Only a few studies have examined the effects of social support on blacks and hypertension, and these have been poorly controlled and largely atheoretical (James 1984b). That social support is important for racial and ethnic minorities is suggested by the role that extended families are thought to play in the lives of minority group members (Jackson 1981). Exploration of the effects of social support systems on hypertension development and progression in blacks is therefore a critical area for future research.

APPLIED ISSUES

Health psychology issues in the treatment of essential hypertension among blacks will be discussed in this section. Two issues will be addressed: compliance with medical treatment regimens and nonpharmacologic treatments.

Compliance with Treatment Regimens

Much of the research on patient compliance to hypertensive therapy has been summarized by Blackwell (1979). In summarizing this literature, Blackwell noted several factors which tend to decrease adherence to medical management, including the complexity of their treatment regimen and the degree of behavior change required of the patient. Factors that tended to increase patient adherence were patients' perception of the seriousness of their disease, family stability, and close supervision of compliance behavior by the physician. Although compliance with medical management is considered a problem among black hypertensives, very little research has focused on ways of improving compliance in this group. Cook (1984) has made several suggestions for improving compliance among black hypertensives. He emphasized factors such as the use of repeated motivational sessions, prompt scheduling of reappointments, the inclusion of significant others, follow-up visits, and periodic telephone contacts. Of course, many of these factors may be important in improving patient compliance regardless of race. Future research should be directed toward evaluating the efficacy of existing adherence strategies with black hypertensives, particularly low SES patients.

Nonpharmacologic Treatment

Health psychologists have been involved for a number of years in the treatment of essential hypertension through the use of relaxation training techniques such as progressive relaxation, autogenic training, mediation, and yoga. The goals of these relaxation techniques are to reduce mental and physical stress that may contribute to elevated blood pressure. Additionally, various forms of biofeedback have also been evaluated either alone, or in conjunction with relaxation training.

Outcome studies of relaxation and biofeedback have not to date included sizeable numbers of black patients. There is a great need to evaluate the effectiveness of relaxation and biofeedback in black hypertensives. To the degree that environmental stress contributes to blood pressure elevations in blacks (cf. Harburg et al. 1973), relaxation training could play a role in attenuating these noxious effects. From physiological perspective, however, it is unclear whether relaxation or biofeedback will affect significantly the pathophysiology of hypertension in blacks. For example, it has been suggested that relaxation techniques work to decrease blood pressure through reducing sympathetic nervous system activity (Lehmann and Benson 1982). As noted previously, hypertension in blacks may be characterized by an inhibition in some aspects of the sympathetic nervous system. Indeed, pharmacologic studies suggest that medications which act to decrease sympathetic nervous system activity, such as beta blockers, are significantly less effective in blacks as compared to whites (Veterans Cooperative Study 1982). Identifying pathophysiological predictors of response to relaxation training in both black and white hypertensives is clearly an important direction for future research.

Besides relaxation training and biofeedback, clinical health psychologists can have an impact on hypertension in blacks in numerous other ways. For example, there is strong epidemiologic evidence of a relationship between obesity and the prevalence of hypertension (Kannel et al. 1967). The prevalence of obesity is significantly higher among black women compared to white females and black and white males (U.S. Department of Health and Human Services 1980). Given the high prevalence of obesity among blacks, the evaluation of behavior modification techniques by health psychologists with this population seems warranted. Psychologists should be cognizant, however, of the potential racial differences in the effectiveness of weight reduction programs as a means of controlling hypertension. For example, two large-scale epidemiologic studies from Evans County, Georgia (Tyroler, Heyden, and Hames 1975) and the Charleston Heart Study, (Boyle et al. 1967) indicate that changes in weight result in greater changes in blood pressure among whites than in blacks.

Numerous studies have found an association between sodium intake and elevated blood pressure in both laboratory animals and humans (Dahl 1972). Despite ancedotal observations to the contrary, Gillum (1979) notes that there is little objective documentation of higher sodium intakes among black Americans as a contributor to the high rates of essential hypertension. Epidemiologic studies have found the sodium intake of blacks and whites to be either similar or less among blacks (Grim et al. 1970; Langford, Watson, and Douglas 1968). Yet, from the biological studies reported earlier, it is important to remember that renal sodium *conservation* may be greater in blacks as compared to whites. This suggests that given the same or equal amounts of sodium intake, the effects on blood pressure may be greater among blacks. Therefore, the need to develop effective techniques for regulating dietary sodium intake is a potentially fruitful avenue for health psychology clinicians and researchers.

Summary and Conclusions

The goal of this chapter was to illustrate, through a representative example, a health psychology perspective on major health problems in racial and ethnic minority groups. Essential hypertension in black Americans was the health problem selected as an example. The four dimensions summarized— biological, behavioral, social/environmental and applied—were felt to be particularly relevant to researchers and clinicians in health psychology. Although a great deal of research has been directed toward each of these factors in relation to hypertension in general, very little work has been devoted to how these dimensions operate among black hypertensives in particular.

Unfortunately, it is a case where the group most at risk has been the least studied. The research that has been done is suggestive of important racial differences in the expression of these dimensions. The field of health psychology, because of its multidimensional orientation toward health care, can be influential in understanding and integrating the aspects of essential hypertension in blacks as outlined in this chapter. A similar approach should be taken with other health problems in other racial and ethnic minority groups.

REFERENCES

Abboud, F. M., and J. W. Eckstein. 1966. Active reflex vasodilation in man. *Federation Proceedings* 25 : 1611–17.

Adair, John, and K. Deuschle. 1970. *The people's health.* New York: Appleton-Century-Crofts.

Alexander, F. G. 1939. Emotional factors in essential hypertension: Presentation of a tentative hypothesis. *Psychosomatic Medicine* 1 : 175–79.

American Public Health Association. 1982. *Health of minorities and women: Chartbook* (Publication no. 072). Washington, D.C.

Anderson, N. B.; M. Muranaku; R. B. Williams, Jr.; and J. D. Lane. 1986. *Peripheral vasoconstriction to cold stress in black and white males.* Unpublished manuscript. Durham, NC: Duke University Medical Center, Department of Psychiatry.

Anderson, N. B., R. B. Williams, J. D. Lane, and S. A. Houseworth. 1986. Family history of hypertension and cardiovascular responses in young black women. Paper presented at the annual meeting of the Society of Behavioral Medicine, San Francisco, CA.

Anderson, R., J. Kravits, and O. Anderson, eds. 1975. *Equity in health services: Empirical analyses in social policy.* Cambridge, MA: Ballinger.

Baquet, C. 1985. *Subcommittee on cancer in minorities report* (Cancer Control Applications Branch, Division of Cancer Prevention and Control, National Cancer Institute). Washington, D.C.: National Cancer Institute.

Baum, A., J. E. Singer, and S. E. Taylor, eds. 1984. *Handbook of psychology and health.* Vol. 4: *Social psychological aspects of health.* Hillsdale, NJ: Erlbaum and Associates.

Berkman, L. F. 1985. The relationship of social networks and social support to morbidity and mortality. In *Social support and health,* edited by S. Cohen and L. Syme, 241–62. New York: Academic Press.

Blackwell, B. 1979. The drug regimen and treatment compliance. In *Compliance in health care,* edited by R. B. Haynes, D. W. Taylor, and D. L. Sackett. Baltimore: Johns Hopkins Press.

Boyle, E., Jr.; W. P. Griffey, Jr.; M. Z. Nichaman; and C. R. Talbert, Jr. 1967. An epidemiologic study of hypertension among racial groups of Charleston County,

South Carolina: The Charleston heart study, phase II. In *The epidemiology of hypertension,* edited by J. Stamler, S. Stamler, and T. N. Pullman, 193–203. New York: Grune and Stratton.

Brod, J., V. Fencl, Z. Hejl, and G. Jorka. 1959. Circulatory changes underlying blood pressure elevation during acute emotional stress (mental arithmetic) in normotensive and hypertensive subjects. *Clinical Science* 23:339–49.

Brunner, H. R., J. E. Sealey, J. H. Laragh. 1973. Renin as a risk factor in essential hypertension: More evidence. *American Journal of Medicine* 55:295–302.

Bullough, B., and V. L. Bullough. 1972. *Poverty, ethnic identity, and health care.* New York: Appleton-Century-Crofts.

Charvat, J., P. Dell, and B. Folkow. 1964. Mental factors and cardiovascular diseases. *Cardiologia* 44:124–41.

Cook, C. A. 1983. *Working group noncompliance in black male hypertensives: Summary report.* Unpublished manuscript. Washington, D.C.: Dynamic Programs, Inc.

———. 1984. Antihypertensive drug compliance in black males. *Journal of the National Medical Association* 76:40–46, supplement section.

Dahl, L. K. 1972. Salt and hypertension. *American Journal of Clinical Nutrition* 25:231–44.

de Champlain, J., D. Cousineau, L. Lapointe. 1980. Evidences supporting an increased sympathetic tone and reactivity in a subgroup of patients with essential hypertension. *Clinical Experimental Hypertension* 2:359.

Esler, M., S. Julius, O. Randall, E. Harburg, H. Gardiner, and V. DeQuathlo. 1977. Mild high-renin essential hypertension: Neurologic human hypertension? *New England Journal of Medicine* 296:405–11.

Fredrikson, M. (forthcoming). Racial differences in reactivity to behavioral challenge in essential hypertension. *Hypertension.*

Fredrikson, M., U. Dimberg, M. Frisk-Holmberg, and G. Strom. 1985. Arterial blood pressure and general sympathetic activation in essential hypertension during stimulation. *Acta Medica Scandinavica* 217:309–17.

Gentry, W. D., A. P. Chesney, H. E. Gary, R. P. Hall, and E. Harburg. 1982. Habitual anger-coping styles: Effect on mean blood pressure and risk for essential hypertension. *Psychosomatic Medicine* 44:195–202.

Gillum, R. T. 1979. Pathophysiology of hypertension in blacks and whites: A review of the basis of racial blood pressure differences. *Hypertension* 1:468–75.

Goldstein, D. S. 1981. Plasma norepinephrine in essential hypertension: A study of the studies. *Hypertension* 3:48.

Grim, C. E.; J. McDonough, Jr., L. K. Dahl; and C. G. Hames. 1970. On the higher blood pressure of blacks: A study of sodium and potassium intake and excretion in a biracial community. *Clinical Research* 18:593.

Guyton, A. 1981. *Textbook of medical physiology.* Philadelphia: W. B. Saunders Co.

Hamburg, D. A., G. R. Elliott, and D. L. Parron, eds. 1982. *Health and behavior: Frontiers of research in the biobehavioral sciences* (IOM Publication no. 82–01). Washington, D.C.: National Academy Press.

Harburg, E. 1978. Skin color, ethnicity and blood pressure in Detroit blacks. *American Journal of Public Health* 68:1177–83.

Harburg, E., E. H. Blakelock, and P. J. Roeper. 1979. Resentful and reflective coping with arbitrary authority and blood pressure: Detroit. *Psychosomatic Medicine* 41:189–202.

Harburg, E., J. C. Erfurt, L. S. Hauenstein, C. Chape, W. J. Schull, and M. A. Schork. 1973. Socioecological stress, suppressed hostility, skin color, and black-white male blood pressure: Detroit. *Psychosomatic Medicine* 35:276–96.

Harwood, A., ed. 1981. *Ethnicity and medical care.* Cambridge, MA: Harvard University Press.

Hastrup, J., K. C. Light, and P. A. Obrist. 1982. Parental hypertension and cardiovascular response to stress in healthy young adults. *Psychophysiology* 19: 615–23.

Helmer, O. M. 1967. Hormonal and biochemical factors controlling blood pressure. In *Les Concepts de Claude Bernard aur le Milieu Intérieur,* 15–128. Paris: Libraries de l'Academie de Medicine.

Henry, J. P., and J. Cassel. 1969. Psychosocial factors in essential hypertension: Recent epidemiologic and animal experimental evidence. *American Journal of Epidemiology* 90:171–200.

Hollenberg, N. K., G. H. Williams, and D. F. Adams. 1981. Essential hypertension: Abnormal renal vascular and endocrine responses to a mild psychological stimulus. *Hypertension* 3(11): 17.

Hypertension Detection and Follow-up Program Cooperative Group: Race, education and prevalence of hypertension. 1977. *American Journal of Epidemiology* 106:351–61.

Iscoe, I. 1982. Toward a viable community health psychology: Caveats from the experiences of the community mental health movement. *American Psychologist* 37:961–65.

Jackson, J. J. 1981. Urban black Americans. In *Ethnicity and medical care,* edited by A. Harwood, 37–129. Cambridge, MA: Harvard University Press.

James, S. A. 1984a. Socioeconomic influences on coronary heart disease in black populations. *American Heart Journal* 108 (no. 3, pt. 2): 669–71.

———. 1984b. Coronary heart disease in black Americans: Suggestions for research on psychosocial factors. *American Heart Journal* 108 (no. 3, pt. 2): 833–38.

———. 1984c. Psychosocial and environmental factors in black hypertension. In *Hypertension in blacks: Epidemiology, pathophysiology, and treatment,* edited by W. Hall, E. Saunders, and N. Shulman. Chicago: Year Book Publishers, Inc.

James, S. A., S. A. Hartnett, and W. D. Kalsbeek. 1983. John Henryism and blood pressure differences among black men. *Journal of Behavioral Medicine* 6: 259–78.

James, S. A., E. H. Wagner, D. S. Strogatz, S. A. Beresford, D. G. Kleinbaum, C. A. Williams, L. M. Cutchin, and M. A. Ibrahim. 1984. The Edgecombe County (NC) high blood pressure control program: II. Barriers to the use of medical care among hypertensives. *American Journal of Public Health* 74:468–72.

Johnson, E. H., and C. L. Broman. 1985. *Anger expression and health problems among black Americans: A report from the national survey of black Americans.* Unpublished manuscript. Department of Internal Medicine, University of Michigan.

Jones, D. H., C. A. Hamilton, J. L. Reid. 1978. Plasma noradrenaline, age and blood pressure: A population study. *Clinical Science and Molecular Medicine* 55:73, supplement 4.

————. 1979. Choice of control groups in the appraisal of sympathetic nervous activity in essential hypertension. *Clinical Science* 57:339.

Jorgensen, R. S., and B. K. Houston. 1981. Family history of hypertension, gender, and cardiovascular reactivity and stereotype during stress. *Journal of Behavioral Medicine* 4:175–89.

Kannel, W. B., N. Brand, J. J. Skinner, Jr.; T. R. Dawber; and P. M. McNamara. 1967. The relation of adiposity to blood pressure and development of hypertension: The Framingham Study. *Annals of Internal Medicine* 67:48–59.

Kasl, S. V. 1984. Social and psychologic factors in the etiology of coronary heart disease in black populations: An exploration of research needs. *American Heart Journal* 108 (no. 3, pt. 2): 660:69.

Krantz, D. S., N. E. Grunberg, and A. Baum. 1985. Health psychology. *Annual review of psychology* 36:349–83.

Langford, H. G., R. L. Watson, and B. H. Douglas. 1968. Factors affecting blood pressure in population groups. *Transactions of the Association of American Physicians* 81:135.

Lehmann, J. W., and H. Benson. 1982. Nonpharmacologic treatment of hypertension: A review. *General Hospital Psychiatry* 4:27–32.

Light, K. C., J. P. Koepke, P. Obrist, and P. Willis. 1982. Psychological stress induces sodium and fluid retention in men at high risk for hypertension. *Science* 220:429–31.

Luft, F. C., C. E. Grim, J. T. Higgins, and M. H. Weinberger. 1977. Differences in response to sodium administration in normotensive white and black subjects. *Journal of Laboratory Clinical Medicine* 90:555.

Luft, F., C. Gurin, and M. Weinberger. 1985. Electrolyte and volume hemostasis in blacks. In *Hypertension in blacks: Epidemiology, pathophysiology, and treatment,* edited by W. Hall, E. Saunders, and N. Shulman. Chicago: Year Book Medical Publishers, Inc.

McDonald, R. H. 1984. Summary of workshop II: Working group on risk factors. *American Heart Journal* 108 (no. 3, pt. 2): 703–6.

Manuck, S. B., and J. M. Proietti. 1982. Parental hypertension and cardiovascular response to cognitive and isometric challenge. *Psychophysiology* 19:481–49.

Matarazzo, J. D. 1980. Behavioral health and behavioral medicine: Frontiers for a new health psychology. *American Psychologist* 35:807–17.

Michaels, D. 1983. Occupational cancer in the black population: The health effects of job discrimination. *Journal of the National Medical Association* 75:1014–18.

Miller, N. E. 1983. Behavioral medicine: Symbiosis between laboratory and clinic. *Annual review of psychology* 34:1–32.

Myers, H. F. 1984. Summary of workshop III: Working group on socioeconomic and sociocultural influences. *American Heart Journal* 108 (no. 3, pt. 2): 706–10.

National Center for Health Statistics. 1984a. *Health indicators for Hispanic, Black*

and White Americans. (DHHS Publication no. 84–1576). Washington, D.C.:
U.S. Department of Health and Human Services.

Obrist, P. A. 1981. *Cardiovascular psychophysiology: A perspective.* New York:
Plenum Press.

Page, I. H. 1960. The mosaic theory of hypertension. In *Essential hypertension,*
edited by K. Bock, and P. Cottier. Berlin: Springer.

Roberts, J., M. Rowland. 1981. Hypertension in adults 25–74 years of age: United
States, 1971–1975. Vital and Health Statistics, series 11, no. 221. DHHS Publication no. PHS 81–1671. Washington, D.C.: Government Printing Office.

Rowlands, D. B., J. Giovanni, R. McLeary, R. Watson, J. Stotland, and W. Littler.
1982. Cardiovascular response in black and white hypertensives. *Hypertension*
4:817–20.

Saunders, A., and R. Williams. 1975. Hypertension. In *Textbook of black-related
diseases,* edited by R. A. Williams. New York: McGraw-Hill.

Sever, P. S., W. S. Peart, T. Meade, I. B. Davies, R. D. G. Tunbridge, and D. Gordon.
1979. Ethnic differences in blood pressure with observations on noradrenaline
and renin. 2. A hospital hypertensive population. *Clinical and Experimental
Hypertension* 1:745.

Shiloh, A., and I. Selavan, eds. 1973. *Ethnic groups of America: Their morbidity,
mortality and behavior disorders.* Vol. 1: *The Jews.* Springfield, IL: Thomas.

Stone, G. C. 1982. Health Psychology, a new journal for a new field. *Health Psychology* 1:1–6.

Surwit, R. S., R. B. Williams, and D. Shapiro. 1982. *Behavioral approaches to
cardiovascular disease.* New York: Academic Press.

Tyroler, H. A., A. Heyden, and C. G. Hames. 1975. Weight and hypertension: Evans
County studies of blacks and whites. In *Epidemiology and control of hypertension,* edited by O. Paul. New York: Stratton Intercontinental Medical Book.

U.S. Department of Health and Human Services. 1980. *Health of the Disadvan-
taged: Chart Book II* (DHHS Publication no. [HRA] 80–633). Public Health
Service, Health Resources Administration. Washington, D.C.: U.S. Government
Printing Office.

———. 1985. *Report of the Task Force on Black and Minority Health,* vol. 1. Washington, D.C.: U.S. Government Printing Office.

Veterans Cooperative Study Group. 1982. Anti-hypertensive agents: Comparison of
propranolol and hydrochlorothiazide for the initial treatment of hypertension.
I. Results of short term titration with emphasis on racial differences in response.
Journal of the American Medical Association 248:1196–2003.

Vick, R. 1984. *Contemporary medical physiology.* Menlo Park, CA: Addison-Wesley.

Weaver, T. 1970. Use of hypothetical situations in a study of Spanish American illness
referral systems. *Human Organization* 29:140–54.

Wisenbaugh, P. E., J. B. Garst, C. Hull, R. J. Freedman, D. N. Matthews, and M.
Hadady. 1972. Renin, aldosterone, sodium and hypertension. *American Journal
of Medicine* 52:175.

Wolinsky, F. D. 1982. Racial differences in illness behavior. *Journal of Community
Health* 8:87–101.

Woolander, S., D. U. Himmelstein, R. Silber, M. Bader, M. Harnly, and A. A. Jones. 1985. Medical care and mortality: Racial differences in preventable deaths. *International Journal of Health Services* 15:1–22.

Young, J. L., L. G. Ries, and E. S. Pollack. 1984. Cancer patient survival among ethnic groups in the United States. *Journal of the National Cancer Institute* 73: 341–52.

20

Child Health Psychology

Ronald B. Kurz

Pediatric Psychology and Child Health Psychology

Child health psychology is a broad field of practice, education, training, and research concerned with the relationship between psychological and physical health of children. The area is generally agreed to have been launched with the publication of a seminal paper by Wright (1967) in which the term "pediatric psychology" was first introduced. With the development of the field of health psychology, child health psychology has become synonymous with pediatric psychology. Among its concerns have been the behavioral and emotional aspects of disease and illness, the role of psychology in pediatric medicine, and the promotion of health and prevention of sickness in children. Although child health psychology traces its roots to both clinical and developmental psychology (Tuma 1982), its link to child clinical psychology by virtue of its training methods and settings, its personnel, and its methodology (Kurz 1983; Tuma and Grabert 1983) is clear and occasionally troubling to those who insist on sharp differentiations. Tuma (1982) has provided data indicating that the trainers of child health psychologists predominantly consider child health psychology to be a subspecialty of child clinical psychology. Certainly, the two fields have considerable overlap, but there are enough differences to permit one to discuss child health psychology as an entity within general health psychology without taking sides in the issue of its distinctness.

The typical function of child clinical psychologists has been their work with psychiatric patients in either a private practice or child guidance setting. The traditional work of the child clinical psychologist as a member of the child guidance team consisting of a psychologist, a psychiatrist, and a social worker involved little collaboration with pediatricians. In contrast, the child health psychologist is typically a member of a health care team rather than a mental health team. Health team members differ from psychiatrists and social workers in training, professional terminology and working style, and child health psychologists must adapt themselves to this new setting. Lavigne and Burns (1981) have noted that pediatricians are oriented to working on a short-term basis involving active intervention which is often quite different from the slower, verbal and indirect methods of the mental health specialist. Child health psychologists are often more concerned with rapid assessment, crisis intervention, prevention, and consultation with professionals in other disciplines. In the role of consultants, child health psychologists are often viewed by their medical colleagues as the experts on child development and education, child rearing practices, and the emotional needs of children (Lavigne and Burns 1981). Of major significance in the definition of child health psychology is the patient population with which its practitioners work. Child health psychologists are more likely to work with children who have psychological problems related to a medical condition. This may involve physical problems that have stress-related components, physical problems that may be helped by psychological intervention, and problems in emotional and cognitive functioning resulting from a physical handicap or a chronic illness.

The Child Health Psychologist in the Pediatric Setting

Many child health psychologists work in pediatric hospitals, departments of pediatrics, and other medical settings. Relatively few of these persons have been specifically trained for their positions as child health psychologists (Kurz 1983; Tuma 1982) and are likely to have been trained in child clinical or general clinical psychology (Drotar 1982). Much of the traditional clinical psychology training is applicable to the pediatric setting, including an understanding of personality and psychopathology, facility with a range of psychosocial assessment and treatment techniques, experience in consultation with professionals in other disciplines, a grasp of basic psychological theory, data and research techniques, and concern for the suffering of others. Such training and experience is particularly appropriate if it occurs with children in a pediatric setting. However, psychologists who work in pediatric settings quickly find that the traditional clinical skills are not enough and that the traditional psychopathological framework is a handicap. The child health psychologist working in a medical setting quickly discovers that the usual concepts from his or her training in psychopathology may not apply to conditions involving chronic illness, psychosomatic problems, chronic pain, behavior problems of infancy and early childhood, and developmental disabilities (Drotar 1982). An understanding of the effects of stress on family interactions, the psychological consequences of physical and cognitive impairments, and the role of coping and adaptation techniques of children and their families will often be more useful than a DSM-III diagnosis. Similarly, assessment techniques that focus on the cognitive and motor capabilities of infants and young children, the family dynamics of the young child, as well as treatment approaches that emphasize short-term behavioral techniques, biofeedback, stress management, and family approaches are often more suited to the needs and rhythms of the pediatric hospital than are the detailed projective evaluation and long-term individual psychotherapy which are more common in psychiatric settings.

In addition to learning specific clinical skills, psychologists in pediatric settings must adapt to an environment that is often hostile, or at a minimum, quite different from their graduate training in universities and from their experiences in community mental health or psychiatric settings. In the minds of the medical staff the psychologist's role is often vaguely defined as a "consultant," or rigidly and narrowly fixed as a "tester." Rather than reject such vague or rigid roles, many child health psychologists use them as entry points into the medical system which enable the psychologists to establish relationships with medical colleagues and to educate them on the range of diagnostic, treatment, consulting, educational, and research activities that are possible with their collaboration. There are also unique sources of stress for the child health psychologist in the medical setting arising from the vagueness of the role of the psychologist, the high degree of patient suffering, and the helplessness of the staff to relieve much of that pain. Drotar (1982) has noted that the medical staff may frequently misconstrue human suffering as psychopathology and therefore make inappropriate referrals to psychologists. It is the psychologist's responsibility to reshape such referrals in collaboration with medical colleagues without threatening or alienating them.

Patient care in pediatric settings is often approached according to the acute illness model (Drotar 1982) in which the illness is within the child, treatments are prescribed, and the child takes them in order to get well. Such an approach is usually in conflict with the psychosocial model of the psychologist, which involves longer term assessment and treatment and with a transactional perspective that at least includes the child's family and frequently the school and other community resources. The skillful child health psychologist learns to adapt his or her psychosocial model to the acute illness model of the medical colleagues, but this adaptation must be recognized as a potential source of conflict and stress.

Psychological Factors in Pediatric Illness

In attempting to understand the contribution of psychological factors in children's physical illness and health, it is necessary to understand the contributions of psychological factors to the etiology, maintenance and treatment of the illness, and the psychological impact of the illness itself. In regard to the psychological contributions to the illness, the psychosomatic model has generated numerous hypotheses about causation and a variety of treatment approaches (Tuma 1982) to a wide variety of pediatric problems. Perhaps the most important lesson to be learned from the voluminous psychosomatic literature is that it must not be used simplistically (Lipowski 1977). It is important to acknowledge that there are multiple psychological and physical factors interacting in the development of illness and the maintenance of health and that the specific unilinear hypotheses involving specific personality types and unconscious motivations (Alexander 1950) are not fruitful. Furthermore, what has been conceived of as a psychological etiology has often turned out to be a psychological consequence of the illness rather than an antecedent (Wright, Schaefer, and Solomons 1979).

The complexity of psychological factors in pediatric illness and health and the need to avoid early foreclosure on cause and effect are well illustrated in the common pediatric condition, asthma. This disease is a useful example of the principle of the complex interaction of physical and psychological factors; certainly other pediatric conditions such as diabetes, brain injury, encopresis and enuresis, chronic pain, and the spectrum of the eating disorders, to name only a few, could be substituted to serve as examples. Psychologists and pediatricians have long proposed that emotional conflicts may cause or exacerbate the disorder (Wright, Schaefer, and Solomons 1979) and it has become a favorite disease for child health psychologists to study. In addition to suspected psychological factors in the etiology and prolonging of the attacks, it has been hypothesized that the disorder itself generates psychological problems. Wright, Schaefer, and Solomons (1979) have exhaustively reviewed the various causative hypotheses and the research supporting them. One class of proposed psychogenic factors are maternal variables, ranging from the "suppressed cry" of French and Alexander (1941) in which the asthmatic child is posited to have experienced unmet dependency needs which results in an inhibited cry (asthmatic wheezing) for the mother, to the rejecting mother (Miller and Baruch 1957), to the overprotective mother (Long et al. 1958). Despite backlash against the notion that there is an asthmatogenic mother, Wright et al. (1979) cite several research studies demonstrating that mothers of asthmatics do tend to have a variety of personality characteristics hypothesized to have a relationship with asthma in particular and with childhood emotional disturbance in general.

Heightened anxiety has been demonstrated in several studies as a causative factor in asthma attack. Enclosing a patient in a body plethysmograph (Stein 1962), presenting emotional stimuli from the patient's past (Dekker and Groen 1956), and the sound of the mother's voice (Owen 1964) have all been found to bring on asthmatic attacks. It is, however, often difficult to determine whether the anxiety and other emotional responses are antecedent or consequential. For example, Smith (1962) found psychological differences were more pronounced in older than in younger asthmatics, with higher anxiety being characteristic of older asthmatics. Wright et al. (1979) cite a number of studies finding no differences between asthmatics and other children with chronic illnesses on a variety of psychological measures and emotional indicators. Certainly, behavioral and life-style variables have been correlated with asthmatic symptomatology. For example, exertion and exercise have been noted as factors in causing asthmatics attacks (Katz 1970), as well as geographic location of the child and degree of exposure to allergic substances; but even where physical and environmental factors are known to be important correlates, emotional and behavioral factors must often be considered. Khan, Staerk, and Bonk (1974) found that even highly allergic subjects could be provoked to have asthmatic attacks by emotional factors.

Other commonly considered psychosomatic diseases of childhood and adolescence, such as ulcerative colitis, have also been intensely studied from an emotional or behavioral perspective. What impresses broad investigators most is the recognition that psychological processes have a highly complex influence on the time of onset of the illness, the duration and course of the illness, and how the illness affects the child's daily functioning. However, as Money (1984) has pointed out, we still do not have a systematic psychology of syndromes in child health psychology. For the major pediatric conditions, we do not know, except in a very general way, the specific psychological functions affected by the condition, the role of the developmental level of the child in determining his or her psychological reactions, and the effect of the child's psychological reactions on the course of the pediatric condition. Future research will probably reveal that for some pediatric disorders there are very specific psychological effects, while for others there will be general effects, shared by large groups of pediatric problems. Money has suggested that until this kind of systematic research is carried out, we will not have a truly unique scientific basis for child health psychology. We will continue to work in a field with concepts borrowed from child clinical and developmental psychology, and the identity of the field will be based not on a unique body of theory and data, but upon the age of the clients and the location of the activity in pediatric settings.

Money's criticisms notwithstanding, there are several research areas that are beginning to help define child health psychology. Pediatric science has advanced greatly in recent years, resulting in the survival of many infants and young children who only a few years ago would have died. Some current psychological research therefore concerns helping children to cope with survival in the face of chronic illness and perhaps with a lifetime of physical pain, stressful treatment, and the social implications of being "different" because of illness. In the area of childhood cancer, researchers have established that most survivors of childhood malignancies have serious emotional and behavioral problems (O'Malley et al. 1979) and that they are viewed by their teachers as having concentration problems and difficulties with peer interactions (Deasy-Spinetta and Spinetta 1980). Childhood cancer has also been found to be strongly associated with parental disharmony (Lansky et al. 1978), school phobia (Lansky et al. 1975), and a large number of social and occupational problems in family members (Kalnins, Churchill, and Terry, 1980).

Although chronic and life threatening illness are dramatic psychological events in a child's life, acute illness has as well been shown to have important effects on children. Mattson and Weisberg (1970) provide data demonstrating that most young children have a temporary loss of age-appropriate behavior such as self-help skills and increases in thumb sucking. The age of the child was an important variable in predicting the child's reaction to the illness. Two-year-olds were more clingy and dependent, while over the age of three they seemed increasingly self-centered.

The effects of hospitalization and other medical procedures on children has been studied by child health psychologists. Probably the most stressful aspect of hospitalization is the separation of children from their parents. Shaw and Routh (1980) showed that even brief procedures in the pediatrician's office, such as injections, were more stressful for children when the mother was absent than when she was present. The pain of the procedures is also a variable that has been investigated. Children are, indeed, fearful of injections (Eland and Anderson 1977) but have been found to respond positively to peer models who show good coping with painful medical procedures (Vernon 1974). Illnesses may also cause restriction of the child's play activities and peer contacts, with resultant deterioration in social interests and skills and increase in rocking (Klaber and Butterfield 1968). Such observations have been important in the development of hospital life programs to provide the needed stimulation and social interactions for the children.

Finally, the prediction of the later psychological status of high-risk children and families has been the object of much research. For example, research on child abuse and neglect has found a relationship between child abuse and socioeconomic status variables, such as income level and type of housing (Garbarino and Crouter 1978), and with family stress (Gaines et al. 1978). The best predictor of child abuse has been the mother's history of having been abused herself (Altemeier et al. 1979). Closely related to child abuse and neglect research, are investigations of the causes and correlates of accidents in children. Although natural environmental dangers and poor engineering of the child's environment are certainly factors, significant family variables have been found in accident potential. Sobel (1970) found the incidence of accidental poisoning to be highly related to psychopathology in the mother or father, marital difficulty, and other family stressors. Thus, future research on parenting skills and the amelioration of family and parental problems is considered by many to be critical in the development of adequate prevention approaches with high-risk children.

Child Health Psychology Assessment Techniques

Kurz et al. (1982) have shown that psychological assessment is performed in settings involving child patients more frequently than in settings where adults are primarily seen. This is understandable when we consider that the pediatric population is mostly a school-age group for whom matters pertaining to abilities, learning styles, and capacities for properly socialized and rewarding interpersonal behavior are crucial for development. Even when the patients are preschool age, psychological assessments are frequently called for to predict later cognitive, emotional, and interpersonal behavior in order to determine what kind of interventions may be necessary. Because of the very wide age range involved in the pediatric population and the very large and rapid developmental changes involved, child health psychologists must master a broad array of assessment techniques. This is complicated further by the special problems in assessment which the pediatric patient often brings to the assessment enterprise. Infants and young children with pediatric conditions, for whom accurate assessment of abilities could be critical in the development of an infant stimulation program, a proper preschool environment, and an early learning disabilities intervention, do not have sufficiently developed sensory, motor, cognitive, and verbal systems to permit accurate long-range prediction.

Assessment practices in child health psychology are at the same time diverse and highly specialized, but the purpose of such assessment is always to help determine the level of cognitive, emotional, and social functioning of children with pediatric conditions and developmental problems for purposes of planning interventions or monitoring their effectiveness. The techniques employed cover the full array of psychological functions of interest in child development and include well-known and standardized tests of intelligence, projective techniques, developmental scales, specialized instruments for assessing specific cognitive, motor or sensory capacities, neuropsychological tests, as well as structured and unstructured interviews. Some assessment approaches focus on the child only, some on the parents and, increasingly, some on the family. Whatever procedure is used, child health psychologists usually find that the involvement of the family in the assessment process is a virtual necessity (Magrab and Lehr 1982).

Child health psychologists must constantly be mindful of the special sensory, cognitive, and motor capabilities of their young patients. Assessment with pediatric patients is unlike routine psychological testing of school children, or even the usual child guidance clinic population. Children with hearing losses are commonly encountered. Psychologists must not only be knowledgeable about special tests that are available for the assessment of such children, but they must also understand the effects deafness may have on the development of verbal abilities and concepts at different developmental levels. It is a common practice for psychologists to administer nonverbal tests, or portions of tests, such as the WISC-R Performance Scale, which were normed on a hearing population. Such a practice may be acceptable if the ultimate comparison the psychologist wishes to make is with a hearing reference group, but it would be inappropriate if the decision for which the testing is performed is to place the child in a school for the deaf. In the latter case, an instrument such as the Hiskey-Nebraska Test of Learning Aptitude would be more appropriate because it provides norms for deaf and hard of hearing children. Similar knowledge regarding test selection and clinical sensitivities about handicapping conditions are necessary in assessing children with other sensory deficits, such as blindness and motor impairments such as cerebral palsy.

Child health psychologists are often called upon to assess children with intact sensory and motor capacities, but who present special problems in testing because of motivational, attitudinal, and behavioral problems. Assessment of hyperactive children, or those with attention deficit disorders, require special efforts on the part of the examiner to maintain their concentration and attention. Chronically ill children similarly may lack interest or motivation and therefore may appear dull. Careful psychological assessment in such instances can be invaluable in educational planning and in determining the level at which to gauge explanations of the disease and treatment (Magrab and Lehr 1982).

The Kaufman Assessment Battery for Children (K-ABC) (Kaufman and Kaufman 1983) is a recent cognitive assessment tool which shows much promise in the field of child health psychology. The Kaufmans cite a number of research studies supporting its use in the diagnosis of learning disabilities, an area of great importance in the practice of child health psychology. Based on neuropsychological research suggesting dichotomous processes in cognitive functioning, the K-ABC enables the child health psychologist to characterize a child's problem-solving ability in terms of sequential ability (information processing that makes use of temporal order and requires integration of stimuli and intuitive approaches). The Kaufmans cite research indicating that learning disabled children often have difficulty with sequential processing, but the differentiation is far from clear-cut (Kaufman and Kaufman 1983). Other features of the K-ABC important to child health psychologists are the separation of basic cognitive ability from academic achievement and the capacity to derive a measure of cognitive ability that is relatively free of verbal expressive ability. Thus, for a learning disabled child or one who has missed significant amounts of school because of prolonged illness, it is possible to understand the basic information processing skills, relatively free of the influence of the amount and quality of prior academic learning. Similarly, for children who have problems in verbal expression, it is possible to get a measure of mental processing that is relatively free of verbal expressive processes. The K-ABC is a well-conceived instrument that will certainly generate much research into its effectiveness as a child health psychology assessment tool.

Neuropsychological assessment in child health psychology is becoming increasingly important as a means of describing brain-behavior relationships. Principles that have been well established in adult neuropsychological evaluation are only now being developed regarding children (Boll 1984), and there are a number of significant research problems for child health neuropsychologists. Yet to be clearly spelled out by neuropsychologists are the effects of type of brain lesion, age of onset and developmental level of the child, duration of the cortical illness, and lateralization on behavior at different ages and levels of development (Boll 1983). Perhaps even greater need for research data lies in the area of neuropsychological status of children with serious and chronic illness or physical anomalies. We are only now beginning to understand the neuropsychological implications of disorders such as kidney disease, asthma, diabetes, cystic fibrosis, and leukemia as well as the effects of treatment for these disorders on brain behavior relationships (Boll 1983).

Behavioral assessment is yet another relatively recent development which has great promise for adding to our understanding of the behavioral correlates of childhood illness. This area includes the many rating scales and checklists that can be administered to parents, teachers, nurses, and others who have opportunities to observe children in depth, structured interviews with children, and direct observation of children. Among the important advantages of these approaches has been their sound basis in behavior theory and research and their close association with treatment goals (Robinson and Eyberg 1984), but there are still many research challenges regarding the development of norms for children of varying ages, social and cultural backgrounds, types of disease, and cognitive abilities.

Child Health Psychology Treatment Approaches

There are several distinct goals of psychological treatment with children in the pediatric population. As noted earlier, psychological stress has been implicated as both an antecedent and a consequence of physical illness; therefore a major goal in treatment is to alleviate such stress. If, for example, family dysfunction is seen as an important factor in the maintenance of anorexia nervosa, then treatment of the family dynamics or structure is appropriate. Similarly, anxiety, body image distortions, or the misregulation of self-esteem resulting from chronic pediatric conditions often require intervention to break the cycle of stressful exacerbation of the medical conditions. Often the focus of the intervention is on matters of compliance. Children with pediatric conditions such as diabetes sometimes are uncooperative or unmotivated to participate in their own treatment, and intervention is necessary, either to deal with the noncompliance as a serious direct byproduct of the physical illness, or as a developmental or personal problem in the realm of an oppositional disorder in its own right. Furthermore, chronically ill and handicapped children frequently have adjustment problems which may vary depending on the nature of the illness or handicap, the age of onset, and the current developmental stage. Such problems require treatment to permit the child to have the most satisfactory adjustment relative to other family members, the schools, and with peers in the community. The ordinary developmental issues may be more stressful than usual for the medically ill child and his or her family, and the child health psychologist is frequently called upon to engage in management of psychological crises and emergencies. For example, a sixteen-old with end-stage renal disease caused a major crisis in his family when he announced he intended to get a driver's license. Immediate intensive treatment was needed to sort out the realities of the child's abilities, the symbiosis that had developed over the years between him and his parents, and the conflict between the parents over whether he was ready to drive. This case nicely illustrates the interplay between normal developmental issues and problems unique to the pediatric population so frequently encountered in psychological interventions in this group. Furthermore, it points up the role of family issues in intervention. It is common for treatment to focus primarily on the family to aid the members to adjust to the special stresses of the child's illness and to foster an understanding of the child's psychological and physical capabilities. With terminally ill children the family focus usually shifts to dealing with issues of death and dying and to consultation regarding when to terminate life supports for brain dead children. Hospitalized children commonly present nurses and physicians with management problems, and a frequent role for the pediatric psychologist is in advising the staff on ward management techniques. Finally pediatric psychologists are usually involved in consulting with schools regarding the special adjustment problems and academic placement which are so frequent in children with medical illnesses.

The intervention techniques employed by child health psychologists are derived from traditional child clinical psychology, but they have the special flavor of the pediatric population. Individual verbal psychotherapy is among the most frequently used techniques (Johnson 1979) and has been found useful in helping children deal with such diverse issues as death and dying (Kubler-Ross 1974), fears of sexual inadequacy and body image problems in renal transplant patients (Drotar 1975), and meeting the needs for emotional support in children who are burn victims (Seligman 1976). Bruch (1977) has reported on the successful use of verbal individual therapy with adolescents suffering from anorexia nervosa. Play therapy, both group and individual, is as popular in pediatric psychology practice as it is in traditional child clinical practice. It seems particularly suited to preparation of young children for surgery and other medical procedures (e.g., Petrillo and Sanger 1980) and to developing trust in abused children (Beezley, Martin, and Alexander 1976). Perhaps the most frequently employed set of therapeutic techniques with the pediatric population are the various forms of behavior therapy. These techniques seem particularly suited to the work of child health psychologists because they are short-term and most appropriate with younger and nonverbal children (Routh 1977). Behavioral treatment has been demonstrated to be particularly effective with enuresis (Doleys and Ciminero 1976; Azrin and Foxx 1974), encopresis (Wright and Walker 1976), eating disorders (Linscheid 1978; Barcai 1971), self-control in Tourette's syndrome (Friedman 1980), and relaxation in the treatment of psychosomatic disorders (Bauer 1975). Family therapy (e.g., Minuchin 1974) and parent training (e.g., Patterson and Guillion 1968) have been used by child health psychologists with a wide variety of disorders such as anorexia nervosa, psychophysiologic disorders such as asthma, and to gain control of conduct disturbances in a wide variety of medically ill and oppositional children. Finally, indirect intervention, through consultation with physicians and nurses in the medical setting and with the schools has become an important aspect of psychological treatment for pediatric problems (Mesibov and Johnson 1982).

Prevention and Child Health Behavior

Efforts of child health psychologists in prevention of illness have taken two major thrusts. The older, but still current, method is intervention with high-risk infants and their families. The second is promotion of positive health behaviors and attitudes in all children, regardless of risk potential.

In working with high-risk children, the child health psychologist identifies factors in the child's physical, behavioral, or environmental status which may increase the potential for developing illnesses or psychological problems at some later date, following which interventions are applied. For example, children of low IQ parents have been provided with intensive day care experiences and have been demonstrated to show IQ gains when compared with a control group that did not have the day care treatment (Heber 1978). In Heber's study, day care was supplemented with home training of the mothers in child care and other domestic skills. Parent training alone was shown by Maisto and German (1979) to have positive effects on cognitive and language development in high-risk infants. Premature infants, who are at risk for physical, psychological, and cognitive defects, as well as for child abuse, have been provided with infant stimulation programs, parent training, and attempts to increase parent-child bonding in the neonatal period. Scarr-Salapatek and Williams (1973) demonstrated increased IQs, when compared with control children, for premature infants who received special sensory stimulation and weekly home visits for one year. In the area of child abuse, Zigler and Hunsinger (1978) have stressed the role of the child health psychologist as child advocate for these at-risk children. Promotion of children's rights, discouragement of devaluation of children through corporal punishment, and advocation of equal opportunities for all children are emphasized as important concepts in the prevention of child abuse.

Writing from the perspective of self-regulation theory, Karoly (1982) discusses prevention in the form of the development of positive health behaviors and attitudes. As yet, there is little empirical data relating to the developmental model of health self-regulation, but Karoly draws on the literature of cognitive and social development to support his ideas. Health self-regulation is defined as the "ongoing process by which individuals gather, evaluate, and act upon data relevant to their physical health and formulate long-term and provisional health 'objectives'" (Karoly 1982, p. 47). The child's stage of development is key to his or her health activities. Clearly, infants depend upon parents for health regulation and preventive activities. For preschool children, imitation of parental models and other socializing agents in the community are prominent, while school-age children are likely to be influenced by peers. Such modeling at the various stages of development is seen as critical for the development of safety attitudes and the avoidance of accidents which account for forty-five percent of childhood mortality. Imitation of models, however, is seen by Karoly as only part of the socialization of health attitudes and behaviors. Internalization is also necessary and is hypothesized to develop when socializing agents utilize incentive, affective, and informational functions in combination with one another in inculcating positive and lasting health behaviors. Karoly's model seems promising, particularly because it ties pediatric prevention to general developmental psychology theory.

Conclusions

With concepts borrowed heavily from child clinical psychology and developmental psychology, child health psychology has been delineating areas of theory, research, and practice concerning the psychological aspects of children's health and illness, assessment and treatment of cognitive and emotional problems, both antecedent and consequent to physical illness, and the prevention of illness and promotion of health-supporting behaviors and lifestyles. Areas of past and current research have been described, and important fields of future research have been indicated. Although it is undoubtedly trite to state, the psychological and physical health of future generations of adults will depend upon the quality of today's child health psychology. We have made important beginning steps in the development of child health psychology, and with the recent development of training programs and tracks in psychology graduate programs and internships, there is every reason to be optimistic regarding the future viability of this field.

REFERENCES

Alexander, F. 1950. *Psychosomatic medicine*. New York: Norton.

Altemeier, W. A., P. M. Vietze, K. B. Sherrod, H. M. Sandler, S. Falsey, and S. O'Connor. 1979. Prediction of child maltreatment during pregnancy. *Journal of the American Academy of Child Psychiatry* 18:205–18.

Azrin, N. H., and R. M. Foxx. 1974. *Toilet training in less than a day*. New York: Simon and Schuster.

Barcai, A. 1971. Family therapy in the treatment of anorexia nervosa. *American Journal of Psychiatry* 128:186–290.

Bauer, R. 1975. Treatment strategies in psychosomatic disorders. *Pediatric Psychology* 3:4–5.

Beezley, P., H. P. Martin, and H. Alexander. 1976. Comprehensive family oriented therapy. In *Child abuse and neglect: The family and the community*, edited by R. E. Helfer and C. H. Kempe. Cambridge, MA: Ballinger.

Boll, T. J. 1983. Neuropsychological assessment of the child: Myths, current status, and future prospects. In *Handbook of clinical child psychology*, edited by C. E. Walker and M. C. Roberts. New York: John Wiley & Sons.

———. 1984. Pediatric neuropsychological assessment. In *Psychological and behavioral assessment: Impact on pediatric care*, edited by P. R. Magrab. New York: Plenum Press.

Bruch, H. 1977. Anorexia nervosa and its treatment. *Journal of Pediatric Psychology* 2:110–12.

Deasy-Spinetta, P., and J. J. Spinetta. 1980. The child with cancer in school: Teacher's appraisal. *American Journal of Pediatric Hematology/Oncology* 2:89–94.

Dekker, D. M., and J. Groen. 1956. Reproducible psychogenic attacks of asthma. *Journal of Psychosomatic Research* 1:58–67.

Doleys, D. M., and A. R. Ciminero. 1976. Childhood enuresis: Considerations in treatment. *Journal of Pediatric Psychology* 1:21–23.

Drotar, D. 1975. The treatment of severe anxiety reaction in an adolescent boy following renal transplantation. *Journal of the American Academy of Child Psychiatry* 14:451–62.

———. 1982. The child psychologist in the medical system. In *Child health psychology*, edited by P. Karoly, J. J. Steffen, and D. J. O'Grady. New York: Pergamon.

Eland, J. M., and J. E. Anderson. 1977. The experience of pain in children. In *Pain: A source book for nurses and other health professionals*, edited by A. K. Jacox. Boston: Little, Brown.

French, T. N., and F. Alexander. 1941. Psychogenic factors in bronchial asthma.

Psychosomatic Medicine, Monograph IV. Washington, D.C.: National Research Council.

Friedman, S. 1980. Self-control in the treatment of Gilles de la Tourette's syndrome: Case study with 18-month follow-up. *Journal of Consulting and Clinical Psychology* 48:400–402.

Gaines, R., A. Sandgrund, A. H. Green, and E. Power. 1978. Etiological factors in child maltreatment: A multivariate study of abusing, neglecting, and normal mothers. *Journal of Abnormal Psychology* 87:531–40.

Garbarino, J., and A. Crouter. 1978. Defining the community context for parent-child relations: The correlates of child maltreatment. *Child Development* 49:604–16.

Heber, F. R. 1978. Sociocultural mental retardation: A longitudinal study. In *Primary prevention of psychopathology,* vol. 2, *Environmental influences,* edited by D. G. Forgays. Hanover, NH: University Press of New England.

Johnson, M. R. 1979. Mental health interventions with medically ill children: A review of the literature, 1970–77. *Journal of Pediatric Psychology* 5:81–92.

Kalnins, I. V., M. P. Churchill, and G. E. Terry. 1980. Concurrent stresses in families with a leukemic child. *Journal of Pediatric Psychology* 5:81–92.

Karoly, P. 1982. Developmental pediatrics: A process-oriented approach to the analysis of health competence. In *Child health psychology: Concepts and issues,* edited by P. Karoly, J. J. Steffen, and D. J. O'Grady. New York: Pergamon Press.

Katz, R. M. 1970. Exercise induced brocho-spasms in childhood. *Annals of Allergy* 28:361–66.

Kaufman, A., and N. Kaufman. 1983. *The Kaufman Assessment Battery for Children: Interpretive Manual.* Circle Pines, MN: American Guidance Service.

Khan, A. U., M. Staerk, and C. Bonk. 1974. Hypnotic suggestibility compared with other methods of isolating emotionally prone asthmatic children. *The American Journal of Clinical Hypnosis* 17:50–53.

Klaber, M. M., and E. C. Butterfield. 1968. Stereotyped rocking—A measure of institutional and ward effectiveness. *American Journal of Mental Deficiency* 73:13–20.

Kubler-Ross, E. 1974. The language of dying. *Journal of Clinical Child Psychology* 3:22–24.

Kurz, R. B. 1983. The predoctoral internship in pediatric psychology. National Working Conference on Education and Training in Health Psychology. *Health Psychology* 2 (5), supplement section.

Kurz, R. B., M. Fuchs, R. F. Dabek, S. M. S. Kurtz, and W. T. Helfrich. 1982. Characteristics of predoctoral internships in professional psychology. *American Psychologist* 37:1213–20.

Lansky, S. B., N. U. Cairns, R. Hassanein, J. Wehr, and J. T. Lowman. 1978. Childhood cancer: Parental discord and divorce. *Pedatrics* 62:184–88.

Lansky, S. B., J. T. Lowman, T. Vats, and J. E. Gyulay. 1975. School phobia in children with malignant neoplasms. *American Journal of Diseases of Children* 129:43–46.

Lavigne, J. V., and W. J. Burns. 1981. *Pediatric psychology.* New York: Grune and Stratton.

Linschied, T. R. 1978. Disturbances of eating and feeding. In *Psychological man-*

agement of pediatric problems, edited by P. R. Magrab. Baltimore: University Park Press.

Lipowski, Z. J. 1977. Psychosomatic medicine in the seventies: An overview. *American Journal of Psychiatry* 134:233–44.

Long, R. T., J. H. Lamont, B. Whipple, L. Bandler, G. E. Blom, L. Burgin, and L. Jessner. 1958. A psychosomatic study of allergic and emotional factors in children with asthma. *American Journal of Psychiatry* 114:890–99.

Magrab, P. R., and E. Lehr. 1982. Assessment techniques in pediatric psychology. In *Handbook for the practice of pediatric psychology,* edited by J. M. Tuma. New York: Wiley.

Maisto, A. A., and M. L. German. 1979. Variables related to progress in a parent-infant training program for high-risk infants. *Journal of Pediatric Psychology* 4:409–19.

Mattson, A., and I. Weisberg. 1970. Behavioral reactions to minor illness in preschool children. *Pediatrics* 46:604–10.

Mesibov, G. B., and M. R. Johnson. 1982. Intervention techniques in pediatric psychology. In *Handbook for the practice of psychology,* edited by J. M. Tuma. New York: Wiley.

Miller, H., and D. W. Brach. 1957. The emotional problems of children and their relation to asthma. *American Journal of Diseases of Childhood* 93:242–45.

Minuchin, S. 1974. *Families and family therapy.* Cambridge, MA: Harvard University Press.

Money, J. 1984. Service and science in pediatric psychology. *Newsletter of the Society of Pediatric Psychology,* October 15.

O'Malley, J. E., G. Koocher, D. Foster, and L. Slavin. 1979. Psychiatric sequelae of surviving childhood cancer. *American Journal of Orthopsychiatry* 49:608–16.

Owen, F. W. 1963. Patterns of respiratory disturbance in asthmatic children evoked by the stimulus of the mother's voice. *Acta Psychotherapeutica et Psychosomatica* 11:228–41.

Patterson, G. R., and M. E. Gullion. 1968. *Living with children.* Champaign, IL: Research Press.

Petrillo, M., and S. Sanger. 1980. *Emotional care of hospitalized children.* Philadelphia: Lippincott.

Robinson, E. A., and S. M. Eyberg. 1984. Behavioral assessment in pediatric settings: Theory, method, and application. In *Psychological and behavioral assessment: Impact on pediatric care,* edited by P. R. Magrab. New York: Plenum Press.

Routh, D. K. 1977. Postdoctoral training in pediatric psychology. *Professional Psychology* 8:245–50.

Scarr-Salapatek, S., and M. L. Williams. 1973. The effects of early stimulation on low birth weight infants. *Child Development* 44:94–101.

Seligman, R. 1976. Emotional responses to burns in children. In *Modern perspectives in the psychiatric aspects of surgery,* edited by J. G. Howells. New York: Brunner/Mazel.

Shaw, E. G., and D. K. Routh. 1980. Children receiving injections cry more often when mother is there. *Bulletin of the Psychonomic Society* 13:255.

Smith, J. M. 1962. Prevalence and natural history of asthma in school children. *British Medical Journal*, (no. 5277): 711–13.

Sobel, R. 1970. The psychiatric implications of accidental poisoning in childhood. *Pediatrics Clinics of North America* 17: 653–85.

Stein, M. 1962. Etiology and mechanism in the development of asthma. In *Psychosomatic medicine*, edited by J. H. Moyer. Philadelphia: Lea & Febiger.

Tuma, J. M. 1982. Pediatric psychology: Conceptualization and definition. In *Handbook for the practice of pediatric psychology*, edited by J. M. Tuma. New York: Wiley.

Tuma, J. M., and J. Grabert. 1983. Internship and postdoctoral training in pediatric and child psychology: A survey. *Journal of Pediatric Psychology* 8: 245–60.

Vernon, D. T. 1974. Modeling and birth order in response to painful stimuli. *Journal of Personality and Social Psychology* 29: 794–99.

Wright, L. 1967. The pediatric psychologist: A role model. *American Psychologist* 22: 323–25.

Wright, L., A. B. Schaefer, and G. Solomons. *Encyclopedia of pediatric psychology.* Baltimore: University Park Press.

Wright, L., and C. E. Walker. 1976. Behavioral treatment of encopresis. *Journal of Pediatric Psychology* 1: 35–37.

Zigler, E., and S. Hunsinger. 1978. Our neglected children. *Yale Alumni Magazine* (February), 41.

21

Older Persons and Health Psychology

Margaret Gatz, Cynthia Pearson, and Wendy Weicker

There has been surprisingly little recognition of the natural overlap between health psychology and the psychology of the adult development and aging—surprising because thirty percent of the health care dollars in the United States go toward treating the health problems of the 11.3 percent of our population that is sixty-five years of age and older (Kovar 1980). Three instances illustrate how professionals have been forced to notice the overlap: health psychology researchers and consultants who find that a significant proportion of their subjects and populations are aged; clinical-aging psychologists who find that their clients' problems also demand medical knowledge and attention; and community psychologists concerned with deinstitutionalization who have discovered that there are more mental patients in nursing homes than in state mental hospitals (Levine 1981). The advantages of jointly considering issues and knowledge in health and aging can only increase, given the predicted continuing growth of the number of older persons in this country.

We applaud the convergence of expertise implicit in this overlap, particularly insofar as it controverts the temptation to regard the aged as a totally unique population requiring a separate specialty to study and treat them. The pitfalls of such a presumption of uniqueness are described persuasively by Kasl and Berkman (1981) who identify a range of social forces that fairly demand age-grading: the existence of academic specialties focused exclusively on the aged; the use of age as a criterion for targeting federal sources of support; and the obvious losses and adversities faced by large numbers of older persons. However, studying the aged separately risks erroneously concluding that the results pertain only to that group and not equally as well to other population subgroups. Moreover, the number of professionals involved in working with older adults will be unduly restricted by fostering a separate specialty. An approach based on joint consideration would begin with the assumption that psychosocial factors influence health status for all people and would then go on to identify age differences in the nature of these effects or in the efficacy of interventions to reduce their stressfulness. We offer this chapter, therefore, not as a prescription for a health psychology of the aged, but as encouragement for the development of a health psychology that extends across the life span.

In accord with this intent, the first section of the chapter provides a brief introduction to the types of knowledge we regard as important to the overlap of aging and health. We highlight background information in three interrelated domains—biological, psychological, and social. Within each, we mention both normal, age-related changes that bear on work with older adults, as well as age differences in some of the most common disorders or adversities. The section ends with a set of conceptual and methodological considerations that arise from life-span developmental research but in practice pertain to translating health psychology expertise into interventions with aged. The second section of the chapter offers an assortment of examples of applications to research, practice, and policy. While certainly not comprehensive, they should serve to suggest a role for sound extrapolation in an emerging joint enterprise.

Background Factors
PHYSICAL CHANGES

The physical health of the aged population reflects both normal biological changes and increased incidence of many major diseases. Although aging does not affect all physiological systems uniformly, virtually all show some decrement (i.e., respiratory, cardiovascular, urinary, musculoskeletal, nervous, endocrine, immune) (Kenney 1982). Moreover, the five senses undergo changes which impede the older person's ability to receive information about the environment. Hearing is diminished with age, and there is a decrease in the ability to perceive high frequency sounds (Corso 1977). Vision is also altered, including impaired accommodation for near objects, a decline in visual acuity, and an increased sensitivity to glare (Fozard et al. 1977). For all of these neurobiological processes, a major change is reduced speed of response, with the result that it takes longer to do nearly all tasks and to recover from any type of stress (Blazer and Siegler 1984).

The biological changes that occur are reflected in the health problems of older adults, primarily in increased vulnerability to certain diseases. For example, chronic diseases increase with age: some eighty-six percent of individuals 65 and over living in the community have at least one chronic disease and fifty percent have two or more (Jarvik and Perl 1981). The chronic conditions that most frequently affected the aged are arthritis, hypertension, and heart disease (Siegler, Nowlin, and Blumenthal 1980). Increased vulnerability is additionally reflected in the fact that, although the incidence of acute illnesses decreases with age, the impact is often more severe in older adults and recovery more protracted (Atchley 1977). Common complaints in the aged not necessarily symptomatic of any one disease include foot and back problems, difficulty sleeping, and hoarseness (Brody and Kleban 1981). Importantly, many of the chronic conditions experienced by the elderly result in part from the life-styles and health practices the individual had as a younger person (Siegler and Costa 1985).

Thus, in contrast to younger adult groups, the health problems of the elderly are more often multiple, chronic, and—although treatable—not curable. Essentially, death in very old persons is due to cumulative frailty; eventually the individual is unable to survive a fresh insult such as a broken hip or the flu (Fries 1984). This pattern of ailments is reflected in the use of medical services. For example, the average stay in the hospital for those 65 and older is 11.5 days, in comparison to 5.4 for those 25 to 34 years of age (Crandall 1980). In addition there is greater use of long-term care. At any given time, five percent of those aged 65 to 74, ten percent of those aged 75 to 84, and over a fifth of those 85 and older live in nursing homes, reflecting the more precipitous decline in health status observed after age 75 (Blazer and Siegler 1984). It is important to note, however, that these figures illustrate the error in regarding the majority of even the very old as sick or decrepit.

As more is learned about health maintenance and disease prevention, the distinction between normal aging and disease is constantly undergoing redefinition and modification. Nonetheless, without this distinction, potentially treatable disorders may be regarded as inevitable concomitants of aging, while expectable age changes may be erroneously labeled as illness, leading to fruitless (even potentially harmful) searches for medical remediation.

Psychological Changes

Of the normal age-related psychological changes, cognitive functioning may be most pertinent. There is no simple summary. Studies indicate that some abilities do not appear to decline with age, while others decline at differential rates. Those intellectual abilities which tend to show decline generally involve speed, unfamiliar material, and complex tasks (Botwinick 1977).

Normal cognitive changes are gradual, and precipitous change indicates some pathological processes.

Older people with psychological disorders constitute a small but significant subgroup of the aged. Paralleling physical illness, the distribution of types of mental disorder alters across the life span. The incidence of functional mental illness actually decreases with increasing age, while the frequency of organic mental disorders such as dementia and delirium increases. The prevalence of organic mental disorders in those 65 years of age and older is estimated at five to seven percent for moderate to severe conditions, and fifteen percent if mild conditions are included. Prevalence figures rise to twenty percent and more for those 80 and above. The dementia syndrome presents a diagnostic challenge that demands thorough evaluation in order that potentially treatable processes that may be producing or exacerbating the cognitive symptoms (e.g., side effects of drugs, malnutrition) can be differentiated from irreversible causes, such as Alzheimer's disease (Cummings and Benson 1983). Furthermore, it needs to be recognized that organic mental disorders have an enormous effect on families and on the service system. For example, Christie (1982) reported that dementia accounts for more admissions and for more hospital inpatient days than any other condition in the geriatric age group.

Of the functional mental disorders, depression has received the most attention. Prevalence estimates vary widely, depending on the sample studied and the method of assessment employed. For example, endorsement of depressive symptoms on self-report scales appears to increase with age, while the psychiatric syndrome of depression is less prevalent in older adults than at earlier points in the life span (Blazer 1982). A further consideration is whether depression manifests itself the same way at different ages; if not, symptoms signifying depression at one age may constitute erroneous overdiagnosis at another age, or treatable depressions may be overlooked. To illustrate this point, consider that in the aged depression may foster exaggeration of normal forgetting. Those who are unaware of this phenomenon may mistakenly assume memory complaints and concomitant cognitive changes to represent an organic condition, thus neglecting a reversible depression (Zarit 1980).

SOCIAL CHANGES

Demographic characteristics and economic status help to define the normal social context of the aged. The portion of the older population that is growing most quickly comprises those 75 and over, when increased biological vulnerability tends to become evident. Because women live longer than men, the sex ratio widens increasingly with age, with the result that older women are likely to be widowed (Siegel 1980). Income affects access to transportation, housing, health care, and social interaction. While incomes among the aged are quite diverse and the majority do not live below the poverty line, it is the case that those aged 65 and older constitute twenty percent of the nation's poor (Schulz 1980).

The life transitions confronting an older person constitute a social developmental context. Discrete life events may be rated for their stressfulness, an approach that is of particular interest because of the relationships that have been shown between stress and disease (Krantz, Glass, and Miller 1981). Age differences in the influence of psychosocial stressors on health status have been insufficiently explored, but—despite a pervasive image to the contrary—there is an absence of empirical support for old age as the time of the most stressful life events (Pearlin 1983) or the greatest number of losses (McCrae 1982). Likewise, social networks have received attention as possibly mediating the effects of stress. Yet, there is not a great deal of evidence to suggest that the aged are exceptionally socially isolated and even less reason to suppose that there are age differences in the relationship between social networks and health status (Kasl and Berkman 1981). If, however, it is established that health is affected by stress through the functioning of the immune system, then one might predict that the aged would be more vulnerable and that teaching stress management and interpersonal skills might be potent interventions (Rodin 1980).

The family is the final aspect of the social context. Again despite popular beliefs to the contrary, studies indicate that adult children do not abandon their parents. Older people have substantial contact with their children, grandchildren, and siblings (Shanas 1979). Furthermore, when older persons become ill, family members supply eighty percent of the care that is needed (Smyer 1984).

LIFE SPAN CONSIDERATIONS

The extension of developmental theory to include adulthood and aging has raised several conceptual issues that are relevant to health psychology and research and practice. First is the matter of *cohort,* or generation. The time at which an individual was born, grew up, and grew older exerts an undeniable imprint. For example, today's 65-, 75-, and 85-year-olds could be expected to have decidedly different attitudes toward disease prevention depending on their own age and the age of their children at the time public health problems to inoculate against communicable diseases were implemented. Similarly, future cohorts of elderly, having been exposed to increased public emphasis on health-promoting life styles and environments, will likely make different use of health services than today's elderly, who tend to associate health services with curing acute illness. Thus, the health and psychosocial condition of individuals who belong to the same birth cohort reflects some indisputable, but not readily partitionable, effects of their age and of experiences shared at the same chronological point in their life spans.

A second consideration is *interindividual variability*. It is a mistake to think of older adults as a monolithic group. For one thing, on virtually all objectively measured variables where there is an average difference between young and old, there are some older people who perform better than the younger adult mean and some younger people who perform worse than the older adult mean. In addition, the accumulation of idiosyncratic life experiences over the life course brings individuals into late life with a personal investment in certain abilities, activities, and objects that have acquired enhanced meaning. In short, older adults become more distinctly themselves and less like each other than at any other point in the life span. A further source of variability is the range of ages and cohorts within the group of adults who are now old. Using the most common marker of age 65 and over to define the elderly population implies an age range of 25 years or more—analogous to combining 10-year-olds with 35-year-olds. Thoughtlessly lumping such vast differences together may dilute research findings and obscure opportunities for intervention.

A third consideration is *multiple interaction*. While the matter of needing to deal with a person's physical and mental health within their social and physical environment is hardly unique to the aged, these issues become more obviously interrelated and have greater interactive consequences with advancing age. On the one hand, the functional health and competence of any individual elder reflects some combination of their medical status, their motivation and sense of well-being, and the extent and stability of their social and environmental support. Even transient illness of a spouse or an important member of an informal support system may lead, for example, to compromised nutrition and hygiene, improper use of medication, diminished cognitive capacity, and even precipitous change in residential status for an individual elder. In turn, health is a sufficiently strong factor that it has been found to account for changes in other areas of functioning previously thought to be due to normal age-related changes. For instance, in studies in which the influence of chronological age and health are considered simultaneously, it is health rather than age that seems to explain observed declines in intellectual functioning (Siegler and Costa 1985); and Himmelfarb (1984) has reported that physical health is the primary mediator of the relationship between age and mental health. Thus for purposes of research as well as for assessment, diagnosis and intervention, it is essential to encompass all of these areas of functioning and attempt to account for how each area is affecting the others.

Applications

In this section we will address some selected topics that we think are especially good illustrations of the collaborative potential that exists between health psychology and adult development and aging. Suggestions are offered regarding the following: some attitudinal factors that are thought to influence both the quantity and quality of health care to the elderly; health policy issues affecting service provision; preventive interventions, including the issue of compliance; and the concept of control, which is a theme that cuts across all levels of work with the aged. This list is by no means exhaustive; rather it is intended to be indicative of the relevance of the joint perspectives for current research and practice and for planning for future cohorts of the elderly.

ATTITUDES AND SERVICE USE

It is often observed that those over age 65 account for a disproportionately large portion of health care service use in relation to other age groups, which may be taken to suggest that older people make excessive use of doctors. However, this image is contradicted by studies demonstrating that the aged avoid reporting symptoms and seeking help commensurate with the well-documented number and nature of their health problems (Kovar 1980). Brody and Kleban (1981) found that fifty-six percent of symptoms were not reported to a professional. More significantly, old people often report the symptoms that are annoying but less serious, yet may not complain of ones that indicate serious underlying pathology where timely treatment might make a difference (Haug 1981).

In attempting to account for this pattern of underservice and misservice, explanations have been offered that involve attitudes and beliefs of older people, as well as those reflected in the health care system. Many symptoms may erroneously be deemed normal for someone their age by older individuals and service providers alike. Older people may not want to "bother the doctor" and be perceived as hypochondriacal. They may also fear that a problem might be found that would jeopardize their continuing to live independently (Besdine 1981). Whether valid or misconceived, such beliefs carry implications for when the elderly will seek treatment.

While professionals' attitudes are often cited as reasons for older people's underservice, simply labeling service providers as "ageist" is not an adequate explanation. Some evidence based on attitude scales suggests that those most committed to working with older adults score less positively — and perhaps more realistically—than their colleagues who are not trained in aging (Pavur and Smith 1983). Nonetheless, the lack of professionals interested or trained in aging may reflect perceived lesser rewards from working with individuals whose illnesses are chronic. Likewise, the perspective that only geriatric specialists can treat the aged, rather than an approach to practice that encompasses the life span, may limit the numbers of health care providers available. In this manner, beliefs can interact with the service system to create barriers for older adults.

Interesting similarities exist between physical health and mental health with respect to service use. Although the prevalence of mental health problems does not increase with age in the same way as physical health, evidence of underservice is striking; for example, the 11.3 percent of the population who are aged used only four percent of the mental health services offered by community mental health centers (U.S. General Accounting Office 1982). The beliefs and attitudes invoked to account for mental health underservice are essentially parallel to those for physical problems.

An additional source of mental health underservice has been that physicians are less likely to refer older patients to psychologists than younger patients (Kucharski, White, and Schratz 1979). While the lack of referrals may reflect the presumed predominance of the patients' medical problems, it takes on particular interest because some studies of younger adults have suggested a cost offset involving decreased use of medical services following psychological consultation (Jones and Vischi 1979). A controlled study of psychological referrals of older patients would be of special interest.

It is important to note that speculation far outweighs evidence in our understanding of the influence of attitudes and beliefs on patterns of service use and provision. To the extent that older adults demonstrate a reluctance to see a professional, it may well be primarily a cohort rather than an age effect. In this case, future cohorts of the aged may drastically increase the demand on the health care system (Riley 1981). With less confidence, perhaps we can also predict that the professionals comprising that future system will not be the same either.

HEALTH POLICY

Medicare is the keystone of health care reimbursement for those aged 65 and older. Yet, less than forty percent of the health bill of older persons is covered, and out-of-pocket expenses can place a great strain on those with marginal incomes. Importantly, many relevant services are not reimbursable, such as routine physical examinations, outpatient drugs, eyeglasses, and dentures; moreover, coverage is limited for preventive care, outpatient services, and mental health treatment (Butler and Lewis 1982).

There is debate about whether or not reimbursement policy shapes service use and, if so, how (Kovar 1980). Some assert that help-seeking is based on need and is not determined by reimbursement; others argue that help-seeking is directly influenced, either by blocking individuals from obtaining care that they need or by stimulating overuse of covered services; still others suggest that the greatest effect is through the influence of reimbursement on the availability of professionals, thus indirectly limiting access to care (Haug 1981). Both direct and indirect pathways are likely factors to research and policy attention.

One resource to which policymakers have turned in attempting to meet rising health care costs is the family, especially in promoting family responsibility for long-term care of chronically disabled elders. This solution does not appear to take into account major demographic and social changes that are influencing families' capacity to provide help. There are not only greater numbers of elderly, but also a declining birthrate is reducing the pool of adult children available to provide assistance. Second, competing demands such as work and alternative family styles further limit potential care (Smyer 1984). Thus, it may be that adult children are doing all they can. Available evidence suggests that risk of institutionalization is greatest for those aged who have fewer family and social supports and that the decision to institutionalize is a last resort for families who have exhausted their own resources and for whom no community options are available. Several states have considered tax incentives for family caregiving to compensate for loss of income and costs incurred by the caregiver (Gray 1983). This idea deserves a controlled evaluation study.

Looking farther into the future, projecting health service needs depends on more than simply the predicted numbers of people who will survive into very old age. Fries and Crapo (1981) have proposed a compression of morbidity hypothesis suggesting that, with increased health maintenance and preventive care, people will experience prolonged vitality until their health declines precipitously during the very last years of life. For example, Fries (1984) pointed out that the rate of nursing home use has been constant over the last two decades, but the average age of those residents has increased. Meyers and Manton (1984) are among those who have questioned the evidence for compression. The alternative hypothesis is that there will be a tradeoff between quantity and quality of life as increased longevity brings with it prolonged periods of illness and disability. What is of interest here are the vastly different implications of these two hypotheses, not only for predicting health care costs but also for projecting our own preferences for a dignified death.

PREVENTIVE INTERVENTION AND COMPLIANCE

Preventive health psychology encompasses all aspects of health-related behaviors concerned with the prevention or reduction of disease (Masek, Epstein, and Russo, 1981). From a developmental viewpoint, prevention must simultaneously focus on those who are now old as well as future cohorts of elderly. For example, life-style modifications may represent a different level of intervention and necessitate a different sort of evaluation for a 70-year-old woman and her 45-year-old daughter. Maintaining good nutrition and regular exercise may constitute primary prevention for the younger adult, preventing the occurrence of disease; but for the older adult the same modifications may be part of a prescribed treatment regimen for a chronic health problem and, as such, may be viewed more appropriately as secondary or tertiary prevention. Evidence is conflicting as to whether risk factors for disease increase or weaken in potency with age (Kasl and Berkman 1981). At least one possibility is that older adults, with their lowered homeostatic capacity, may appreciate greater immediate benefits from life-style modifications than the younger adults for whom such health-promotion interventions were initially conceived. A more speculative question about the importance of risk factors would be how modifying one generation's habits affects the prevalence of disease in the next. In any event, extending preventive health research to encompass the life span seems warranted.

Education about aging is another approach to preventive intervention. Information about normal age changes in auditory, visual, and memory functioning can alleviate an elder's unnecessary concern, aid in identifying a potentially serious change, and provide a basis for devising environmental compensation. The phenomenology of aging as eloquently described by Hebb (1978) and Skinner (1983) in their invited addresses to the American Psychological Association is exactly the sort of information that we imagine being helpful in this context. Programs that provide education about life transitions such as retirement, relocation, and bereavement, or groups related to the management of specific illnesses are currently popular, as are interventions involving the family. Support group meetings for relatives caring for Alzheimer's disease patients that include education about the disease, sharing of problems and solutions, and emotional ventilation have been shown to be helpful (Zarit and Zarit 1982), thereby indirectly enabling the impaired elder to appreciate maximal independence.

A critical problem in preventive health care for the aged is compliance, although it is not clear whether adherence to therapeutic directives bears any consistent relationship to age (Kasl and Berkman 1981). Treatment of multiple chronic ailments may require rather substantial changes of lifestyle, from salt-free diets to colostomy bags, as well as the use of an array of medications prescribed by more than one physician. Even these interventions may not effect improvement but serve only to prevent further decline, which offers little motivation for maintaining treatment regimens. Consider further how proximity to death alters motivation to comply with life-style changes that may drastically reduce one's enjoyment of living.

For the older patient, it may be particularly difficult to grasp and retain information and instructions, much less to convey them to family members. For that matter, the family's role in encouraging or undermining compliance is relatively unexplored. Physicians' busy schedules, the cognitive and sensory declines associated with normal aging, and timidity on the part of many elders combine to limit the effectiveness of physician-patient communication and contribute to noncompliance (Butler and Lewis 1982). Straightforward solutions such as having the patient write down instructions and encouraging patient phone calls to verify directives are worth empirical investigation.

A particularly problematic compliance issue is the use of drugs. Those aged 65 and older account for over twenty-five percent of all prescribed drugs (Lofholm 1975). The potential for misuse, abuse, or adverse reactions is magnified by the number of different drugs prescribed to one individual, the fact that many are prescribed on an "as needed" basis, the combination of prescriptions from multiple physicians, the combination of prescription and over-the-counter medications, and the use of drugs previously prescribed or prescribed for someone else. Furthermore, the extent to which physiological changes with age affect drug clearance and hence dosages is often unknown or not taken into account (Lamy 1980). Not surprisingly, especially given the complexity of the medications, estimates are that up to sixty percent of older patients make errors in drug taking, at least a quarter of which are potentially serious (Krupka and Vener 1979). Yet, it is not known what percentage of errors could be avoided simply by taking into account the changes in the aging visual system—for example, one does not enhance compliance by typing instructions in extremely small type, wrapping them around a bottle, and then further obscuring them in the glare of shiny scotch tape.

Sense of Control

A concept that ties together many different kinds and levels of health-related interventions with the aged is the sense of personal control. Indeed, the life situation of the aged fairly invites being interpreted in terms of lessened control. It is helpful specifically to consider sense of control as a mediator in many of the arenas on which we have already touched: the effects of physical illness or disability on the patient's level of distress, the extent of strain induced by events in the older individual's life, ways that communication between patient and physician might ensure better compliance and better care, or how responsibility for a frail older relative can make a family member feel burdened. Analyzing the situations in these terms often can lead the psychologist to find ways to enhance the older person's control.

A number of researchers have demonstrated interventions that successfully increased sense of control. For example, Rodin (1982) has completed several studies where nursing homes residents are given choices, provided with a contingent situation, or otherwise allowed to experience more control in their daily lives. She has found improvement in sense of well-being, alertness, memory performance, participation in activities, physical health, and discharge rates. In community-residing elderly, an outreach program to older citizens that provided information and education about community services was shown to increase their sense of control (Gatz et al. 1982), and support groups for relatives of Alzheimer's patients have been shown to increase the sense of control of participants (Lazarus et al. 1981).

Control may also be enhanced by activities as diverse as soliciting older people's input into health policy formulation; sitting down with a patient and the family to integrate the results of evaluations by numerous professionals; or asking a convalescent care patient about her personal preferences regarding food. In addition, the idea of control is reflected in medical personnel's inviting patients to make informed choices and enlisting patients as more active participants in their own treatment. A caution, of course, is that the patient must retain the choice of declining to be more actively involved in decision making—for example, an individual may elect to defer to professional opinion—otherwise, the giving of control is only illusory.

A further way in which sense of control serves as an integrating concept is provided by recent work identifying physiological mechanisms by which perceived control is related to better health outcomes, in particular, the efficiency with which the immune system responds to stress (Rodin 1982). Thus, not only does it appear possible that sense of control is a key explanatory factor in how stressful environments can affect physical and mental health, but also that the physiological mechanisms associated with perceived control are fundamental aspects of the biology of aging.

Conclusion

We have presented some material indicating that the overlap between health psychology and adult development and aging is only likely to increase. We have also argued that deliberate attention to that overlap is beneficial, especially if we can avoid making erroneous assumptions about the uniqueness of the aged. Such thinking isolates older adults conceptually from the rest of the life span and impoverishes our resources in responding to their problems. We have suggested that there is an existing knowledge base that provides a picture of today's older adults. The concepts of cohort, interindividual variability, and multiple interaction both enhance our understanding of that picture and encourage informed extrapolation, in research and practice, from what is being done with other populations. In presenting a brief indication of that knowledge base and highlighting these three developmental concepts, we have attempted to provide a sufficient background to illustrate the potential fruitfulness, by way of applied examples, of jointly considering health and aging.

For the health psychology practitioner, we have described the ways in which health problems of the aged take on not only a chronic but also a multiple nature, with physical, psychological, and social factors all playing mutually influential roles in determining a person's condition. This complexity may confound diagnostic clarity; at the same time, it offers intriguing diagnostic challenges for assessment and intervention, including the possibility of far-reaching effects in areas outside of the presenting problem. We have also warned that the same disorder may present itself differently at different ages, whereas the same symptoms at different ages may imply different disorders. Moreover, we have cautioned that normal age-related changes may be mistaken for symptoms of a disease, while true disease symptoms may masquerade as normal aging. Finally, we urged application to the aged of what is known in health psychology, while taking the caution of attending to the knowledge base and to the various sources of potential misinterpretation.

For the health psychology researcher, the complexity of the health problems of the aged can interfere with survey research or make recruiting patients for a controlled outcome study of a single illness next to impossible. However, rather than barriers, these difficulties can instead be construed as magnifications of phenomena that are not unique to the aged, thus affording an abundant area for study. The interpretation of observed age differences is never straightforward. As we have indicated, a number of social and psychological variables show no age differences—or rather, apparent differences are not inevitable consequences of aging but in all likelihood are due to physical health differences or cohort differences. Including older adults in health psychology research designs not only would permit testing hypotheses about age differences, it would also allow variables that exert a robust effect on health status across the life span to emerge in greater clarity, thereby enriching our conceptualization of health and illness processes at all ages.

The overriding factor is demographic. Although alternative models refining life expectancy and epidemiological projections for the future raise questions regarding the concentration of various illnesses across the life span, the undisputed prediction is for increased numbers of older adults with substantial physical illnesses. Moreover, because of the interactive nature of their problems, older individuals with social and psychological difficulties will continue to be seen in large numbers in the health system. The health psychologist located in a medical setting is in a special position to bring psychological knowledge to bear on the investigation and treament of these complex problems.

REFERENCES

Atchley, R. C. 1977. *The social forces in later life: An introduction to social gerontology*. Belmont, CA: Wadsworth Publishing Co.

Besdine, R. W. 1981. Health and illness behavior in the elderly. In *Health, behavior and aging* (IOM Publication no. 81–102), edited by D. L. Parron, F. Solomon, and J. Rodin. Washington, D.C.: Institute of Medicine.

Blazer, D. G. 1982. *Depression in late life*. St. Louis, MO: C. V. Mosby Co.

Blazer, D., and I. C. Siegler. 1984. *A family approach to health care of the elderly*. Menlo Park, CA: Addison-Wesley Publishing Co.

Botwinick, J. 1977. Intellectual abilities. In *Handbook of the psychology of aging*, edited by J. E. Birren and K. W. Schaie. New York: Van Nostrand Reinhold Co.

Brody, E. M., and M. H. Kleban. 1981. Physical and mental health symptoms of older people: Whom do they tell? *Journal of the American Geriatrics Society* 29:442–49.

Butler, R. N., and M. I. Lewis. *Aging and mental health: Positive psychosocial approaches.* St. Louis, MO: C. V. Mosby Co.

Christie, A. B. 1982. Changing patterns in mental illness in the elderly. *British Journal of Psychiatry* 140:154–59.

Corso, J. F. 1977. Auditory perception and communication. In *Handbook of the psychology of aging,* edited by J. E. Birren and K. Warner Schaie. New York: Van Nostrand Reinhold Co.

Crandall, R. C. 1980. *Gerontology: A behavioral science approach.* Reading, MA: Addison-Wesley Publishing Co., Inc.

Cummings, J. L., and D. F. Benson. 1983. *Dementia: A clinical approach.* Woburn, MA: Butterworth Publishers.

Fozard, J. L., E. Wolf, B. Bell, R. A. McFarland, and S. Podolsky. 1977. Visual perception and communication. In *Handbook of the psychology of aging,* edited by J. E. Birren and K. Warner Schaie. New York: Van Nostrand Reinhold Co.

Fries, J. F. 1984. The compression of morbidity: Miscellaneous comments about a theme. *The Gerontologist* 24:354–59.

Fries, J. F., and L. M. Crapo. 1981. *Vitality and aging: Implications of the rectangular curve.* New York: W. H. Freeman.

Gatz, M., O. A. Barbarin, F. B. Tyler, R. E. Mitchell, J. A. Moran, P. J. Wirzbicki, J. Crawford, and A. Engelman. 1982. Enhancement of individual and community competence: The older adult as a community worker. *American Journal of Community Psychology* 10:291–303.

Gray, V. K. 1983. Providing support for home caregivers. In *Mental health and aging: Programs and evaluations,* edited by M. A. Smyer and M. Gatz. Beverly Hills, CA: Sage Publications.

Haug, M. R. 1981. Age and medical care utilization patterns. *Journal of Gerontology* 36:103–11.

Hebb, D. O. 1978. Watching myself get old. *Psychology Today* 12:15–23.

Himmelfarb, S. 1984. Age and sex differences in the mental health of older persons. *Journal of Consulting and Clinical Psychology* 52:844–56.

Jarvik, L. F., and M. Perl. 1981. Overview of physiologic dysfunctions related to psychiatric problems in the elderly. In *Neuropsychiatric manifestations of physical disease in the elderly,* edited by A. J. Levenson and R. C. W. Hall. New York: Raven Press.

Jones, K. R., and T. R. Vischi. 1979. Impact of alcohol, drug abuse and mental health treatment on medical care utilization: A review of the research literature. *Medical Care* 17:1–82, supplement section.

Kasl, S. V., and L. F. Berkman. 1981. Some psychosocial influences on the health status of the elderly: The perspective of social epidemiology. In *Aging: Biology and behavior,* edited by J. L. McGaugh and S. B. Kiesler. New York: Academic Press.

Kenney, R. A. 1982. *Physiology of aging.* Chicago, IL: Year Book Medical Publishers.

Kovar, M. G. 1980. Morbidity and health care utilization. In *Epidemiology of aging: Proceedings of the Second Conference,* edited by S. G. Haynes and M. Feinleib. NIH Publication no. 80–969.

Krantz, D. S., D. C. Glass, and N. E. Miller. 1981. *Behavior and health.* Paper for the National Science Foundation commissioned by the Social Science Research Council, New York

Krupka, L., and A. M. Vener. Hazards of drug use among the elderly. *The Gerontologist* 19:90–95.

Kucharski, L. T., R. M. White, and M. Schratz. 1979. Age bias, referral for psychological assistance, and the private physician. *Journal of Gerontology* 34:423–28.

Lamy, P. P. 1980. *Prescribing for the elderly.* Littleton, MA: PSG Publishing Co.

Lazarus, L. W., B. Stafford, K. Cooper, B. Cohler, and M. Dysken. 1981. A pilot study of an Alzheimer patient's relatives discussion group. *The Gerontologist* 21:353–58.

Levine, M. 1981. *The history and politics of community mental health.* New York: Oxford University Press.

Lofholm, P. 1975. Self medication by the elderly. In *Drugs and the elderly,* edited by R. H. Davis and W. K. Smith. Los Angeles: The University of Southern California Press.

McCrae, R. R. 1982. Age differences in the use of coping mechanisms. *Journal of Gerontology* 37:454–60.

Masek, B. J., L. H. Epstein, and D. C. Russo. 1981. Behavioral perspectives in preventive medicine. *Handbook of clinical behavior therapy,* edited by S. M. Turner, K. S. Calhoun, and H. E. Adams. New York: John Wiley & Sons.

Meyers, G. C., and K. G. Manton. 1984. Compression of mortality: Myth or reality. *The Gerontologist* 24:346–53.

Pavur, E. J., Jr.; and P. C. Smith. 1983. Absenteeism, turnover and an inservice program. In *Mental health and aging: Programs and evaluations,* edited by M. A. Smyer and M. Gatz. Beverly Hills, CA: Sage Publications.

Pearlin, L. I. 1983. Role strains and personal stress. In *Psychosocial stress: Trends, theory and research,* edited by H. B. Kaplan. New York: Academic Press.

Riley, M. W. 1981. Health behavior of older people: Toward a new paradigm. In *Health, behavior and aging,* edited by D. L. Parron, F. Solomon, and J. Rodin. IOM Publication no. 81–012. Washington, D.C.: Institute of Medicine.

Rodin, J. 1980. Managing the stress of aging: The role of control and coping. In *Coping and health,* edited by S. Levine and H. Ursin. New York: Plenum Press.

———. 1982. *Aging, control and health.* Presidential address at the Eastern Psychological Association.

Schulz, J. H. 1980. *The economics of aging.* 2d ed. Belmont, CA: Wadsworth Publishing Co.

Shanas, E. 1979. Social myth as hypothesis—Case of the family relations of old people. *The Gerontologist* 19:3–9.

Siegel, J. S. 1980. Recent and prospective demographic trends for the elderly population and some implications for health care. In *Epidemiology of aging: Proceedings of the Second Conference,* edited by S. G. Haynes and M. Feinleib. NIH Publication no. 80–969.

Siegler, I. C., and P. Costa. 1985. Health behavior relationships. In *Handbook of the psychology of aging*, 2d ed., edited by J. E. Birren and K. W. Schaie. New York: Van Nostrand Reinhold Co.

Siegler, I. C., J. B. Nowlin, and J. A. Blumenthal. 1980. Health and behavior: Methodological considerations for adult development and aging. In *Aging in the 1980s: Psychological issues,* edited by L. W. Poon. Washington, D.C.: American Psychological Association.

Skinner, B. F. 1983. Intellectual self-management in old age. *American Psychologist* 38:239–44.

Smyer, M. A. 1984. Supporting the supporters: Working with families of impaired elderly. *Journal of Community Psychology* 12:323–33.

U.S. General Accounting Office. 1982. *The elderly remain in need of mental health services.* (Document no. HRD–82–112). Washington, D.C.: Government Printing Office.

Zarit, S. H. 1980. *Aging and mental disorders.* New York: The Free Press.

Zarit, S. H., and J. M. Zarit. 1982. Families under stress: Interventions for caregivers of senile dementia patients. *Psychotherapy, Theory, Research, and Practice* 19:461–71.

Part Six

Challenges and Opportunities in Training Health Psychologists

Editor: Joseph D. Matarazzo

It is a given that the types and quality of the educational and training offerings available in a discipline constitute some of the most important and relevant features which affect its credibility. However, stating this truism does not address the question of how good quality educational programs are initially crafted and then put into place. The latter, in turn, confronts us with the question of which came first—the chicken or the egg. That question has had to be addressed by every new occupation, academic discipline, and profession since the formal organization of guilds, accomplished before the twelfth century, and of university-based academic programs for the professions which require a doctoral degree, established in Bologna in the year 1182. This philosophic as well as pragmatic issue of chicken versus egg is complicated because it is customarily perceived as downright arrogant for some individuals to assert that they are prepared to offer formal training in an area, field, or discipline in which they themselves have never received such training. Yet since antiquity this lack of formal training traditionally has been a feature of the circuitous route by which programs for the formal and accredited training of barbers, priests, architects, nurses, attorneys, physicians, psychologists, and electricians, as well as others have been established. Although limited space precludes my elaborating here on the complex and interrelated issues involved in this historical aspect of the sociology of professions, a fuller discussion is presented in Matarazzo and Abdellah (1971) and Matarazzo (1983).

The purpose of the present section is both to provide another small segment in the history of the sociology of professions and, especially, to try to focus on some of the relevant issues as they apply today to initiatives directed toward training an emerging breed of psychologist—namely, a health psychologist. The establishment of clinical psychology as a more formalized discipline took root with the Shakow Committee Report of 1947 and the

Boulder Conference of 1949. An excellent historical description of that evolution is provided in Paul Nelson's chapter. The psychologists of the 1949 era (who were not themselves formally trained in clinical psychology) pragmatically resolved the "chicken versus egg" problem when they began to offer—by fiat and mere declaration—accredited training in clinical psychology; their situation suggests clear parallels for today's psychologists (from many areas of psychology) who are beginning in increasing numbers to offer formal education and training programs in health psychology.

For example, in the chapters which follow, Belar, Boll, Strickland, Nelson, and Istvan and Hatton each provide valuable and complementary sets of insights into the issues involved in overhauling and retooling our existing graduate school faculties, graduate curricula, and apprenticeship internship programs, as well as our profession's apparatuses of accreditation, to make each more applicable to the emerging predoctoral and postdoctoral program offerings in health psychology. Although each of these authors states this opinion in different ways, all espouse the view that the health psychologist being educated and trained today must be a *psychologist* first—one who is sufficiently familiar with the knowledge base of psychology to then apply that core of knowledge to the health arena. Furthermore, and although the focus of their respective chapters is the *postdoctoral* segment of the currently prescribed education and training experience, Friedman, Matarazzo, Sechrest, and Fordyce and Meier are in agreement with the view of the other authors that quality postdoctoral education and training in health psychology can probably best be utilized, at present, by trainees whose predoctoral education was that of a generic psychologist with a minor or related extras in health psychology rather than by a graduate whose predoctoral program sacrificed that core and breadth for specialization as a health psychologist too early on. That is, there is a unanimity of belief espoused within each of the chapters in this part that the postbaccalaureate program of training for a career in health psychology (either as service provider, researcher, or both) should begin with acquisition in the predoctoral years of the core knowledge of psychology. This serves as a base for apprenticeship-acquired attitudes, professional and ethical standards, and the broad range of proficiencies which, collectively, by the end of a mandated two-year, postdoctoral program of considerably more in-depth training, coalesce into a psychologist competently prepared to provide service or do research in today's emerging specialty area of health psychology.

Furthermore, for those individuals who now wish to respecialize and who did not follow this integrated training sequence, which is coordinated from the beginning of predoctoral through the end of postdoctoral training, but first trained for work in other areas of psychology (e.g., experimental, clinical, social, etc.), the to-be-added teaching and fieldwork components should be no less rigorous than for the psychologist who is more cost-effectively trained from his or her first postbaccalaureate days for a career in health psychology.

REFERENCES

Matarazzo, J. D. 1983. Education and training in health psychology: Boulder or bolder? *Health Psychology* 2:73–113.

Matarazzo, J. D., and F. G. Abdellah. 1971. Doctoral education for nurses in the United States. *Nursing Research* 20:404–14.

22

The Current Status of Predoctoral and Postdoctoral Training in Health Psychology

Cynthia D. Belar

As a field grows, so does the focus on the credentials of those professing expertise in the area. Issues of standard setting become prominent, and the kind of training experiences necessary to call oneself a specialist are discussed and delineated. So it has been with health psychology. Yet these discussions do not occur in a vacuum. Before setting standards, information about current training experiences and models are shared both informally and formally through published position papers, program examples, and surveys of training opportunities. The purpose of this chapter is to summarize these kinds of data in order to provide an overview of the current status of predoctoral and postdoctoral training in health psychology. Issues of continuing education and respecialization are dealt with in other chapters in this book. In beginning, however, it might be of interest to review the kinds of training obtained by those individuals who currently call themselves health psychologists.

Morrow, Carpenter, and Clayman (1982) conducted a survey of the American Psychological Association Division of Health Psychology membership in 1981 in an attempt to obtain information on training backgrounds. Completed surveys were returned by 1,477 (57.2%) members of the Division. Almost half (46.1%) reported having obtained a Ph.D./Psy.D. degree in clinical psychology; another 15% reported a doctoral degree in counseling psychology. A background in social psychology training accounted for 8% of the responents, 6.2% were trained as experimental psychologists, and 3.4% were trained in physiological psychology. Other areas of psychology (e.g., community) accounted for the remainder, although 3% reported degrees in disciplines other than psychology. The authors also asked respondents to indicate where they had obtained formal training in health psychology: predoctoral courses, predoctoral practica, predoctoral internship, postdoctoral and/or continuing education workshops/seminars. Morrow et al. concluded that irrespective of degree areas, the primary way the majority of respondents had obtained health psychology training was through continuing education. Almost three-fourths of the respondents had obtained formal training in this manner, while only 20 to 30% had obtained formal training at the predoctoral level. Interestingly, only 38% of the clinical psychologists had obtained formal health psychology training as interns. Obviously there are currently few health psychologists who could meet the standards for training that have been proposed by the recent National Working Conference on Education and Training in Health Psychology (Stone 1983). This is perhaps as it should be in a rapidly evolving area such as health psychology. In fact, it is interesting to note in this connection that Matarazzo (1983, p. 87) reports that today's leaders in health psychology received their doctorates with study in *every area* of psychology, including social, counseling, experimental, and others. Furthermore, he offered his opinion that it was just such *diversity* which had provided the impetus and vitality to the recent advances in health psychology as a discipline.

Obtaining accurate information about the current status of training has been difficult. Many of the surveys cited below reported return rates of 50 to 65%. The surveys supported by the Division of Health Psychology (Belar, Wilson, and Hughes 1982; Belar and Siegel 1983) employed a second mailing in an effort to reconfirm self-report data via signed statements from the training directors. In addition, the public dissemination of the predoctoral and postdoctoral training directories has made many programs eager to be included. Nevertheless, there have been notable omissions and undoubtedly errors of fact. The most interesting methodologic issue, however, was discovered during the first survey. When some of the respondents were contacted by representatives from the American Psychological Association about the training opportunities in health psychology, several denied having any (despite having rather extensively and affirmatively completed the survey questionnaire). This may have been due to the fact that when the American Psychological Association telephoned, questions were phrased utilizing the term "health psychology," which was apparently unfamiliar to many training directors. The Division 38 survey utilized an operational approach, namely the Division of Health Psychology's *definition* of the term, when inquiring about training opportunities. This phenomenon is unlikely to be witnessed again.

Predoctoral Training

Recent publications contain several descriptions of different kinds of training programs with an emphasis on health psychology, as does chapter 30 by

Istvan and Hatton in this volume. Belar (1980, 1982) describes training within a clinical psychology program and discusses differences in both applied and research areas from traditional clinical psychology training.

The author, herself, developed training tracks in medical psychology at predoctoral, postdoctoral, and internship levels at the University of Florida's Department of Clinical Psychology doctoral program. That predoctoral program curriculum is consistent with that of other Boulder model (see chaps. 23 and 26 by Boll and Matarazzo for a description of this model) clinical psychology programs, with emphases on core psychology, research methods, and basic clinical skills. In addition, that University of Florida medical psychology track requirements include: (1) a course in pathophysiology; (2) a seminar in medical psychology including theories of psychobiological functioning, methodologic issues in research, critical reviews of particular content areas such as compliance, pain, etc.—students select an area for review and concurrently spend at least one half-day per week as an observer on a ward or clinic relevant to the topic chosen; (3) a practicum in applied medical psychology, including ongoing seminars focusing on professional issues and case presentation, plus direct supervised experience with inpatient and outpatient consultation and therapy with a wide variety of patients referred from various medical and surgical specialties; and (4) an elective course (e.g., psychopharmacology, neuroanatomy). The student is concurrently involved in health psychology research. The administrative structure of the Department of Clinical Psychology, with its integration into a major interdisciplinary academic health center, facilitated the development of this program. Departmental faculty and research collaborators include neurologists, rheumatologists, endocrinologists, oncologists, etc. Although emphasizing training for research careers which integrate studies involving behavior and the basic sciences instead of clinical work, the Ph.D. program offered in a second health sciences university, presented by Matarazzo (1983, pp. 101–5), takes advantage of many of the same strengths of a large academic health center as does the Florida program.

Evans (1982) details a social psychology program providing training in behavioral medicine research in a combined university and medical school program. The focus is on prevention of cardiovascular disease. Social psychology seminars which relate social psychological concepts to program development in health behavior provide the theoretical training. Physiological components of risk factors and orientations to cardiovascular disease are learned via seminars available with the Baylor College of Medicine National Heart and Blood Vessel Research and Demonstration Center (of which social psychological research is a component) and the Baylor National Heart

Center (which includes the long-range adolescent smoking prevention project). Since program evaluation skills are highly emphasized, seminars in this area, as well as other aspects of research methodology, are required. Trainees become involved in research areas such as the evaluation of strategies for increasing compliance, for enhancing physician-patient communication, for dealing with life-style changes of patients, and for modifying coronary-prone behavior.

Still another kind of program is described by Stone (1979). The Graduate Group in Psychology at the School of Medicine, University of California, San Francisco, began in 1970 to develop the first explicitly labeled specialized program in health psychology. This program stresses basic courses in social, personality, and cognitive psychology, as well as research methods and physiological aspects of health. In addition, emphasis is placed on becoming knowledgeable about the social and biomedical aspects of health care systems. A research placement within the health care system fosters the development of skills in interdisciplinary collaboration and provides experience in developing a research project in a field setting such as a coronary care unit, a community medicine department, a VA hospital, a department of epidemiology, a family planning clinic, an adolescent health unit, etc. Each of the programs noted places emphases on learning basic human physiology and developing an awareness of the sociopolitical aspects of health care systems, as well as firm grounding in the core of psychology. For the interested reader, Matarazzo (1983) provided the actual, year-by-year curriculum for the Ph.D. program offered at four universities. This material is updated and extended to nine additional programs in chapter 30.

Also available in the literature are survey data on training opportunities in specific content areas within health psychology, such as applied psychophysiology and clinical neuropsychology (Feuerstein and Schwartz 1977; Golden and Kuperman 1980a). However, the most complete and current data on doctoral training come from a Division of Health Psychology survey (Belar, Wilson, and Hughes 1982). Forty-two programs were identified in thirty-eight institutions representing essentially four different models of training. Six programs described a primary focus, i.e., a specialized degree in the area (three in health psychology, two in behavioral medicine, one in neuropsychology). Of the remaining programs, the predominant model (70%) was that of training as a track within another specialty in psychology. The models of "individually designed course of study" and "selected opportunities available" were equally represented (14%). In two-thirds of the programs, health psychology was offered within the context of clinical, counseling, and/or school psychology specialties. The most frequently mentioned orientation available was behavioral (60%), followed by psychodynamic, eclectic, cognitive, and psychophysiological (26–36%). Most importantly, only half of the programs reported having an interdisciplinary faculty (medicine being the most commonly mentioned discipline). Nearly 70% of the programs reported that funding was available in terms of trainee support.

Internship Training

Gentry, Street, Masur, and Asken (1981) found that forty-eight of sixty-five respondents to an APA approved internship program survey ($n = 128$) offered formal training in medical psychology, although in only nineteen was such training required of all interns. Assessment and intervention were rather equally emphasized, with neuropsychological assessment represented as frequently as personality assessment. (A survey of APA approved internships specifically designed to investigate training in *clinical neuropsychology* identified eighty-six or ninety-eight respondents as offering experience in this area, although only thirty permitted specialization (Golden and Kuperman 1980b). Eighty-four institutions providing intern-level training in health psychology were noted by Belar et al. (1982) in their survey of the Association for Psychology Internship Centers (APIC) membership, which includes both APA and non-APA approved internship programs. Petty and Rakowsky (1983) also surveyed APIC members and reported that practical clinical experience with the following presenting problems were the most common: chronic pain, diet/weight management, death/bereavement, substance abuse, compliance, and cardiovascular problems. Over half of the fifty-two internships identified by Petty and Rakowsky reported involvement with special medical services such as neurology, general medicine, pain clinics, oncology, and rehabilitation.

In general, it appears that internship training in health psychology occurs primarily within hospital-based programs in clinical and/or counseling psychology. Nevertheless, special issues of training in a *rehabilitation* setting are discussed by Gold, Meltzer, and Sherr (1982), who delineate the professional role functioning requirements in those settings and highlight the needs in training for learning to deal effectively with patients who have suffered dramatic violations of their physical integrity. Both Gold et al. and Belar (1980) have emphasized the need for sensitivity to students' needs and concerns as they confront their emotional responses to disease and disability and their preexisting prejudices in interdisciplinary functioning. Gold et al. suggest more training in brain-behavior assessments, in evaluating the reality-based depth of mourning reactions, in assessing personal and environmental assets, and in dealing with issues of dependence-independence.

Behavioral medicine internship training at a VA medical center is described by Swan, Piccione, and Anderson (1980). Within that setting in Palo Alto, a rotation in behavioral medicine follows the scientist-practitioner model and provides training in stress and pain management, adherence programs, life-style adjustment (e.g., cardiac rehabilitation, coping with cancer), treatment of addictive behaviors, and behavioral dentistry.

More recently, Tuma and Grabert (1983) have reported on internship and postdoctoral training in *pediatric psychology*. Their survey attempted to delineate differences between pediatric and clinical child training programs, but the authors conclude that the similarities are more numerous than the differences in training. "Pediatric psychology can thus be considered the clinical child psychology entry into health psychology (p. 258)." Curricula differences for the pediatric psychologist include more medically related seminars, more emphases on evaluation procedures, and greater emphasis on behaviorally oriented treatment interventions than usually found in clinical child programs.

There are as yet no systematic data on the opportunities for training at the internship level in schools of public health, industrial consulting firms, and/or health policy organizations. Although such opportunities exist, the development in such settings of what might be more appropriately called apprenticeships in health psychology is rudimentary at best.

Postdoctoral Training

Forty-three programs offering postdoctoral training in health psychology were identified by Belar and Siegel (1983). The overwhelming majority emphasized applied research (90%) and/or clinical experience (70%), while public health and/or community and public policy were represented in 32% and 12% of the programs, respectively. None of the programs indicated an emphasis on industrial health psychology. Issues related to children, adolescents, and adults were addressed in approximately 75% of the programs, while half had training related to the aged. Trainee groups tended to be interdisciplinary. While more than three-fourths offered training in assessment and intervention, only half provided opportunities in primary prevention/health promotion.

Heterogeneity was apparent both across and within programs. In 1983, the University of Florida at Gainesville (Department of Clinical Psychology) offered six postdoctoral positions; three were primarily clinical positions (adult medical psychology, pediatric psychology, and neuropsychology), while three were primarily research oriented (behavioral dentistry). The School of Medicine's Department of Medical Psychology at the Oregon Health Sciences University likewise currently offers six postdoctoral fellowships supported by the National Heart, Lung, and Blood Institute—again, three with a combined basic science and clinical focus and three in the area of basic research in animal models of cardiovascular disease. The University of Houston Department of Psychology offered four postdoctoral traineeships to train researchers in social psychology as applied to the prevention and control of cardiovascular diseases. With a grant from the National Institute of Mental Health, the University of California (San Francisco) program supports both predoctoral and postdoctoral trainees. Alcohol research characterizes the postdoctoral program at the Department of Psychiatry, University of Connecticut Health Center.

Sources of funding for postdoctoral programs were also varied and frequently multiple: 55% reported funding via federal training grants; 26% obtained private training grants; and 19% operated with state training funds. Patient fees supported 22% of the programs.

Overview

Since none of the surveys previously cited made independent attempts to confirm the accuracy of responses, these data should be considered as unvalidated self-report. There have also been no attempts to assess *quality* of training in health psychology in these programs (the criteria for such evaluation being nonexistent until the National Working Conference on Education and Training in Health Psychology began the process of establishing guidelines). Thus, the current state of training in the area of health psychology is one lacking both designation and accreditation of programs at all levels. Nevertheless, programs continue to expand and to multiply in this field, which was a priority area for NIMH clinical training grant support in 1983. While Matarazzo (1983) has elsewhere articulated a series of issues relevant to this evolution, which were subsequently addressed by delegates to the National Training Conference, this author will make a few observations on the current status of training in this area. Those observations are based on the literature previously cited, the perspective gained as chair for The Division of Health Psychology Education and Training Committee, and nearly ten years of experience in developing such training programs at predoctoral, internship, and postdoctoral levels.

First, there appears to be a dearth of training in industrial health psychology. This training emphasis was not noted in any of the doctoral or post-doctoral programs identified, although the other traditional applied areas (school, counseling, clinical) were represented. Yet many psychologists are involved in activities such as reducing job stress, screening for health behavior risk factors, and preventive health programs. Indeed, the theme of the 1983 Annual Meeting of the Society of Behavioral Medicine was "Behavioral Medicine in Industry"; program materials reflect the breadth of current psychologists' roles in this area. Although not yet formalized, occupational settings do offer unique opportunities for apprenticeship training in industrial health for psychologists. Also underrepresented is the important area of public policy.

My second observation concerns the lack of interdisciplinary faculty in many of the current training programs. With the exception of the health psychology training programs supported by NIH and NIMH training grants in schools of medicine and health sciences universities, the need for such collaboration in order to learn about relationships with other health professions, as well as to obtain knowledge fundamental to research and practice in health psychology, appears especially unfulfilled at the predoctoral level. In addition, a number of the programs identified in the Belar surveys appear quite dependent upon one or two staff members to deliver the health psychology training component. Lack of program breadth and stability are potential problems for these educational settings.

A third observation has to do with training in the *applied* area of health psychology. On occasion the specialty emphasis appears to have preceded the general practitioner model of training even within health psychology. There has been a tendency in some programs to divide people's health problems into chunks of behavior (smoking, weight, tension reduction, exercise) without attention to the person in his or her total emotional and social environment and to train students in limited interventions prior to more general clinical training in interviewing, assessment of emotional, psychosocial and behavioral factors, and intervention skills. Those of us who have spent years fighting notions of mind-body dualism held by physicians are frequently disturbed when hearing from our own discipline that it is possible to treat health problems psychologically without regard to personality and mental health issues. The philosophic position adopted on this issue has great implications for the development of applied training programs.

Summary

In summary, the current state of training in health psychology is best described as vibrant, heterogeneous, and still evolving. Four models account for training at the predoctoral level, the most common one being a track within some other subarea of psychology. Across predoctoral and postdoctoral programs, clinical training is emphasized in over two-thirds, but even here there is considerable variability among programs. In this evolving field, this heterogeneity has been welcomed. As the field matures, criteria and guidelines can be developed, a process begun by the recent National Working Conference on Education and Training in Health Psychology.

References

Belar, C. D. 1980. Training the clinical psychology student in behavioral medicine. *Professional Psychology* 11:596–604.

———. 1982. Current patterns and issues of doctoral training in health psychology. Paper presented to the Annual Meeting of the American Psychological Association, Washington, D.C., August.

Belar, C. D., and L. J. Siegel. 1983. A survey of postdoctoral training programs in health psychology. *Health Psychology* 2:413–25.

Belar, C. D., E. Wilson, and H. Hughes. 1982. Health psychology training in doctoral psychology programs. *Health Psychology* 1:289–99.

Evans, R. I. 1982. Training social psychologists in behavioral medicine research. In *Social psychology and behavioral medicine*, edited by J. Richard Eiser. New Jersey: John Wiley & Sons.

Feuerstein, M. and G. E. Schwartz. 1977. Training in clinical psychophysiology. *American Psychologist* 32:560–67.

Gentry, W. D., W. J. Street, F. T. Masur, and M. J. Asken. 1981. Training in medical psychology: A survey of graduate and internship training programs. *Professional Psychology* 12:224–28.

Gold, J. R., R. H. Meltzer, and R. L. Sherr. 1982. Professional transition: Psychology internships in rehabilitation settings. *Professional Psychology* 13:397–403.

Golden, C., and S. K. Kuperman. 1980a. Graduate training in clinical neuropsychology. *Professional Psychology* 11:55–63.

———. 1980b. Training opportunities in neuropsychology at APA-approved internship settings. *Professional Psychology* 11:907–17.

Matarazzo, J. D. 1983. Education and training in health psychology: Boulder or bolder? *Health Psychology* 2:73–113.

Morrow, G. R., P. J. Carpenter, and D. A. Clayman. 1983. A national survey of health psychologists: Characteristics, training and priorities. *The Health Psychologist* 5 (2):6–7.

Petty, N. E., and G. W. Rakowsky. 1983. Health psychology training in predoctoral APIC internships. Unpublished manuscript. Western Michigan University.

Stone, G. C. 1979. A specialized doctoral program in health psychology: Considerations in its evolution. *Professional Psychology* 10:596–604.

———, ed. 1983. Proceedings of the National Working Conference on Education and Training in Health Psychology, May 23–27. *Health Psychology*, 2 (5): 1–153, supplement section.

Swan, G. E., A. Piccione, and D. C. Anderson. 1980. Internship training in behavioral medicine: Program description, issues, and guidelines. *Professional Psychology* 11:339–46.

Tuma, J. M., and J. Grabert. 1983. Internship and Postdoctoral training in pediatric and clinical child psychology: A survey. *Journal of Pediatric Psychology* 8 (3): 245–60.

23

Predoctoral Education and Training in Health Psychology

Thomas J. Boll

Origins of Psychology Training

The history of education in general psychology and more particularly clinical and finally health psychology has been reviewed in some detail by Matarazzo (1983); Belar (1980); and Matarazzo, Carmody, and Gentry (1981). Matarazzo (1983) documents the very interesting historical beginnings of what we now consider to be graduate education. The first university degrees began with the awarding of the Doctor of Philosophy (Ph.D.) degree, wherein the title "Doctor" was drawn from the Latin word "doctorem," meaning a teacher. At about the same time, a similar guild formation occurred in Paris which entitled its university teachers to call themselves "masters," from the Latin word "majester," and to award this same doctoral-level degree to their successful students. It was just 100 years ago that the first Ph.D. in psychology was conferred in the United States by Johns Hopkins University in 1886. The growth of programs offering doctoral degrees in psychology ever since has resulted in tens of thousands of individuals entering the discipline and profession of psychology.

Health Psychology Organization

This history of the field of health psychology, outlined in chapters 2 and 3, underlines how very rapidly the emergence and identification of health psychology as an area of interest and professional pursuit developed from its

The working group on predoctoral education/doctoral training was comprised of Nancy Adler, Mary Ellen Olbrish, Judy Hall, Jan Woodring, Camille Wortman, Lauren Weiss, Nathan Perry, Theodore Millon, and Carl Thoresen. These individuals provided the past experience and background knowledge, current sophistication, and drive toward the future necessary for the development of the initial document from the National Conference on Graduate Education and Training in Health Psychology. It is from this document and from the readings, background materials, and outstanding discussions that occurred in preparation for, during, and following this conference that the current chapter has developed.

first formal organizations in the late 1970s to its first formal training conference in the early 1980s. It also demonstrates what a long lag there has been between the recognition of the importance of psychology to the field of medicine and vice versa in 1911, the emergence of psychologists in any reasonable number in medical centers in the 1950s, and the formal development of an organizational structure entitled health psychology in the 1970s and 80s.

Issues of Generic and Service Provider Training

What training then do we provide? Two issues seem to float to the top of almost any discussion despite the fact that there are many issues that could be and often are discussed. One issue is that of the overall nature of exposure to generic psychological science. The other is the discussion of whether or not individuals should be prepared to provide or deliver service and whether or not two tracks, for service providers and nonservice providers, should be developed.

With regard to the first issue, the participants in the National Working Conference on Education and Training in Health Psychology were unanimous in endorsing the guidelines for defining a doctoral degree in psychology as developed by the Conference on Education and Credentialing in Psychology in 1977. The statement from that group with regard to the issue of a core and irreducible amount of training in the area of general psychology is described in chapter 14. The specifications do not represent requirements for specific courses but rather for areas of integrated knowledge and skill. A number of course requirements are detailed in chapter 15. Training in advanced research and design, methodology and statistics, and knowledge and skill in areas specifically relevant to health psychology such as field research, epidemiology, comparative methods, longitudinal design, biostatistics, survey research and time series analysis, experimental designs, and small and large N designs were strongly emphasized. In addition to the central areas of knowledge and skill, four core areas in psychology each requiring a minimum of three semester hours of course work were adopted. These included: (1) biological bases of behavior, such as psychophysiology, comparative psychology, neuropsychology, and psychopharmacology; (2) cognitive-affective bases of behavior, such as learning, memory, perception, cognition, thinking, and motivation; (3) social bases of behavior, such as social, cultural, ethnic, group, organization, systems psychology, and psychology of women; and (4) individual differences (psychological bases of behavior), such as personality theory, human development, psychopathology, individual differences, and psychology of the handicapped. It was the opinion of the 1983 Arden House Conference that programs entitled Health Psychology must meet these minimum standards and criteria in the field of generic psychology.

Millon (Millon, Green, and Meagher 1982) has provided an excellent discussion of the nature of clinical health psychology and many of the difficulties encountered in establishing an adequate curriculum for the education of individuals in this area. He proposed to use the basic sciences of psychology (e.g., social, developmental, etc.) as stepping stones in a manner designed specifically to show the relevance of these areas to health psychology. A curriculum then could be constructed so that each of these areas was covered in such a way that each course would, in turn, relate to the underlying purpose of the overall curriculum, namely to educate in the field of health psychology. This proposal is consistent, efficient, and has an obvious parsimony that is certainly appealing and may well represent an excellent approach to the utilization of the basics of psychology in the education of health psychologists.

An alternate approach is one oriented toward somewhat greater breadth and possibly toward longer range preparation of individuals. Such an approach would recognize that what knowledge from the basic psychological sciences is relevant for health psychology in the twenty-first century may or may not be that which is most apparent today. One could educate more broadly in the several areas with no undue or specially developed focus on health so that the fullest appreciation of the basic psychological fields is obtained. This approach, rather than an early (premature?) selection (by others) of what is and what is not contributed from each basic psychological area to health psychology, might well provide for a degree of increased breadth in the overall educational program of the student and avoid premature closure. This is especially important in such a rapidly developing field. It might also tend to provide the kind of education that would allow the student to develop psychological research and intervention approaches that draw upon his or her own appreciation and understanding of what the basic sciences have contributed. Learning would occur as issues and problems arise and are connected by the creativity of the individual students rather than students receiving them in a more structured fashion through the creativity of an individual professor. This approach would allow the broadest, rather than the most focused, coverage of the basic psychological sciences. While less immediately and obviously relevant in a student's eye, it may provide the kind of background for future growth and development espoused routinely as the sine qua non of education in health psychology.

The second issue relates to the amount of professional (applied, small "c" clinical) training that is needed and what the focus of that training should be for health psychology students who wish to pursue training in the area of direct service delivery in addition to the other health psychology and general psychology training that they are to receive. The argument has been put forth by Neal Miller (1983) and Stanley Schneider (1983) that a minimum amount of what is generally considered to be traditional clinical psychological training is necessary and appropriate in the training of an applied health psychologist. Both Miller and Schneider point out that the patient population which applied health psychologists will be dealing with are not those with primary psychiatric pathology. Rather they are normal individuals who have become ill and for whom the relevant behavior is, in one way or another, an aspect of their illness. As such behavior is becoming a concern to a greater percentage of ill patients, most of whom would not be classified as "psychiatric" in nature, the need to focus training on traditional mental health approaches to assessment and intervention should be appropriately reduced. Millon et al. (1982) would add that the reduction in traditional mental health intervention and assessment procedures should be offset by an increase in training in assessments specific and relevant to health behavior and in intervention strategies specific to dealing with patients in the context of medical illness in a medical setting.

Not opposed but somewhat distinct from this position is a discussion presented by Belar (1980) that addresses both a practical issue of program accreditation as well as a conceptual analysis of the need for basic clinical training. With regard to the practical issue, despite the strong interest in the establishment of specialties within the American Psychological Association and the active discussion that is being pursued in this regard, the American Psychological Association has yet to identify any area as a formal specialty (see chaps. 26 and 29 by J. Matarazzo and P. Nelson in this volume for further details on this point). Moreover and more to the point, the accreditation committee of the Education Training Board of the American Psychological Association presently recognizes accreditation only in the areas of clinical, counseling, and school psychology. Thus, if one is to train an applied health psychologist from a program recognized by the American Psychological Association and accreditated by its accrediting arm, qualifications must be achieved that meet the requirements for recognition in one of those three areas. As the largest single employer of psychologists in the United States, the Veterans Administration system now prescribes against the hiring of psychologists whose degrees are not from such accredited programs. Therefore, to fail to provide for one's applied students such accreditation is to graduate them with a significant occupational handicap. If that is the choice of the training program certainly even a modicum of consumerism would require appropriate warning labels on that graduate program. Then, students and consumers alike would recognize what was and was not being provided to participants in that program and what could and could not be expected from those participants following their graduation.

Belar (1982) developed a more content-based argument for "traditional" clinical training bolstered by considerable weight of evidence. She points out that one of the major areas of increased awareness developed by the field of health psychology is the relationship between psychological problems and psychological stress and physical illness. Individuals with psychological problems, who are under significant psychological stress and subject to significant amounts of life change, do have an increased incidence of physical illness. In the same context Belar points out that fifty to sixty-five percent of medical patients show some affective disturbances. I have pointed out elsewhere (Boll 1983) that individuals with neurological illness are six times more likely to experience psychiatric symptoms, and patients with physical disabilities without neurologic symptoms are three times more likely than the normal population to have psychiatric illness. The association of any chronic illness with increased risk for emotional-psychological disruption is well recognized in the literature of those illnesses. Belar goes on to ask how, if one's medical patient population is at high risk for being either pre- or postmorbidly involved with some degree of psychopathology and, if the presence of psychopathology can influence the course of an intervention, can these risks be ignored? How can they be recognized unless training in this area has been received. Belar adds, "It does not follow that just because some clinical psychologists are not trained in a particular area that a specialty in psychology without any consistent applied training is more appropriate. . . . It is my opinion that anytime one utilizes the technology of psychology in an attempt to intervene in a patient's life, one needs an understanding of the whole person. This requires skills in interviewing, assessment of emotional, psychosocial and behavioral factors, and intervention skills" (Belar 1982, 3).

On the basis of these and other discussions, the Health Psychology Training Conference recommended, regarding professional applied training for work as a health psychologist, the adoption of the training models and curricula contained in the section of the "Criteria for Accreditation of Doctoral Training Programs and Internships in Professional Psychology" contained in the American Psychological Accreditation Handbook (1983). In recommending these guidelines, it was recognized that they have been developed in relation to existing professional areas. Fortunately they have been written broadly enough to encompass the types of skills and knowledge that professional psychologists in the field of health psychology should have. In terms of their application to the training and education in health psychology they should be viewed in terms of their applicability to the activities in which health psychologists will be engaged and in relation to emerging techniques and procedures in assessment, intervention, consultation, and evaluation relevant to health psychology problems and populations most broadly considered. The four areas of professional practice which must be addressed are assessment, intervention, consultation and evaluation.

Specific sections adopted from the accreditation manual are reproduced in Appendix A to this chapter. It was the further consensus of the group that the formal practicum/clerkship experience was central to professional preparation for health psychologists. Toward that end, the criteria of the American Psychological Association Accreditation Handbook (revised 8 March 1983) were adopted and are reproduced here in Appendix B of this chapter. It should be noted in this context that the practicum, field experience, and formal internship are to be specifically identified with the field of health psychology and that the experience encountered should be appropriate to that area.

The discussion so far has provided a training and curricular model for the generic or psychological bases of behavior and for the professional applied or clinical bases of behavior, education and training. These are seen as integral to and basic for the development of specialty knowledge and skill in the area of health including both basic science and applied activities. Numerous authors (Millon, Green, and Meagher 1982; Stone, Cohen, and Adler, 1979; Filskov and Boll 1981) recognize that in order to function in health care environment (medical school, hospital, private practice, biobehavioral research laboratory, health education and training program, wellness center, etc.) knowledge of at least three different types must be obtained.

First, reasonable knowledge and skill must be obtained about basic bodily functions underlying biochemical and physiological and anatomical processes and organization. This includes awareness of disease systems which the psychologist must have to participate in other than a woefully naive fashion in research or clinical pursuits with physically ill patients and with other providers of physical health care.

Second, knowledge of psychological theory and research findings as it relates to intervention and assessment with physical illness is core to all health psychology training. This includes knowledge about psychological factors related to health and illness and knowledge about psychologically based research methodologies. This is crucial for pursuing investigating of these issues and for the development of interventions, including interventions aimed at prevention of illness and enhancement of health.

Third, knowledge must be had of the system and the environment in which all aspects of health care are carried out. The health care environment is not an academic department of psychology nor a mental health clinic. The behaviors and sociopolitical understandings and interpersonal relationships appropriate to those settings more traditionally occupied by psychologists will stand one in very poor stead in attempting to get along and take one's place along side colleagues in the health care environment. No matter how good one's research or applied product, if the purveyor of product doesn't know the territory, very few sales are going to be made.

With regard to health psychology, the National Training Conference also outlined what was considered a minimum amount of knowledge in the area of health psychology. This knowledge is appropriate to any health psychologist, be they trained in the pure researcher model or in that of the scientist practitioner professional. In addition to basic courses in psychological bases of behavior and in applied psychological techniques for prevention, courses in health promotion, interventions, assessment, consultation and evaluation called for in every doctoral program in psychology, and didactic and practicum experience leading to knowledge and skills at an advanced level must be included.

For research oriented psychology programs not providing professional applied training, it is particularly appropriate that students begin their research activities at the earliest possible opportunity and pursue these activities consistently throughout the entire program. The equivalent of one year in an apprenticeship in a health-related environment should be obtained. For individuals aiming toward exclusively research-oriented careers, experience involving a breadth of research strategies which exposes them to the environment in which the delivery of health care is provided and in which both applied and basic research is conducted should be integral to their training. This last requirement says, with reasonable directness, that even nonclinicians must be exposed, beyond a practicum/clerkship level, to patients, patients' problems, and the real life difficulties of the health care environments. With this exposure, their research and their interactions and behaviors while conducting research will be appropriate to the constraints of the situation being investigated and not developed in an artificial environment with no identifiable relationship to the situation in which the issues being addressed actually occur. While it is obvious that clinical/applied psychologists must obtain this kind of training, it was held and unanimously endorsed that nonapplied researchers in the health field should gain this training. This clerkship type experience should be a required part of the basic training of researchers as well as applied health psychology professionals.

Breadth and Depth

The final issue is one of breadth versus depth. Stone (1979) and Miller (1983; and chap. 1 in this volume) have expressed the concern that, in the process of teaching in each of these highly desirable areas of knowledge and skill in the context of a four-year training program, insufficient time is available and something will have to give. One approach, commonly referred to as the "let 100 flowers bloom" strategy (Matarazzo 1983), is to provide for decreased breadth in order to allow for increased depth of investigation and training during the predoctoral years. While any single individual trained in this manner might be less broadly able to deal with the complexities of a health care environment, the totality of the training skills provided to a significant number of students would, in fact, provide that breadth. Interaction among several of these psychologists would lead both to individual depth and to investigative breadth for the group. Miller, among others, fears that, if we do not take this approach, the amount of knowledge students have in any particular area will be insufficient to allow them to draw upon their training adequately to bring it to bear in the best possible fashion on problems of health psychology. Stone (1979) raises an additional problem of the boundaries of the field. He points out, as have many others before and since, that psychology is an extremely broad undertaking in the area of human knowledge. When one identifies oneself as a psychologist, others tend to expect knowledge of everything from dream interpretation to the effect of TV violence to cognitive rehabilitation and memory enhancement. No single psychologist can possibly provide competent service, or even opinions, in all of those areas. Therefore, some limitation of the field such that others may recognize "what kind of psychologist" is being dealt with would obviously be of some value. This issue has been explicitly addressed by Matarazzo in chapter 26 of this volume. While recommending training in generic psychology at the predoctoral level, he urges, with considerable vigor, that only through *postdoctoral* training can one arrive at an adequate skill level for journeyman entrance into the activities of health psychology—be they in the research or applied realm.

It is the purpose of the present chapter to put forward a view which does not in any way oppose postdoctoral training but which indicates that predoctoral training can be modeled to provide what doctoral training is designed to do: to prepare a student to begin the lifelong process of self-education. Students would commence their careers with sufficiently sophisticated tools for that endeavor in the area of both process (skill training) and content (statistics, methodology, research design, and a core understanding of the theoretical development of the body of psychological knowledge currently existing). In that way a continued self-education can be pursued throughout a lifetime. Miller, who on the one hand argues for decreased breadth and increased depth in training because of the fear that students can simply not learn enough about all there is to know, also points out that students should not be expected to learn all there is to know. Rather they are merely embarking upon a lifelong educational process. He says eloquently "we should bear in mind vividly that health psychology hopefully will continue to develop fast enough so that what we teach today will be out of date a decade from now when most of our students will still have thirty years of their career ahead of them" (Miller 1983, 2). If, in fact, the field is both hopelessly broad and rapidly changing then it is probably safe to say that even in-depth training may be characterized by a very limited half-life. It is fraught with the risk that depth may be obtained in an area soon to be dramatically changed or found no longer relevant. Too much focus at the expense of breadth could leave the student in the position of having no background at all in the new and emerging areas. The student would then be faced with the need for a complete retraining process rather than a switch in reliance from one set of skills learned early on to yet another set of skills which can more rapidly be brought up-to-date as the current scientific and clinical situation demands. Broadest education in basic sciences of psychology, basic knowledge in the area of health and human behavior, and basic skills in the area of professional assessment, intervention, consultation and evaluation should produce a viable psychologist. Viable does not just mean something that works for the present. Viable also means something capable of future growth and development. It should be our goal to produce not a finished product but a *viable* one.

In fact, our current educational and occupational situation is designed quite well in this regard. First in the area of professional activities, according to the recommendations of the National Conference, the applied psychologist must, following four years of formal postbaccalaureate education and training in the university setting, take an additional two years of applied residency to further hone and develop skills in that area (see chap. 26 in this volume). Second, employment settings have been, and undoubtedly will continue to be, the place in which the vast majority of health psychologists have developed their breadth and their depth. To date, at least in most instances, the psychologist's initial experience with health psychology issues, which have served to define the field, has come after so-called formal training has been completed.

If a product of either a broad or a specialized psychology program obtains employment in a setting hostile to the advancement of knowledge, the likelihood of this individual flourishing is small. If the employment situation is neutral, then development of a research program will take time, persistence, and resourcefulness. If the environment is encouraging and supportive the ideal setting will have been found. Clearly, even in the latter situation, however, research and scholarly productivity are difficult to predict and ensure. Much depends on individual characteristics, most notably hunger to achieve and drive to do what is necessary—that means long hours, the pursuit of long- rather than short-range goals, delayed gratification, toleration for unfunded proposals, unavailable and unpredictable research populations, and the introduction of clinical confounds into the scientific effort, to mention only a few. No one has yet identified a psychological or other assessment tool capable of predicting who will and who will not actively pursue the advancement of knowledge following the completion of formal training. No one can predict who will and who will not dependably and actively pursue the maintenance of knowledge following departure from the formal educational environment. Teachers always have been, and continue to be, limited to doing that which is in our power and not spending huge amounts of time obsessing about things over which we have no control. What we can do is provide intellectual sophistication and a style of critical thinking. What we can do is provide a certain amount of content and skill training very probably limited in part by the realities of the available instructional environment and the knowledge and skill of the professors on hand. The other thing that we must do is protect our public. The way we can do that is to see to it that psychologists in the health psychology field are recognizable, have a core of overlapping training and skill and are aware, in sufficient breadth, of the issues, technologies, and professional practices that make up the corpus of health psychology. By our so doing, a patient or a research consultee seeking aid from someone appropriately labeled health psychologist can be assured of a constancy of training in that individual at least equivalent to that assured when a health psychologist approaches individuals in other professions such as law, medicine, etc.

An individual conscientiously trained in this model of general psychology, health psychology and (where appropriate to practice goals) professional psychology is in a position to teach, investigate, and practice. Such a person is also prepared to benefit from a variety of growth opportunities. This level of training and preparation for current investigational and professional activity, coupled with an adequate awareness of one's limitations and a desire to continue to grow (be viable) represents a good model for journeyman preparation. Upon this preparation further specialized training can be built, not just for one or two additional years but throughout one's life as a health psychologist.

APPENDIX A

Appendix A contains the relevant sections from the *American Psychological Association Accreditation Handbook* (1983) with regard to practicum, clerkship, externship, and/or preinternship field experience.

D. For competent professional functioning, professional psychologists require training in specific skills related to their specialties in areas such as psychodiagnosis, psychological assessment (group and individual), intervention procedures (group and individual psychotherapy and behavioral therapy), consultation, program evaluation, etc. Training must provide skills which encompass several types of assessment and intervention procedures, rather than being restricted to a single type. Every student must become familiar with major assessment and intervention techniques and their theoretical bases.

E. The values of professional and scientific responsibility and integrity should be conveyed to all students. Appropriate APA policies should be brought to their attention: APA Ethical Standards, APA Standards for Providers of Psychological Services, APA Standards for Educational and Psychological Tests, etc.

J. In order to assess students' competence to practice, programs must develop an explicit, comprehensive system for evaluation. The evaluation of practice competence must be the responsibility of the practitioners on the faculty, augmented, if desired, by practitioners from the community. In these evaluations, it is prudent to assess competence in those areas which are required by licensure regulations and/or other formal standards for psychological practice (ABPP, etc.). The specific competencies of graduates may vary with the goals of the program. Programs should have particularly stringent standards for the evaluation of those skills emphasized. For example, programs training for practitioner roles will have higher requirements for practicing skills while those emphasizing other roles may have higher standards for other skills.

L. Students should be made aware of policies, standards and regulations promulgated by such organizations as the state board of psychology examiners and state and local psychological associations.

M. Various models of training exist. A diversity of philosophies, goals and practices from program to program and from individual student to individual student must be permitted. Each program must specify its training model and goal in writing. The responsibility for definition of its model and goals rests with the faculty of the training program. Student participation in this definition should be encouraged. The goals of training should be clearly articulated and made available to students and applicants. The abilities and skills expected of graduates should be specified, the experience designed to develop those abilities and skills should be described, and the methods for assessing the outcome skills should be identified. Each program must develop training models consistent with the principles of social responsibility and respect for cultural and individual differences, as discussed in Section II.

Programs are evaluated in terms of the model endorsed, the goals stated and the success in meeting these goals. The training model and goals are evaluated in terms of their relevance to available resources and to local, regional and national needs.

The goals of professional training may be achieved through a variety of formal and informal curricula. A primary emphasis should be on helping the student acquire proficiency in the broad area of professional practice at a high level of skill. A commitment to lifelong professional development should be incorporated as a basic value to be adopted by faculty and students.

APPENDIX B

Appendix B provides the APA accreditation guidelines for approval of a program in any area of professional psychology. Currently, only programs formally designated as either clinical, counseling or school psychology may be accredited. There is a task force currently working on guidelines for expansion of accreditation beyond these three areas.

VII. Practicum and Internship Training

Doctoral programs in clinical, counseling, and school psychology include systematic intensive training in the application of psychological principles and skills to human problems. This field training is generally graded in intensity and responsibility and is offered sequentially through practicum and internship experiences. The specific structure of practica and internship experiences varies with the psychological specialty and, to some extent, within each specialty. The doctoral program will actively direct its students toward field settings providing training appropriate to its model whether in its own facilities and by its own faculty or in other, independent settings. Whenever and by whomever the training is provided, the applied services rendered should be responsive to the needs of the people residing in that geographical area.

Practicum training is field experience, usually taken for academic credit, often on campus. The practicum provides for student experiences with client problems and learning of relevant psychological skills. The practicum is intended to prepare the student for the internship and is prerequisite to it.

A formal internship is required as a means of training advanced students to meet the range of problems the professional psychologist may expect to confront (in consonance with both the student's and the program's objectives). The nature of the internship, its locus, the populations served, the experiences provided, the qualifications and skills of the faculty and staff, and other relevant considerations must be appropriate to the graduate program's training model.

Close liaison should be maintained between the doctoral training program and the practicum or internship agency for the purpose of the evaluation of the students' preparation for field experience, their progress in the field, practicum, or internship program, and their evaluation of the field experience.

A. Practicum

Practicum training may occur either on or off campus. Whatever the geographical locale of the practicum setting, close liaison between the working professionals of the practicum setting and the faculty of the graduate training program is particularly important as the student begins the experience. Practicum sites should be service installations with training as one of their major functions. Psychological services in the practicum settings should conform to all relevant APA standards and guidelines.

Practicum training should facilitate the development of the following important capacities: (1) understanding of and commitment to professional and social responsibility as defined by statutes of the ethical code of the profession; (2) the capability to conceptualize human problems; (3) awareness of the full range of human variability along the dimensions stated in Section II; (4) understanding of one's own personality and biases and of one's impact upon others in professional interaction; (5) skill in relevant interpersonal interactions such as systematic observation of behavior, interviewing, psychological testing, psychotherapy, counseling, and consultation; and (6) ability to contribute to current knowledge and practice.

Achievement of these objectives in the practicum setting will require a high degree of access to professional psychologists who will serve as appropriate role models. Such contact is intended to facilitate the student's development of a professional identification and skills as a practicing psychologist.

Practice training should begin as early as feasible in the doctoral training program. The experiences of students should be appropriate to their level of training. Choice of particular facilities should be based primarily upon their quality and their relevance to the training objectives of the program. This training should be coordinated by an active faculty member, or by an adjunct professor associated with the practicum facility. The minimum practicum experiences is 400 hours, of which at least 150 hours is in direct service experience and at least 75 hours is in formally scheduled supervision. Other recommended practicum activities include attending case conferences and writing reports and clinical notes.

REFERENCES

American Psychological Association. 1983. *American Psychological Association accreditation handbook.* Washington, D.C.: APA.

Belar, C. D. 1980. Training the clinical psychology student in behavioral medicine. *Professional Psychology* 11:620–27.

———. 1982. Current patterns and issues of doctoral training in health psychology. Paper presented at the annual meeting of the American Psychological Association, Washington, D.C., August.

Belar, C. D., E. Wilson, and H. Hughes. 1982. Health psychology training in doctoral psychology programs. *Health Psychology* 1:289–99.

Boll, T. J. 1983. Neuropsychological assessment of the child: Myths, current status, and future prospects. In *Handbook of clinical child psychology,* edited by C. E. Walker and M. C. Roberts, 186–208. New York: John Wiley and Sons.

Filskov, S., and T. J. Boll, eds. 1981. *Handbook of clinical neuropsychology.* New York: John Wiley & Sons.

Knowles, J. H. 1977. The responsibility of the individual. In *Doing better and feeling worse: Health in the United States,* edited by J. H. Knowles. New York: Norton.

Matarazzo, J. D. 1980. Behavioral health and behavioral medicine. *American Psychologist* 35:807–17.

———. 1982. Behavioral health's challenge to academic, scientific and professional psychology. *American Psychologist* 37:1–14.

———. 1983. Education and training in health psychology: Boulder or bolder? *Health Psychology* 2:73–113.

Matarazzo, J. D., T. P. Carmody, and W. D. Gentry. 1981. Psychologists on the faculty of United States schools of medicine: Past, present and possible future. *Clinical Psychology Review* 1:293–317.

Miller, N. E. 1983. *Letter in briefing book.* National Working Conference on Education and Training in Health Psychology.

Millon, T., C. Green, and R. Meagher, eds. 1982. *Handbook of clinical health psychology.* New York: Plenum.

Olbrisch, M. E., and L. Sechrest. 1979. Educating health psychologists in the tradition of graduate training programs. *Professional Psychology* 10:589–94.

Report of the working group on predoctoral education/doctoral education. 1983. *Health Psychology* 2 (5):123–30.

Schneider, S. F. 1983. Some issues in training in health psychology. Briefing Book for the National Working Conference on Education and Training in Health Psychology.

Stone, G. C. 1979. A specialized doctoral program in health psychology: Considerations in its evolution. *Professional Psychology* 10:596–604.

Stone, G. C., F. Cohen, and N. E. Adler. 1979. *Health psychology: A handbook.* San Francisco: Jossey-Bass.

24

Apprenticeships in Health Psychology

Bonnie R. Strickland

The apprenticeship has a long and honorable history in psychology. Advanced graduate study has almost always been conducted under the tutelage of experienced mentors. Undergraduate study, as well, has often demanded "hands-on" laboratory experience. Apprenticeship is defined as: "one bound by legal agreement to serve another for a certain time with a view toward learning an art or trade in consideration of instruction; one who is learning, especially by practical experience." This model has been adopted for students learning scientific methods in psychology as well as for students who are pursuing professional activities.

In the early days of the development of psychology, almost every major American figure went abroad to study with a special mentor. A preponderance of early psychologists traveled to Germany to become involved with Wilhelm Wundt in his newly founded laboratory. In fact, in the late 1800s, scholars from all over the world served apprenticeships with Wundt. J. McKeen Cattell, Wundt's first American assistant, worked with him for three years before joining Galton in Cambridge, England.

Both William James at Harvard and Stanley Hall at Johns Hopkins developed laboratories in this country for instruction in experimental psychology and served as mentors to numerous students interested in this new field (Robach 1952). The opportunity for students to become involved in clinical apprenticeship opportunity began in 1896 with the establishment of Lightner Witmer's psychological clinic at the University of Pennsylvania.

Psychology had, of course, been taught for many years in the classrooms of colleges and universities in the United States. Moral philosophy and mental science, often taught by theology faculty, were required courses for many undergraduates. As psychology began to gain credibility among the sciences, however, it became incumbent upon students to have the opportunity to engage in practical work in laboratories and clinics; it was important that each student be involved in actual "hands on" experience under the close supervision of experienced scientists and practitioners.

In the early 1900s, students and scholars traveled to Europe for yet another kind of apprenticeship in clinical practice. Many of the early figures in psychoanalytic theory went to Vienna to work with Sigmund Freud. Others joined Jung in Switzerland; still others worked with students or disciples of Freud, most often in Germany. These practical experiences were in keeping with clinical interests focused on attempts to understand the nuances of disturbed behavior and how one might change neurotic or dysfunctional personal styles through psychoanalysis. Here again, though, the predominate mode of inquiry was through the actual "experience" of psychodynamic theory, either through seminars with practitioners or on the couch in psychoanalysis.

As psychology developed in this country, the apprenticeship model was readily incorporated into both graduate study and clinical practice. In contemporary psychology, students in general areas of psychology are still expected to receive close supervision in their research endeavors by experienced psychological scientists. Within the professional practice of psychology, the apprenticeship model has developed into formal practica and internship experiences. These are demanded in all accredited clinical, counseling, and school psychology programs and continue to serve as an integral part of practitioner training.

The Development of Internships

At the American Psychological Association (APA) Conference on Graduate Education and Clinical Psychology held in Boulder, Colorado, in 1949, Robert H. Felix, the Director of the National Institute of Mental Health, noted in some introductory remarks that "the broad scope of the work included under clinical psychology can be readily understood when one thinks for a moment of the functions such a person is expected to perform. These include diagnosis, therapy, research, training, and consultation. Each of these functions . . . requires careful training and supervised experience . . . although the best possible didactic and laboratory work is very necessary, the techniques and attitudes learned in clinical clerkships, ward walks, internships, and residencies leave a lasting impression and are the shapers of attitudes and concepts which, for better or for worse, last a lifetime" (Raimy 1950, xvi).

These remarks were apparently taken quite seriously by participants at the Boulder Conference, who then devoted a major portion of their recommendations to field training. Participants agreed that closely supervised practical experience in a clinical setting was necessary in the training of clinical psychologists. They recommended that students be involved in practical clinical experiences during their graduate training, including a nine-month predoctoral internship. "Extensive and intensive experience *with* people is held to be essential if the student is to acquire proper perspective and the ability to apply effectively the scientific facts and techniques which he has acquired in the academic setting. . . . The major contribution of the internship is the provision of extended practical experience of gradually increasing complexity under close and competent supervision" (Raimy 1950, 230, 231).

Following the Boulder Conference, the Committee on Accreditation of the Education and Training Board of APA began to evaluate internships, and by the early 1970s, over 100 internships had been accredited or provisionally approved. At the time of the Arden House Conference on Training in Health Psychology in 1983, around 250 internships were accredited or provisionally approved (APA Committee on Accreditation 1983). These internships are predominately clinical in nature although placements for counseling and school psychologists are also available. The Veterans Administration (VA) has been one of the major sponsors of both clinical and counseling accredited internships. In the 1950s, following the Boulder Conference, stipends were made available for clerkships and internships within the VA and provided, along with Public Health Fellowships, the majority of support at that time for the education and training of clinical psychologists.

More than half of the internship placements currently available in professional psychology are APA approved (Kurz 1983–84). Twelve clearly discernible types of internship settings have been noted: children's facilities, children's hospitals, community mental health centers, consortium, prison systems, general hospitals, medical centers, military service, private psychiatric hospitals, state mental hospitals, university counseling centers, and Veterans Administration hospitals (Kurz et al. 1982). Comprehensive medical facilities, including university hospitals and Veterans Administration hospitals, comprise about half of the internship settings.

From these data, it would seem that considerable opportunity is available for students with an interest in health psychology to work with medically ill patients. On the other hand, it must be noted that the majority of these internships are in clinical psychology and the broad focus of most of these placements is on assessment, therapy, and consultation with patients or clients most generally characterized as mentally or emotionally distressed. Some programs do offer broad-based experience with medical patients and rotations across specific medical areas. In a survey conducted in the late

1970s, three quarters of the sixty-five internship programs which responded reported having formal training in medical psychology. "These included consultation/liaison services to medical/surgical clinics, biofeedback and other types of behavioral intervention services to medical patients, and a full range of clinical services on pediatric and neuropsychological wards. In 39% of these programs, such training was required of *all* interns; in the remaining programs, such experiences were elective" (Gentry et al. 1981, 227). No doubt additional opportunities have been developed since this time and the student in health psychology should be alerted to these possibilities. In addition to the organized and formal predoctoral settings, apprenticeship experiences for students interested in health psychology may also be available in a variety of other settings, such as public policy consultations, legislative activities, and public service agencies.

Apprenticeships Specific to Health Psychology

The participants at the Arden House Conference clearly endorsed the scientist/practitioner model as the appropriate training mode for health psychologists and recommended that apprenticeship experiences be a necessary component of such training. Thus, apprenticeship opportunities for the health psychologist must encompass both research and applied practical experiences.

For the training of the scientist and practitioner in health psychology, it is imperative that research opportunities of specific relevance for health psychology be available. These may occur under the guidance of university faculty or through committee or consortium arrangements in which additional research supervisors are available from relevant health settings. Obviously, there should be no limitations on the areas of inquiry which are open to the students nor the empirical methods that may be used. At this time in the evolving science and profession of health psychology, it may be necessary to develop additional research opportunities for graduate students that are not now available. A number and variety of practica and internship experiences should also be further developed.

During the Arden House Conference, a subgroup of participants examined the role of the apprenticeship in the education and training of health psychologists.[1] This working group made the following general comments and recommendations, which are quoted in their entirety:

1. The members were D. D. Altman, J. Cahn, C. M. Dingus, R. Kurz, L. Temoshok, E. Trickett, and recorder M. Follick.

Current State of Apprenticeship Opportunities

Apprenticeship experiences may now be obtained in a variety of settings (e.g., universities, research agencies such as NIMH, schools, churches, corporations, medical centers, and government and community agencies). These experiences include field placement, practica, externships and internships. Many of these apprenticeship opportunities, especially within the area of health care services, are well established, whereas others are evolving. Internships which provide formal opportunities for supervised experiences within organized health care settings have been particularly well developed in clinical and counseling psychology. Two-hundred-thirty-nine internship placements are now approved by the Accreditation Committee on the Educational and Training Board of the American Psychological Association.

Apprenticeship positions for the newly developing areas of psychology as well as industrial/organizational (I/O) health psychology, public policy, public health, and community psychology are more emergent than actualized. In many cases, the field supervisors will not be trained as psychologists. While this has the advantage of providing an inter-disciplinary approach to health-related issues, the core experiences within psychology may need improved structure.

Present opportunities for supervised experiences in the I/O areas include affiliation with health promotion programs, employee assistance programs, and the opportunity for program evaluation involvement. These apprenticeships may be seen as involving both clinically related activities, such as may be found in employee assistance programs, and activities designed to promote goals of the organization per se. In the latter, organizational assessment/diagnosis would constitute one important source of experiential learning for the apprentice. Examples of potential practitioner roles may include interventions designed to decrease stress in the workplace and the design of educational programs to inform employees about health practices.

Apprenticeships in the area of public policy are contingent upon the development of access to persons and programs relevant to the formation and/or implementation of health policy at a variety of local, state, and national levels. Knowledge of policy formation, research design to assess the impact of policy, and the development of comprehensive conceptualization of the economic, political, legal, social, and cultural issues are examples of substantive areas useful to the health psychologist working in the policy areas. Examples of potential practitioner roles may include use of information deriving from health impact studies, gathering and presenting data to health policymakers, and analysis of health policy legislation. There are many areas of health psychology that offer potential quality training opportunities of which psychologists have not taken advantage. Currently, many psychologists are not involved in public policy because they lack knowledge of the availability and appropriateness to psychologists of these apprenticeship experiences. Such positions include White House, Congressional, and Judicial fellowships; the NIMH grant associate program; local, state, regional, and national government appointments; "think tanks" (e.g., Rand, Brookings, Hasting); regulatory commissions (e.g., JCAH); insurance corporations; labor management trust funds; and lobbyists.

Apprenticeships in the public health/community area provide the opportunity to develop skills in ecological assessment, needs assessment, epidemiological assessment, or assessment of social system dynamics. For example, possible apprenticeships may include such activities as being a content expert working with a community organization concerned with children's health issues in the community, developing a health program with a county health officer, and working with the mass media on an educational campaign.

Overall, we now find formal, structured apprenticeship activities within certain traditional areas of psychology which have long demanded broad and relevant supervised clinical and counseling experiences. Other important areas of psychology with special links to health psychology provide flexible and creative avenues of experience but are not organized in a fashion that allows easy access for public awareness and evaluation.

Conceptualization and General Recommendations

Apprenticeship activities are necessary for the education and training of health psychologists and are conceptualized as supervised "hands on" experience. These activities are dependent upon and related to the educational and training goals of health psychology. Health psychologists are trained for two primary roles: the scientist and the scientist/practitioner. Although these roles are overlapping, there are also distinct features that must be accommodated in apprenticeship training experiences appropriate to each. All health psychologists who will be providing direct health care services to individuals or groups are further required to complete apprenticeship activities focusing on health and illness in an organized, inter-disciplinary health service training program. Based upon a number of assumptions, listed below, the following recommendations are made:

1. Health psychologists should have an apprenticeship component in their training related to health and illness issues.
2. Apprenticeship activities should begin early in the educational process and extend throughout the student's training.
3. Apprenticeship experiences should be appropriate and relevant to the student's level of research and professional development.
4. Apprenticeship experiences should be coordinated with other components of the training program.
5. The timing, nature, and extent of apprenticeship activities are dependent upon the goals and objectives of the training program or track as well as upon the student's specific career goals and objectives.
6. A specific goal of the apprenticeship is the integration of basic knowledge in health psychology and application/practice.
7. Apprenticeship activities may occur in a wide range of laboratory and field settings.
8. Apprenticeships should sensitize students to the diverse needs and values of different cultural, ethnic, and social groups.
9. Apprenticeships should include a consideration of ethical, legal, and professional issues.
10. Apprenticeship supervision should be done by appropriate mentors who have expertise in the activities in which the student is involved.
11. Quality control and coordination of program demands and training activities are a joint function of the field supervisor and the faculty of the health psychology program.

Recommendations for Basic Research Apprenticeships

Basic research apprenticeships should provide experiences in: (1) posing questions and formulating hypotheses; (2) using a variety of research methodologies; (3) implementing research; (4) analyzing data; (5) publishing results in appropriate outlets; (6) preparing grant proposals.

Recommendations for Applied Research Apprenticeships in Field Settings

Applied research apprenticeships in field settings should include all of the above criteria for basic research apprenticeships as well as the following:

1. Awareness and understanding of the roles, values, and vocabularies of others in the system
2. Understanding the social, cultural, and environmental context
3. Systems theory and analysis
4. Ability to communicate effectively with other members of the system
5. Consideration of the immediate and long-term impact of the health psychologist's activities on the setting
6. Experience in the use of appropriate methodological and statistical techniques
7. Assessment and intervention skills appropriate to the applied setting

Apprenticeships in the emerging areas such as public health, public policy, community and industrial/organizational psychology include all of the criteria listed in the prior recommendations.

Recommendations for Direct Health Care Provider Apprenticeships

Apprenticeships for direct health care providers should include all the criteria from the basic and applied research areas as well as clinical research and practice concerns specific to the delivery of health psychology services. With regard to practice and clerkship activities for direct care training, apprenticeship experiences should occur in settings in which a psychologist holds an appointment to the professional staff or its equivalent. At the internship level, these apprenticeships must occur in inter-disciplinary programs that meet the professional standards for accreditation of the APA. Necessary experience includes assessment, intervention, evaluation, and consultation activities as well as experience in designing, implementing, and interpreting clinical research.[2]

Issues and Problems

In many ways, the status of the emerging field of health psychology can be compared to that of clinical psychology at the time of the Boulder Conference in 1949. Psychologists with interests in health are being trained in university programs, and some apprenticeship opportunities are available. The training programs are quite diverse, however, in goals and mission as well

2. From the Proceedings of the National Working Conference on Education and Training in Health Psychology, by Bonnie Strickland, Michael Follick, David Altman, Jerry Cahn, C. Mary Dingus, Ronald Kurz, Lydia Temoshok, Edison Trickett. In *Health Psychology* 2(5): 131–34, supplement section. © 1983 by *Health Psychology*. Reprinted by permission of the publisher and authors.

as curriculum requirements. The apprenticeship opportunities, as well, are varied in both breadth of coverage and quality of training in specific health issues. Standards for the education and training of health psychologists are only now being developed.

Some major differences between the status of clinical psychology in 1949 and that of health psychology today should also be noted. The proposal of the scientist/practitioner model at the Boulder Conference was a unique development. No other profession has attempted to train scholars to be both scientists and practitioners. We now have some three decades of history to consider whether such a training model was appropriate and viable for clinical psychology. Most would agree that the model was an extremely successful one, but some would maintain that a professional model is now preferred for the education and training of clinical psychologists. Some will also surely question whether health psychology in the 1980s is not beyond the necessity for training in both science and practice. They would point to the fact that clinical psychologists trained in the scientist/practitioner model do little research but rather respond to critical needs for service. They would argue that the health practitioner as well can build on an already extant base of psychological theory and provide competent services that are in high demand by consumers.

Another major difference is that we now have a substantial proportion of psychologists in professional practice. Psychology is also regulated by licensing laws in fifty states and, although not in statute, at least four traditional specialties are identified by the profession itself with numerous new interest areas seeking recognition. Clinical psychology was faced with the necessity of relating with the other major mental health disciplines—psychiatry, nursing, and social work. Health psychology is faced with the complex issues and problems of how it will relate both intraprofessionally with already extant health service providers (and scientists) in psychology as well as interprofessionally with physicians from a variety of specialties, public health specialists, social workers, nurses, and a broad range of other health specialists.

Since apprenticeships are so heavily dependent on opportunities within major medical facilities as well as newly emerging community, industrial, and public policy settings, the development of standards and the establishment of field training will face a different set of problems than was evident in the past. The Boulder Conference was called in response to the public need for competently trained mental health practitioners to serve emotionally distressed veterans returning from the Second World War. Considerable resources were made available in support of clinical training programs and graduate student stipends. Resources are now more limited. And, although politicians and the public are becoming increasingly aware of the intimate links between health and behavior, a specific and focused need for health promotion and maintenance has not been articulated with corresponding support.

But whatever the similarities and differences in the development of clinical and health psychology, surely psychologists have learned some important lessons of quality control. We must continue to ensure that selected students are given the opportunity to study with competent and experienced teachers. Appropriate core knowledge in psychology must be covered. We must develop and monitor the establishment of relevant practica activities and apprenticeship experiences. And, we must continually remind ourselves that the development of health psychology is not only for the advancement of knowledge and the application of psychology to health and illness, but is also a commitment to our concern for human welfare.

REFERENCES

APA Committee on Accreditation. 1983. APA-Accredited predoctoral internships for doctoral training in clinical and counseling psychology. *American Psychologist* 38:1373–78.

Gentry, W. D., W. J. Street, F. T. Masur, and M. J. Asken. 1981. *Professional Psychology* 12:224–28.

Kurz, R. B., ed. 1983–84. *Directory: Internship programs in professional psychology.* 12th ed. Washington, D.C.: Association of Psychology Internship Centers.

Kurz, R. B., M. Fuchs, R. F. Dabet, S. M. Kurtz, and W. T. Helfrich. 1982. Characteristics of predoctoral internships in professional psychology. *American Psychologist* 37:1213–20.

Raimy, V., ed. 1950. *Training in clinical psychology.* New York: Prentice-Hall.

Robach, A. A. 1952. *History of American psychology.* New York: Library Publishers.

Working Group on the Apprenticeship. 1983. National Working Conference on Education and Training in Health Psychology. In *Health Psychology* 2(5): 131–34, supplement section.

25

Postdoctoral Training for Research

Howard S. Friedman

For those newly educated psychologists intending to conduct health psychology research, postdoctoral training will likely become the norm. As in the other life sciences, the degree of sophistication needed to conduct independent research in health psychology can rarely be achieved in a doctoral program alone. The challenge of and need for advanced training is especially great in health psychology for two reasons. First, most research problems in health psychology, whether on pain control or coronary-prone behavior or substance abuse or stress, necessitate knowledge of both biological *and* social factors. Second, much research in health psychology will at some point involve human patients, with the attendant clinical, ethical, legal, institutional, and policy issues. The researcher with postdoctoral experience in health psychology should have the necessary breadth of scientific knowledge and breadth of practical experience to function independently alongside other well-trained biomedical and public health researchers.

The major issue to be faced in the establishment of rigorous and general postdoctoral research training programs involves the insufficiency of existing organizational structure in health psychology. Currently, postdoctoral training programs are more likely to be located in mental health institutes, in departments of psychiatry, behavioral medicine, or behavior therapy, or in other medical school departments than in departments of psychology (Belar and Siegel 1983). This state of affairs is understandable given the history of medical psychology and, some might argue, desirable given the interdisciplinary nature of the field. However, this is in striking contrast to the predoc-

Several points in this chapter were developed from insightful comments made by participants in the working group on postdoctoral training at the 1983 National Working Conference on Education and Training in Health Psychology. In addition to the author, members of that group were Joan Borysenko (chair), Christine Dunkel-Schetter, Richard Evans, Neil Schneiderman, Gary Schwartz, Shelley Taylor, and Retha Wellons.

toral situation, in which the training of psychologists is directed by and mostly provided by psychologists. Although there is no doubt that health psychology researchers will sometimes need to undertake advanced training in related biomedical fields such as immunology or epidemiology, the core training of health psychologists should be grounded in the concepts and methods of psychology (National Working Conference 1983). Regular channels for such postdoctoral training need to be established.

Postdoctoral research training requires substantial resources. Scientific research is a multipronged and unpredictable enterprise. It is often unclear where and when the payoff will come. On the other hand, health service delivery generally provides tangible, immediate results. Hence there is a danger that health psychologists, in a rush to establish standards for practice, will pay insufficient attention to the needs for research support. However, if indeed health psychology is "a generic field of psychology, with its own body of theory and knowledge" ("Conference consensus" 1983), then the health of health psychology ultimately depends upon the quality and quantity of that theory and knowledge.

Types of Training Programs

Most postdoctoral research training involves the conduct of independent research under the general supervision of a more senior collaborator. This can sometimes be accomplished by joining a health psychology research team. However, given the relatively small number of card-carrying health psychology researchers presently in existence, postdoctoral training must often be under the supervision of a more traditionally trained psychologist, usually in a medical setting (cf. Olbrisch and Sechrest 1979). For example, a postdoctoral fellow may be supervised by a university-affiliated social or clinical psychologist while studying psychological reactions to breast cancer, to birth defects, to chemotherapy, to pain, or to a host of other social and clinical issues (cf. DiMatteo and Friedman 1982b). An important fringe benefit of such an arrangement is that the postdoctoral trainees can provide necessary links among university professors, medical personnel, and predoctoral students.

Other psychologists intending to become health psychologists may need more formal postdoctoral training, including extensive coursework. For example, traditionally trained research psychologists who become interested in health psychology often need to learn new jargon, read new journals, master new measurement tools, make new contacts, find new funding sources, and acquire a broad range of information about the structure of the health care system and how it works. Postdoctoral programs providing such opportunities are limited in number. In fact, presently no complete listing has been compiled that provides information about the number and form of postdoctoral health psychology training programs (Belar and Siegel 1983), although some information is available from relevant federal agencies (Matarazzo 1982, 14).

Formal interdisciplinary training efforts are also sometimes appropriate. For example, psychologists may benefit from Master of Public Health (M.P.H.) programs (which generally require a doctorate as a prerequisite) or from advanced formal training in psychoneuroimmunology. On the other hand, physicians or dentists or other health professionals may need postdoctoral research training in health psychology. The possibilities for programs of these types should be explored by organized health psychology (see also Matarazzo 1983).

Assorted insights about mechanisms for advanced training in health psychology can also be gleaned from the fields of gerontology and geropsychology (e.g., Niederehe 1981; Special section 1981) which underwent dramatic growth over the past decade. For example, these fields warn against overspecialization. Interestingly, perhaps the firmest conclusion that can be drawn about research in the field of aging is that the amount of research, the type of research, and the methods of research changed rapidly in a short period of time (Hoyer, Raskind, and Abrahams 1984). Or, as Neal Miller put it in describing health psychology training: "To prepare our students for such changes, we must motivate and educate them for a lifetime of continued learning. Thus, during their training we must give them the opportunity and require them to demonstrate the ability to learn new things completely on their own" (Miller 1983, 13).

Skills

The National Working Conference's committee on postdoctoral research training listed five kinds of skills to be refined in postdoctoral training (Borysenko et al. 1983). These are: (1) the application of behavioral research techniques to the study of health and disease, including particularly strong emphasis on the specific applications of methodology, design, statistical analyses, and computer skills; (2) the acquisition of relevant assessment and intervention skills that may be appropriate to research; (3) the development of behavioral models related to health and disease; (4) communication at the interface between health psychology and related disciplines (including detailed knowledge of the health care system); and (5) understanding of and sensitivity to ethical and legal issues involved in the conduct of both human and animal research.

The skills of theory construction and of research design and analysis are of course the key characteristics of a health psychology researcher (cf. Taylor and Raven 1980), as of any scientist, and characterize current research training in all subfields of psychology. The research health psychologist, however, also must acquire expertise in working in the health care system (broadly construed) and with other health researchers and health care professionals. More concretely, this means: an ability to work with physicians, nurses, and other healers; a knowledge of relevant biological processes; facility of movement in hospitals, HMOs, and government health agencies; and an understanding of the special ethical and legal considerations involved in working with patients. So, for example, an experimental or clinical or social psychologist who might be able to go to an airport and conduct a good study regarding travelers' perceptions, cognitions, attitudes, and/or reactions to air travel cannot simply walk into a cardiology clinic and conduct a study of psychological aspects of heart disease.

The particular content of the training will of course depend heavily on the topic being researched and on the long-term professional goals of the trainee. For example, meaningful research on cooperation with treatment regimens among the elderly requires substantial knowledge of gerontology, the Medicare system, and doctor-patient communication and influence patterns. Nevertheless, it may be possible to develop lists of content areas of high priority for the field, to which all researchers should be exposed during their training. For example, a survey of faculty concerning the importance of various topics for inclusion in a course on social psychology and health (DiMatteo and Friedman 1982a) found agreement on the special importance of face-to-face interaction in medical settings and of psychosomatic issues (such topics as communication skills, patient cooperation, attitude change, life change events, psychosomatic illness). The provision of such information may help insure that at least some researchers are being trained to conduct research in the areas of highest need and may facilitate the future employment of the trainees.

Given the goal of making training in health psychology comparable to and competitive with training in other sophisticated biomedical fields, the nature of any clinical component of the training emerges as an important issue. Much biomedical research is conducted by physicians, who are generally clinically and legally prepared to work with patients. Although a residency program modeled on medical schooling may work for training health psychology service providers, it has significant disadvantages for postdoctoral research training. Many health psychology researchers, focused on research issues, will have insufficient inclination and clinical experience to take on total responsibility for the management of a patient. Yet some degree of clinical work is inevitable in much health psychology research. Therefore, supervised contact with patients should be a part of most postdoctoral research training. Extensive contact is probably most easily achieved in those psychology programs based in medical schools (e.g., Thompson and Matarazzo 1984). However, the precise nature of such clinical work depends upon the goals of the research. For example, an intensive research program on coronary-prone behavior will likely provide postdoctoral trainees with important clinical experience with heart disease patients.

Credentialing

Traditionally, health psychology researchers and professors have not become licensed psychologists unless they were trained in clinical psychology. However, there are a number of reasons for this situation to change and for licensing preparation to become part of postdoctoral research training. First, the process of becoming licensed directs attention to the ethical, legal, and clinical issues which the researcher is likely to encounter in research with patients. For example, a researcher studying how children cope with chronic illness would, in the course of preparing for licensure, become better informed about child abuse reporting laws and about available children's services. Second, health psychology researchers may routinely work in hospitals, clinics, county health departments, and similar settings, where all professionals are expected to be licensed for either real or perceived legal purposes, insurance purposes, or purposes of professional respect.

A third reason for licensing is to help insure researchers' knowledge about the limits of their abilities. Licensing laws and exams generally make clear the restrictions on working outside one's area of competence. Just as a research physician would probably not attempt heart surgery, a licensed research psychologist would probably not attempt health service delivery or psychotherapy without first obtaining the relevant training. Fourth, licensing for all health psychologists may help eliminate questions on the part of physicians, nurses, and patients about who or what is a "legitimate" health psychologist.

Fifth and finally, health psychology professors will be in the position of supervising the research of fellows who intend to work in a clinical setting. For example, a professor studying biofeedback in a university's department of psychology may supervise a fellow who intends to conduct pain control research on chronic pain patients in a hospital clinic. The fellow will eventually need to become licensed. If the professor were licensed, at least two sorts of benefits would ensue. Most importantly, the various clinical, legal, and ethical issues of service delivery are more likely to become known and be discussed. Also, on a more practical level, the licensed professor may be more likely to be recognized as a qualified supervisor by licensing authorities.

With the generic licensing in most states, most health psychology researchers are eligible for licensure after two years of supervised postdoctoral research. (Under generic licensing, any licensed psychologist may practice in his or her area of training and expertise.) The extent of supervised clinical work, if any is deemed necessary, is a matter to be decided by doctoral programs in health psychology. But decisions about licensing should not be taken lightly. There are dangers. Licensing for health psychology researchers might be viewed as or might even actually become a threat to academic freedom, although research physicians (who are required to be licensed when they undertake independent clinical research) have thus far retained their autonomy. Additionally, professional licensing in general may come to protect the economic and political interests of the professionals rather than to serve the consumer (e.g., Hogan 1983). However, given the entrenchment of the licensing system in American health care, it appears that health psychologists, including those in research, will have to construct a workable arrangement or else risk being excluded from the major challenges of the field. Now is the time to incorporate safeguards which will work to protect both freedom of inquiry and the public welfare against the potentially detrimental side effects of regulation.

Financial Support

Funding opportunities for postdoctoral researchers in health psychology appear promising. There are a number of potential sources of support. These include public and private general research support, federal training grants, and public and private individual fellowships. Large federal research grants (e.g., from NIH and NSF) to principal investigators allow support for postdoctoral positions, and such awards are common in the biomedical sciences. Federal agencies (e.g., NIMH) also award broader institutional training grants in psychology, and these currently emphasize postdoctoral training. On the individual level, the National Institutes of Health offer individual postdoctoral fellowships (National Research Service Awards) for training in "biomedical and behavioral research." Senior fellowships are also available. On the more applied side, postdoctoral internships and fellowships are sometimes offered in medical departments, such as in pediatric psychology (Tuma 1982; also Roberts and Wright 1982).

Private health foundations are a good source of research training funds but seem relatively untapped by psychologists. For example, the American Cancer Association and the American Heart Association and some of their state affiliates offer individual postdoctoral research fellowships; in addition, funds for such positions can usually be budgeted in their research grants. Other private sources can probably be developed as well, if a vigorous effort is made. For example, employer-sponsored programs or fees from patients themselves might finance postdoctoral fellows conducting applied research on the development of effective techniques in such areas as weight control, smoking cessation, pain control, and stress management. Health Maintenance Organizations, large corporations, and organized social support groups (such as those for patients facing cancer and their families) are likely candidates to provide such funding.

Financial support for trainees is not enough. A problem in developing postdoctoral training programs arises from the fact that many universities, especially public universities, are structured for the support of undergraduate and graduate students but make little provision for postdoctoral trainees (cf. Stone 1979). Furthermore, federal support programs often limit funds primarily to the support of trainees, with little or no funding for administrative support and overhead costs. These factors combine to produce the unfortunate situation in which postdoctoral trainees may face severe restrictions on office and research space, computer funds, secretarial support, and conference travel funds. This significant problem is not unique to health psychology and must be addressed together by psychology departments, universities, the organizations representing the profession, and the state and federal governments.

Conclusion

This chapter has considered postdoctoral training for research, as distinguished from postdoctoral training for health service delivery and for policy roles. However, this separation derives from an editorial decision rather than from any existing formal structures. It is clear, generalizing from our graduate programs in health psychology at the various University of California campuses, that many excellent students enter health psychology with the goal of eventually conducting applied research in a hospital or clinic setting;

they will thus be involved with health service delivery as well as with research. It also can be anticipated that many researchers and professors with a broad and deep knowledge of health psychology problems will be called into the service of the government, the private health promotion interests, and health care administration; they will be involved with making health policy. In short, because research in health psychology will often be closely tied to the provision of service to clients or patients, it is hazardous to view postdoctoral health psychology research as a purely academic and nonprofessional endeavor. Finding secure and appropriate homes for postdoctoral research training deserves the immediate attention of organized health psychology.

REFERENCES

Belar, C. D., and L. J. Siegel. 1983. A survey of postdoctoral training programs in health psychology. *Health Psychology* 2 : 413 – 25.

Borysenko, J., H. S. Friedman, C. Dunkel-Schetter, R. Evans, N. Schneiderman, G. Schwartz, S. Taylor, and R. Wellons. 1983. Working group on postdoctoral research training. *Health Psychology,* 2(5): 135 – 40, supplement section.

Conference consensus regarding the status of health psychology. 1983. *Health Psychology* 2(5): 9, supplement section.

DiMatteo, M. R., and H. S. Friedman. 1982a. A model course in social psychology and health. *Health Psychology* 1 : 181 – 93.

———. 1982b. *Social psychology and medicine.* Cambridge, MA: Oelgeschalger, Gunn & Hain.

Gentry, D., J. Street, F. Masur, and M. Asken. 1981. Training in medical psychology. *Professional Psychology* 12 : 224 – 28.

Hogan, D. B. 1983. The effectiveness of licensing: History, evidence and recommendations. *Law and Human Behavior* 7 : 117 – 38.

Hoyer, W. J., C. L. Raskind, and J. P. Abrahams. 1984. Research practices in the psychology of aging. *Journal of Gerontology* 39 : 44 – 48.

Matarazzo, J. D. 1982. Behavioral health's challenge to academic, scientific, and professional psychology. *American Psychologist* 37 : 1 – 14.

———. 1983. Education and training in health psychology: Boulder or bolder? *Health Psychology* 2 : 73 – 113.

Matthews, K. A., and N. Avis. 1982. Psychologists in schools of public health. *American Psychologist* 37 : 949 – 54.

Miller, N. 1983. Some main themes and highlights of the conference. *Health Psychology* 2(5): 11 – 14, supplement section.

National Working Conference on Education and Training in Health Psychology. 1983. *Health Psychology* 2(5): 1 – 153, supplement section.

Niederehe, G. 1981. Postgraduate training of psychologists for work in aging. In *Psychology and the older adult: Challenge for training in the 1980s,* edited by J. Santos and G. VandenBos. Washington, D.C.: American Psychological Association.

Olbrisch, M. E., and L. Sechrest. 1979. Educating health psychologists in traditional graduate training programs. *Professional Psychology* 10:589–95.

Roberts, M., and L. Wright. 1982. The role of the pediatric psychologist as consultant to pediatricians. In *Handbook for the practice of pediatric psychology*, edited by J. Tuma. New York: Wiley & Sons.

Santos, J., and G. VandenBos. 1981. *Psychology and the older adult: Challenges for training in the 1980s.* Proceedings of the Conference on Training Psychologists for Work in Aging, Boulder, CO.

Special Section: Educational programs in gerontology and geriatrics. 1981. *Gerontology and Geriatrics Education* 1:181–212.

Stone, G. C. 1979. A specialized doctoral program in health psychology: Considerations in its evolution. *Professional Psychology* 10:596–604.

Taylor, S. E., and B. Raven. 1980. *Health psychology training at UCLA: First year report.* Unpublished manuscript.

Thompson, R. J., and J. D. Matarazzo. 1984. Psychology in United States medical schools: 1983. *American Psychologist* 39:988–95.

Tuma, J. M. 1982. Training in pediatric psychology. In *Handbook for the practice of pediatric psychology*, edited by J. Tuma. New York: Wiley & Sons.

26

Postdoctoral Education and Training of Service Providers in Health Psychology

Joseph D. Matarazzo

Psychology Predoctoral Education Is Generic

I presented a few opinions on graduate education and training in health psychology in an earlier publication (Matarazzo 1983) and developed two of them in more detail in chapter 4 of this volume. The first of these two is that the *predoctoral* education of all psychologists preparing for a career in psychology as it interfaces with health has been, is today, and very likely will continue for years to consist of study of a *generic* body of knowledge which relevant constituencies in the science and profession of psychology have agreed is the needed minimum (core) of such knowledge. No currently extant predoctoral educational program in psychology has the faculty and requisite health-related resources to educate and graduate fully trained *health* psychologists, per se (Belar, Wilson, and Hughes 1982; Matarazzo 1983; Olbrisch and Sechrest 1979). Even the best of such predoctoral programs can, at the most, only help their students assimilate the bare minimum of core knowledge in generic psychology, train them in the necessary methods of inquiry, begin to infuse them with ethical and professional standards, and provide a rudimentary introduction to the health-related special professional knowledge and skills which they one day will need to function as independent and mature health psychologists.

The second opinion I offered is that along with that common core of knowledge, the "extras" students elect in their predoctoral minor program of didactic courses and in their laboratory and preprofessional apprenticeship training experiences (thesis, dissertation, practicum, and internship) will add a slightly different "track" of minor underpinning for students electively heading for a career in clinical, experimental, health, or other

Preparation of this chapter was supported in part by National Heart, Lung and Blood Institute Grants HL20910 and HL07332.

areas of psychology. Over the years it has increasingly been acknowledged that *postdoctoral* experiences and training are necessary to prepare newly graduated doctoral students for the application of their core knowledge of psychology to more specialty-related problems in one of a number of recognized different arenas and settings and with different populations of individuals. Today no *research specialty areas* are credentialed in psychology (or in any other academic discipline). Postdoctoral "specialty" areas for service providers which currently are formally recognized by the profession of psychology, through credentialing of individuals by the American Board of Professional Psychology, are the applications of psychology in the fields of clinical, counseling, school, industrial-organizational, clinical neuropsychology, and forensic psychology. In 1983 the leadership of Division 40 (Clinical Neuropsychology) of the American Psychological Association (APA), and in 1985 the leaders of the American Board of Forensic Psychology, each concluded negotiations with the American Board of Professional Psychology (ABPP) and added clinical neuropsychology's and forensic psychology's subdiscipline-specific skills, knowledge, and areas of application as professional psychology's fifth and sixth credentialed areas of "specialization." However, as I have written before (Matarazzo 1983; chap. 4), for clinical neuropsychology and forensic psychology, no less than for health psychology, there is a substantial difference between the *wish* to be credentialed as a new specialty and the fact of *de jure* acknowledgement as a bona fide specialty by significant others within and without the discipline of psychology, even after being so credentialed. In my opinion, part of the reason for this continuing "wish versus deed" dilemma in neuropsychology, in forensic psychology, in health psychology, and even in clinical psychology is the still substantial dearth of adequate numbers of mentors, suitable postdoctoral training sites, and stipends to support the present (let alone future) numbers of students receiving this postdoctoral training.

Quality Psychology Postdoctoral Training in Health Service Delivery Is Today Still Relatively Unavailable

Just before the conferees met for the 1949 Boulder Conference on Training in Clinical Psychology there were available in our country only a few settings (and fewer qualified psychologist-mentors) which offered a one-year predoctoral internship and none that were nationally acknowledged by the emerging profession as capable of offering the high-quality postdoctoral professional training that the conferees agreed was a necessary ingredient for training in clinical psychology. Accordingly, the conferees decided to forego the investment of other than a small proportion of their limited resources into developing postdoctoral training and, rather, to first invest these resources of the discipline into building high-quality *predoctoral* internship training sites (Raimy 1950, 77, 109, 194). It took psychology a good part of the ensuing thirty-six years to develop the necessary mentors and facilities which today assure society and the profession, via a well-established accreditation mechanism, that the quality of these predoctoral internships is demonstrably high. In parallel, and with considerably fewer financial resources, psychology concurrently began in 1949 the process of developing what one day hopefully would *become* similarly high-quality postdoctoral professional training sites, again primarily in the area of clinical psychology.

The result is that today the extra predoctoral internship is an integral, well-established, and well-accepted apprenticeship component of the education and training of young psychologists aiming for careers in clinical psychology. However, compared to their counterpart numbers available for teaching in these *predoctoral* internships, there are today both relatively fewer experienced teachers to serve as role models and fewer high-quality training facilities and resources, on the one hand, and also a smaller number of psychology doctoral students aiming for a career in clinical psychology who *apply* for, and actually *avail* themselves of, such *postdoctoral* clinical training, on the other. Two-, three-, and even seven-year postdoctoral residencies are available today and *mandated* by one or another of the twenty-three specialties in medicine which between 1917 and 1979 were credentialed and were acknowledged as bona fide medical specialties by a number of relevent constituencies which make up, or interact with, the health care industry. Although not as well developed, nor yet mandated by the profession, such postdoctoral residencies also have begun to emerge in several specialties in the professions of both dentistry and law. Nevertheless, psychology today does not have a societal or a professional requirement or a mechanism under and through which to begin to *mandate* additional postdoctoral education and training. This lack of a formal mandate requiring postdoctoral training holds today even for those clinical psychologists who are being credentialed by the ABPP to practice as bona fide specialists.

This lack of mandate for postdoctoral training is not due to resistance by the boards which license psychologists in the fifty states plus the District of Columbia. Nor does it reflect resistance from ABPP or, in my opinion, resistance from any other quarter among the constituencies with a power base in professional psychology. An important, although not primary, factor is the scarcity of qualified psychologist mentors who work full time as professional psychologists in facilities deemed appropriate for postdoctoral training. A further obstacle is a dearth of such qualified mentors who are *willing to offer,* and whose institutions *can fund,* fellowships for increasing numbers of graduates in psychology who desire postdoctoral training in clinical, health, or other areas of professional psychology. However, restricted availability of postdoctoral stipends may not be more important than the lack of available, willing, and qualified mentors working in the requisite settings whose other work responsibilities administratively afford them the considerable amount of time required for quality postdoctoral training. I shall return later to the problem of adequate funding. First I wish to discuss the issue of the quality of postdoctoral training independent of its financial feasibility.

Quality of Mentor and Setting: Sine Qua Nons of Postdoctoral Training

There is universal agreement within our profession that whether the postdoctoral training is for a career in clinical psychology, health psychology, clinical neuropsychology, etc., the product will be determined, in the main, by the quality of both the mentors and the training facility. One of the major indices of the quality of these components of postdoctoral training is the inclusion, under several active mentors and role models, of a wide variety of practical experiences selected from the outset to provide professional challenges of gradually increasing complexity under competent supervision that is very close at first and gradually diminishes. As in clinical or general experimental psychology, the building up of an apperceptive mass which gives concrete meaning to the subject matter and to the general principles learned predoctorally quite likely is best accomplished by exposure to both a *volume* and a *variety* of contacts with actual problems, challenges, and issues. Such experiences should be guided by well-prepared health psychologist-mentors in an educationally rich interdisciplinary setting who already are playing important professional roles as co-equals of practitioners from other professions. The families of skills and techniques needed by the provider who is licensed and later credentialed to offer health psychology services to other persons cannot be acquired solely from books, lectures, or related pedagogic experiences. Rather, as has been learned in law, medicine, dentistry, and nursing, more extensive and intensive experience *with* people is another sine qua non if such a future independent-practicing, professional health psychologist is to acquire both the appropriate perspectives and the requisite abilities to apply effectively the scientific facts, principles, understandings, and techniques he or she acquired in the predoctoral academic setting and began to apply in a predoctoral internship.

It is as difficult to gain these elements of the requisite education and training needed by the future professional health psychologist in a primarily academic predoctoral program in psychology with an added "track" in health psychology as it is to accomplish it predoctorally for the would-be fee-for-service practitioner of clinical psychology. Neither the requisite professional standards, ethics, and ideals nor the requisite physical health (or mental health) arena-specific skills can be taught in the abstract in the predoctoral classroom (or even in the limited one-year predoctoral internship). It is at the worksite, in a hospital, in a clinic, or in a multi-professionally staffed state health department, industrial toxic waste prevention setting, or worker risk management program that the professionally more mature postdoctoral (in contrast to predoctoral) student, under supervision, will acquire the knowledge, skills, techniques, experience, and self confidence with patients, former patients, and potential patients necessary to persuade the licensing board of a state that he or she has the minimum preparation to be a licensed, independent practitioner. It also is in such an on-the-job, postdoctoral training site that the professional psychologist-in-training perceives how patients (or nonpatients identified as at risk) present themselves and respond to either an increased risk or to a whole host of physical (medical) disorders which affect every bodily as well as most organ systems.

Additionally, it is in an actual health setting rather than in the classroom that the young, doctorate-holding health psychologist learns, almost by osmosis, the varieties of important contributions which can be made in the service of the same patient by individuals from other professions. In such a process, and in most cases at a subliminal level, the development of interprofessional skills and, as important, intraprofessional attitudes, skills, and identification is accomplished. Obviously, such postdoctoral training will be more easily accomplished today in a well-staffed university or (community) teaching hospital setting where all the above ingredients are already in place than in a nonhospital setting (Belar and Siegel 1983; Matarazzo 1965; Sheridan 1981). Psychologists wishing to develop comparably rich postdoctoral training programs in other settings (small hospitals, health departments, industry, the schools, etc.) may have to develop the needed training resources in such sites (e.g., quality staff and patient resources, plus multidisciplinary consultants, etc.). It also is my opinion, held in common with many other educators in health psychology no less than in clinical psychology, that this complex socialization process leading from novice to full professional cannot be accomplished in less than two postdoctoral years.

Unfortunately, the reality is that there are today too few qualified psychologists (and qualified settings) to offer postdoctoral training in health psychology. There also were too few to offer comparable postdoctoral (or predoctoral) training in clinical psychology just before the Boulder Conference set into motion the forces which in thirty-six years would establish enough of these resources for *predoctoral* training in that first area of special application. Nevertheless the conferees at Boulder performed a highly valuable and much needed service in 1949 by carrying out a balanced appraisal of the status of clinical psychology as an emerging specialty in psychology and added to that their reasoned, collective opinions regarding both the philosophic perspectives as well as a large number of specifics to serve as general pedagogic blueprints for the faculties which soon began doing the actual university and practicum education and training. The conferees at the 23–27 May 1983 Conference on Education and Training in Health Psychology fulfilled a similar role. It is to the opinions offered by the subgroup [1] relevant to this chapter, which I chaired, (and whose opinions were endorsed by the whole Conference), that I turn next. Those of us invited to write chapters for this volume were asked to resynthesize what was recommended at the Conference, to write it in our own words, and add our personal, task-specific and focused views. Therefore, these working subgroup colleagues as well as the other conferees should not be held responsible for any interpretations or even for any of the personal opinions regarding postdoctoral education which follow.

Recommendations

First, training of psychologists for careers as licensed *service providers* in health psychology should be carried out through a two-year postdoctoral residency. Furthermore, the completion of a doctoral degree in generic psychology, preferably with a health psychology focus, and an appropriate applied internship, are each necessary prerequisites to a two-year residency as here proposed.

The rationale for a *two*-year postdoctoral residency rests on an appreciation of: (a) the rapidly developing number of new techniques for health promotion as well as new interventions for ameliorating specific health disorders, coupled with; (b) the rapidly accelerating advances in scientific knowledge within both psychology and within other relevant disciplines,

---

1. The other members of this 1983 Conference working group were Cynthia D. Belar, J. Alan Best, David A. Clayman, Mary A. Jansen, Nelson F. Jones, Dennis C. Russo, and Edward P. Sheridan. The opinions and recommendations of this group are published in Stone (1983, 141–45).

and thus; (c) the magnitude of the training task required to ensure mastery before the young psychologist is entrusted with a license to intervene in the life and well-being of other humans. Although the postdoctoral training of such psychology residents could occur in a variety of venues, under the tutelage of experienced mentors from different fields of psychology and related disciplines, the important ingredient which differentiates this type of postgraduation, professional training from others is that, as discussed above, it would occur in a setting with an *organized* postdoctoral training program which will eventually meet the professional standards for accreditation and where the trainee develops in a multidisciplinary milieu an appreciation of the rights of the individual client or patient, the moral, legal, and personal responsibility of a service provider, and the impact an intervention can have on another human being, including the possibility of untoward and unexpected consequences. Awareness of the limits of one's own knowledge, and thus the necessity to seek consultation actively as necessary, is incumbent on the practitioner in every profession. The influence of cultural diversity on outcome of intervention and a host of other humanistic issues as well as requisite skills must be developed in a sensitive, competent manner. Whereas an introduction to a rudimentary knowledge of physiology, pathophysiology and clinical medicine, plus a few of the relevant professional skills, will have been part of the predoctoral curriculum, it is expected that this knowledge and these skills will be much more finely honed and assimilated as one proceeds through the first and second year of this type of postdoctoral training and emerges as a professional with sufficient training in both health and behavior to function as an independent professional psychologist.

Second, postdoctoral training should not be focused on training highly specialized practitioners who are expert only in one or two skills but, rather, should have as its goal the development of a professional psychologist with a *broad,* general orientation to health service delivery who is highly trained in a number of the specific proficiencies and competencies which are everyday practiced and, thus, demonstrated by role-modeling mentors in that particular training program.

The already rich history in training professional psychologists amassed by our discipline since the Boulder conference suggests that such a two-year "generalist" model of training is sensitive both to the uniqueness of individuals seeking training and to the extensive variety of sites potentially able to offer such training. As is true for training in other currently existing areas of professional psychology, the generalist principal does not imply training every postdoctoral resident across every one of the myriad possibilities offered by the health psychology field. Probably no postdoctoral program will ever possess the potential to cover training in all or most of the knowledge and skills required by a health psychologist. Natural divisions already appear in the split between training to work with children as contrasted to working with adults. However, along with their appropriate professional academic counterparts, acceptable training sites minimally should include university hospitals, medical centers, public health departments and clinics, and public schools and industrial settings,[2] providing they have in place psychologist mentors who themselves are qualified to offer such advanced postdoctoral training in health psychology service delivery, as well as such other resources as adequate numbers and different types of patients and clients, and the high-quality input from professionals from other disciplines recently mandated for service delivery settings in clinical psychology (APA 1981).

From the above discussion it is clearly imperative that postdoctoral training programs should have sufficient breadth and depth so as to foster the development not of one or two but of a variety of skills (proficiencies and competencies) in assessment, intervention, and consultation. It also would appear clear that such training programs should attempt to provide a number of experiences that vary with respect to setting, problem focus, interacting disciplines, level of intervention (i.e., individual, group, system), multiple supervisory models, and related relevant professional issues. Of course, the nature of the setting and faculty resources will determine specific content to some extent, but the quality of training programs will depend upon the ability of such programs to transcend singular or highly limited experiences. For example, if the postdoctoral program were situated in a medical setting it is expected that the resident would interact with a variety of medical subspecialties and, under appropriate supervision, deal with a number of different clinical problems (e.g., noncompliance by diabetic patients or those with other life-threatening disorders, presurgery or prerenal dialysis anxiety, management of chronic pain, care of the terminally ill, amelioration of anxiety, stress, and maladaptive coping in postmyocardial infarction patients, the postsurgery confusion in the intensive care unit shown by a high propor-

2. As is well known, psychology currently has in place a number of predoctoral and postdoctoral training sites for its graduates who are interested in a career practicing psychology in applied clinical settings such as hospitals, clinics, etc. It is my observation that there currently are available no *health psychology* postdoctoral training programs in which to train licensed service providers for careers either in industry or in the public schools. However, Chesney and Feuerstein (1979) and Dwore and Matarazzo (1981) provide a glimpse of the future potential of each of these sites for such training.

tion of patients who have undergone open heart surgery, differential reactions of families, nurses, and other caregivers to the death of a child, young mother, or elderly patient, and so on). There should also be systematic exposure to the different methods of assessing these problems (e.g., by use of the clinical interview or by use of such standardized instruments as the Minnesota Multiphasic Personality Inventory, etc.). In an industrial setting, indirect and direct service training with a variety of appropriately supervised experiences should be required (e.g., risk factor modification, hypertension detection, executive stress management, employee assistance programs, nonstressful reassimilation into the preillness job of the patient who has experienced a heart attack or a serious automobile injury, etc.). Admittedly, assurance of quality postdoctoral training in an industrial or in a school setting would create a somewhat heavier burden than in medical settings where quality assurance procedures already are in place. It is conceivable that, as an initial step in some settings, consortia could be developed that would offer the trainee placement and concurrent training in a well-designed training program made up of *properly supervised* experiences involving a number of components (e.g., industrial or school site plus a medical center, HMO, and family practice center). Because the varieties of settings and, thus, training offered could span a wide range of different training experiences, it is imperative that postdoctoral training institutions clearly inform prospective applicants what specialized knowledge and which health service provider skills are addressed by the postdoctoral program and counsel them about the viability of future employment for individuals with such knowledge and skills.

No matter in which type of setting this two-year training takes place, it is important to underscore a requisite ingredient which must be present in each of them. Because of the complexity involved in learning highly technical new information, skills, proficiencies and competencies, in each specific setting the postdoctoral training of such generalist health psychologists should progress in a systematic fashion from highly structured and supervised activities at the outset to increasingly autonomous activities. The judgment that the postdoctoral experience has led to minimum levels of professional competency should be based upon the trainee's demonstrated capability to discharge responsibility as an independent professional in that particular setting of training. To accomplish this it is the responsibility of the training director to assure that each trainee receives supervision appropriate to her or his own level of development throughout the postdoctoral training experience. Admittedly, this requirement will not be easily met. Nevertheless, as in other fields of professional training, a major component in the evaluation of the trainee's suitability to function as an independent professional (and thus a major index of the quality of the training received) rests on the supervisory judgment or evaluation, at the end of the two-year period, of that trainee's capability to provide ethical, accountable, and effective psychological services in a variety of health delivery settings.

Third, there is a critical need for an input of federal and private sources of new funds to permit the retooling of the necessary numbers of new training institutions, new mentors, as well as to recruit the numbers of new residents needed as service providers in health psychology.

No discussion was included in my introductory remarks as to whether or not there is a societal need for increased numbers of health psychologists. However, perusal of the Surgeon General's 1990 goals for this nation, discussed in detail elsewhere (Matarazzo 1982, 1984a, 1984b), will leave little question of this societal need. The Surgeon General boldly stated an overall goal for our nation of substantially reducing the rapidly increasing human and financial costs associated with life-style dysfunctions which interface health and behavior. Progress toward attaining this goal requires the training of qualified new service providers in a number of health areas, including health psychology. More specifically, improved understanding, detection, treatment, rehabilitation, and prevention of the ten major killers of American citizens, detailed elsewhere (Matarazzo 1984a, 1984b), will depend upon the availability of a sufficient number of well-trained and qualified health psychology service providers, as well as other kinds of health professionals. The recruitment and training of capable service providers from sister professions (e.g., preventive cardiology, health education, epidemiology) are also essential elements of this effort to improve the health of our nation's citizens (Dwore and Matarazzo 1981; Matarazzo 1982). Continuity and stability of the postdoctoral training programs for trainees in each of these disciplines are also essential, as we learned from the drastic consequences of the interruption of federal support of professional training programs that occurred in 1973.

I have already stressed that there currently are in place too few training sites with appropriate resources, too few qualified mentors to provide such training, and little or none of the financial support required to attract the large numbers of new trainees needed to meet the Surgeon General's 1990 goals for this nation. Consequently, it is my hope that providing the resources needed to fund these training institutions, mentors, and trainees will be given a high priority in the future budgets of this nation's teaching hospitals, as well as in the budgets of the NIH, NIMH, NIHR, VA, and other federal, state, and local government agencies and institutions in the private sector (Matarazzo 1980, 1982). It must be recognized by educators in professional psychology and by their universities that a fundamental reordering of the health care system appears to be taking place to achieve improved health for the nation and, thus, the input of the new resources needed to develop such training facilities is quite likely underway (Matarazzo 1980, 1982, 1984a, 1984b).

Fourth, it also needs to be emphasized here that the very nature of health and illness as an arena of application of psychology requires that *different* types of mentors, residents, and didactic training models than currently exist need to be developed so as to better apply the core knowledge of generic psychology to the field of health. Because of the complexities involved in understanding the rapidly accumulating advances in normal physiology and pathophysiology, such psychologist mentors first and foremost should themselves be scientist-practitioners.[3] Instilling in the psychology resident the necessary level of sophistication and subtlety regarding biobehavioral interactions would be difficult to achieve by mentors with other types of training in psychology. Furthermore, even scientist-practitioners recruited only from psychology will be inadequate to provide the breadth of the training which is needed. As emphasized several times above, to qualify the young psychologist for licensure to function as an independent professional, his or her postdoctoral health psychology service delivery training should include a range of mentors drawn from both psychology and other key disciplines central to such a training experience (e.g., family medicine, preventive medicine, and internal medicine and its specialties).

In addition to these psychologist and physician mentors, new didactic components, designed to provide another element of a quality postdoctoral education, also would appear to be necessary to further help insure minimal standards of training for independent practice of health psychology service delivery. Graduates of psychology departments who have taken a minor track in professional psychology still will enter the postdoctoral training programs with varied backgrounds in health psychology. They will still need structured training experiences, including health-specific seminars; internal

---

3. The future development of health psychology will depend upon additions to its research base which are contributed by its scientists. Because another chapter in this volume is devoted exclusively to postdoctoral training for research in health psychology, that subject will not be further addressed here. Suffice it to add here that the area of health psychology is today one of our discipline's most inviting and potentially best financed research areas (Matarazzo 1982, 1984a, 1984b).

medicine and specialty rounds; family medicine; clinical pathology and clinical neuropathology conferences; directed reading courses; specialized training in focused brief psychotherapy and in techniques of biofeedback, relaxation training, etc. Such career-specific educational components will help insure an adequate depth in a minimum number of required knowledge, proficiency, skill and competency areas. In some of these skills and competencies, the skill and knowledge would be general across settings and populations (e.g., biofeedback), in others the specifics will be tailored to fit training opportunities (e.g., the standardized interview for assessing Type A behavior pattern). Examples of other corollary postdoctoral didactic *educational* components, also specific to the application of psychology in a health arena, might include courses and seminars on: (1) normal and pathophysiology of each of the bodily systems and organs; (2) illness behavior; (3) assessment, intervention, consultation, and related psychological proficiencies and competencies appropriate to the particular health setting and population served by that postdoctoral training institution; (4) professional relationships with members of other health service delivery disciplines; (5) legal and ethical issues; (6) advanced biostatistics and research methods; (7) epidemiology; (8) health systems and their administration; (9) program development, implementation, and evaluation; (10) health psychology consultation; and (11) professional standards.

Each of these training and didactic educational components are focused on different, although overlapping, and complementary objectives and, as appropriate in each setting, they will need to be integrated throughout the two-year postdoctoral residency experience.

Fifth, to help the orderly development of postdoctoral training of service providers in health psychology, mechanisms for the designation and the accreditation of these as health psychology postdoctoral training programs should be explored now by the leadership of health psychology in order that, one day, they may be brought under the aegis of the accreditation mechanism of the appropriate constituencies of our discipline. These latter, with input as appropriate from the Council of Graduate Departments of Psychology, include the APA's Education and Training Board, the American Board of Professional Psychology, the National Register, the American Association of State Psychology (Licensing) Boards, and the Association of Psychology Internship Centers.

How most of these constituencies already have worked together effectively toward designating and accrediting programs which offer predoctoral education was detailed in chapter 4, which the interested reader is encouraged to consult for specific details. Although not yet fully accomplished, it has taken the discipline of psychology thirty-six years from the Boulder conference to the present to promulgate the requirement that, to be so designated and accredited in the future, all doctoral degrees earned in a department of psychology must cover a specified and mandated minimum number of *core* areas of knowledge in psychology. Consequently, it is my opinion that it will be at least a decade, if not longer, before mechanisms will have been put in place to both mandate and to accredit in any numbers the type of two-year residency program in health psychology recommended in this chapter. However, as a guide to training faculties seeking to develop postdoctoral training of adequate quality, it is imperative for us to examine some considerations which directly relate to the issue of what is or is not a bona fide specialty in psychology. The debates which currently are in progress on this issue in APA's Divisions 38 (Health Psychology), 40 (Neuropsychology), and subsets of 12 (Pediatric Psychology within Clinical Psychology) are ample proof that there is a considerable difference of opinion as to what subsets of psychology currently are or are not specialties in psychology.

Proficiencies as well as De facto and De jure Specialties

The controversy as to whether clinical neuropsychology, health psychology, or pediatric psychology have today achieved the status of a specialty may be more semantic than substantive. In other related writings (Matarazzo 1965, 1983; also chap. 4) I have offered an opinion that *no* such specialties in psychology are yet well established and widely accepted by significant others in society. That opinion, which has stimulated considerable healthy counterargument, is based on such realities as that only in 1983 has the American Psychological Association Subcommittee on Specialization for the first time been able to publish the steps by which a Division of APA or another subset of psychologists might apply for designation as a specialty within psychology (Sales, Bricklin, and Hall 1983, 1984). Sales (1985) and Sales et al. (1983, 6–8) report that for a number of years the APA has received requests from a number of constituencies of psychologists (i.e., forensic psychology, psychoanalysis, several Divisions of APA) wishing to have their subfield officially declared a bona fide specialty of psychology. Acknowledging that it had no criteria by which to honor or support such requests, the APA, acting through the Committee on Standards of Providers of Psychological Services (COSPOPS) of its Board of Professional Affairs (BPA), established in 1978 a Task Force on Specialty Criteria (TFSC) to fill this void. After five years of work (in August 1983), TFSC produced a *Manual for the Identification and*

Continued Recognition of Proficiencies and New Specialties in Psychology (Sales et al. 1983), which for the first time tried to provide the steps by which to help American psychology chart its course on the path toward officially recognizing the first bona fide "specialties," per se, in psychology. Thus, although beginning with the establishment of the *American Board of Professional Psychology* in 1947, the profession of psychology has recognized special areas for the professional practice of psychology (i.e., clinical, counseling, industrial and school, and in 1983 and 1985 clinical neuropsychology and forensic psychology, respectively), no one of these six areas has ever been *officially acknowledged by APA* to be a "specialty" inasmuch as no criteria for such designation or credentialling had ever been ratified and thus been officially approved by the organization which represents most of the country's psychologists (Sales 1985).

That fact notwithstanding, these "special areas" of psychology were accorded special status by the ABPP and in isolated legislative and judicial actions; and since 1947 they have been evolving into bona fide specialties. Although subsequently appearing to retreat a step or two (Sales 1985; Sales et al. 1984), as a much needed step to clarify what has been an ambiguous situation for all parties involved, the 1983 Manual published by TFSC (Sales et al. 1983) made a distinction between a "proficiency" and a "specialty." This distinction should do much to help clear up the differences of opinion among psychologists, and between APA and some of its Divisions which represent professional psychologists, on what is or is not a specialty in psychology. According to Sales et al., recognition of a *proficiency* such as expertise in relaxation training or competent neuropsychological assessment minimally requires the identification of substantial knowledge and skills in one of the following four relatively unique areas: (a) the client population, (b) services rendered, (c) problems addressed, and (d) settings and services which form the foundation of the specialty. On the other hand, recognition as a bona fide *specialty* of psychology (clinical, health, neuropsychology, etc.) minimally requires the identification of substantial knowledge and skills in *each* of these same four areas (Sales et al. 1983, 129). Thus, the four steps required for an area of psychology to be officially designated as a specialty of psychology appear now to be becoming more clearly defined and should make it much easier for a special area such as health psychology, or clinical, or neuropsychology, etc. to do a self-study, apply for specialty designation and, if approved, better continue its evolution with this newly won, public endorsement.

Sales et al. do not deny the reality that some psychologists already *believe* their area has achieved specialty status. Specifically, the contribution of Sales et al. (1983, 129; Sales 1985) adds to the psychologist's understanding of the complex issues surrounding this process by the insightful distinction between two generic categories of specialization: de facto and de jure. *De facto specialization* is the result of the *informal* process of self-selection (or being influenced to select) a more limited sphere of professional practice which involves a special client area, set of skills and services, problems addressed, and settings for professional services. *De jure specialization,* on the other hand, involves a more *formal,* quasi-legalistic process of certification or recognition indicating that a practitioner is a specialist. Psychology clearly has been moving toward de jure recognition of specialists through the establishment of such bodies as the ABPP and the National Register. However, with few exceptions, none of the fifty state and District of Columbia licensing boards, and few if any state and no federal laws, yet define and thereby officially codify (as by case law in medicine) what is a specialist in psychology. These latter steps quite likely will follow as soon as the APA (like the AMA and its sister national accrediting bodies) begins to formally accredit specialties; a process that might occur in the next several years now that APA has distributed (and to date has not yet rescinded) a manual (Sales et al. 1983) which contains the steps and the criteria to be followed by subsets of psychologists wishing to have their area declared a specialty of psychology.

Although these new terms have been presented here only in capsule form, it appears that much of the recent debate over whether health psychology or clinical neuropsychology (or clinical psychology) are or are not specialties revolves around the differing frame of reference of each of the protagonists. Now that the distinctions between proficiency versus specialty and de facto versus de jure specialties have been clarified, it is quite likely the proponents of the position that there are today no bona fide specialties (such as the present writer) and those arguing that there are (many of my colleagues in health psychology and neuropsychology) will find, to their relief, that they are and have been in agreement. The history of clinical, health, and neuropsychology leaves little question that each subdiscipline has evolved unique proficiencies and also that today each has achieved a fair amount of de facto recognition as a specialty. If this is true then my earlier arguments on this issue thus may soon be replaced by an argument over a narrower and possibly less difficult aspect of the debate. Namely, which of these three areas is now also a de jure specialty by the criteria described in general terms for all professions by Matarazzo (1983) and by Sales et al. (1983) when applied specifically to psychology? Continuing experience and debate will no doubt make it easier for the protagonists to reach a consensus on the answer to this better defined and articulated question.

Summary

For the graduate student wishing a career as a licensed psychologist providing fee-for-service health care there already exists in present APA-accredited predoctoral programs in clinical psychology in our country's departments of psychology a body of knowledge in generic psychology plus a minor track of selected courses related to health which may effectively be applied to patients and other individuals in the health arena who are in need of services embraced by the term "professional health psychology."

Although such predoctoral programs offer the high-quality education to prepare individuals at a journeyperson-psychologist's level, acquisition of the additional needed skills, knowledge, and professional maturity to provide such services independently as an acknowledged health psychologist to persons with medical illnesses (or their prevention) should be accomplished in a postdoctoral, professional health psychology training program that is formally organized as such, is multidisciplinary, is two years in length, and is offered in an appropriate setting under the tutelage of several qualified practicing health psychologist-mentors and physician-mentors.

Teaching hospitals, federal agencies such as NIH, NIMH, NIHR, and the VA, as well as private sources of funding, should put the providing of the necessary resources high on their list of priorities because of the present dearth both of well-suited training institutions and of qualified mentors who have the *time* to help recruit and to train such needed students in these new postdoctoral residency programs.

To facilitate the eventual acceptance by society, by psychology, and by significant others of the numbers of needed graduates from these postdoctoral programs, the leadership in health psychology within the American Psychological Association, working with others within and outside of psychology, recently began to study the steps which will be necessary to designate and accredit both the institutions and the programs offering such two-year postdoctoral training. Consideration is also being given by others to the matter of credentialling the individuals who receive such training as a precondition to launching their careers as independent providers of health psychology services. Once these steps are accomplished the distinctions between proficiency and specialty, and between a de facto and a de jure specialty, will have been better clarified. Health psychology, with its mandated two-year postdoctoral residency, will be a bona fide specialty (i.e., one which is more widely acknowledged as such both within and without psychology).

Probably more than the provider of psychological services in any other arena (including that of traditional clinical psychology) the practitioner of psychology in the acute, hospital, health-illness arena will confront on a daily basis conditions that are associated with death and severe forms of disability and illness as a regular and continuing part of his or her work. Society and the profession of psychology already have in place a number of statutes, as well as quasi-legal and ethical and professional guidelines and other types of formal and informal controls, which govern the work of the already licensed health care professionals who carry out their practices in such a milieu. It is my opinion, after twenty-eight years of training young health psychologists in one such university hospital setting (Matarazzo 1965), that two years of postdoctoral education and training is the minimum amount of time necessary to adequately help prepare them for a life's work as a service provider in health psychology.

REFERENCES

American Psychological Association. 1981. Specialty guidelines for the delivery of services by clinical psychologists. *American Psychologist* 36 : 640–51.

Belar, C. D., and L. J. Siegel. 1983. A survey of postdoctoral training programs in health psychology. *Health Psychology* 2 : 413–25.

Belar, C. D., E. Wilson, and H. Hughes. 1982. Health psychology training in doctoral psychology programs. *Health Psychology* 1 : 289–99.

Chesney, M. A., and M. Feurstein. 1979. Behavioral medicine in the occupational setting. In *Behavioral approaches to medicine: Application and analysis*, edited by J. R. McNamara. New York: Plenum Press.

Dwore, R. B., and J. D. Matarazzo. 1981. The behavioral sciences and health education: Disciplines with a compatible interest? *Health Education* 12 (May–June): 4–7.

Matarazzo, J. D. 1965. A postdoctoral residency program in clinical psychology. *American Psychologist* 20 : 432–39.

———. 1980. Behavioral health and behavioral medicine: Frontiers for a new health psychology. *American Psychologist* 35 : 807–17.

———. 1982. Behavioral health's challenge to academic, scientific and professional psychology. *American Psychologist* 37 : 1–14.

———. 1983. Education and training in health psychology: Boulder or bolder? *Health Psychology* 2 : 73–113.

———. 1984a. Behavioral health: A 1990 challenge for the health sciences professions. In *Behavioral health: A handbook of health enhancement and disease prevention*, edited by J. D. Matarazzo, S. M. Weiss, J. A. Herd, N. E. Miller, and S. M. Weiss. New York: John Wiley & Sons.

———. 1984b. Behavioral immunogens and pathogens in health and illness. In *Psychology and health: Master Lecture Series*, vol. 3, edited by C. J. Scheierer and B. L. Hammond. Washington, D.C.: American Psychological Association.

Olbrisch, M. E., and L. Sechrest. 1979. Educating health psychologists in traditional graduate training programs. *Professional Psychology* 10:589–95.

Raimy, V. 1950. *Training in clinical psychology.* New York: Prentice-Hall.

Sales, B. 1985. Specialization: Past history and future alternatives. *The Clinical Psychologist 38*, no. 3 (Summer): 48–52.

Sales, B., P. Bricklin, and J. Hall. 1983. *Manual for the identification and continued recognition of proficiencies and new specialties in psychology, August 1, 1983 Draft* (135 pp.). Washington, D.C.: American Psychological Association.

———. 1984. *Specialization in psychology: Principles, November 1984 Draft* (20 pp.). Washington, D.C.: American Psychological Association.

Sheridan, E. P. 1981. Advantages of a clinical psychology residency program in a medical center. *Professional Psychology* 12:456–60.

Stone, G. C., ed. 1983. Proceedings of the National Working Conference on Education and Training in Health Psychology. *Health Psychology* 2(5): 1–153, supplement section.

27

Postdoctoral Training in Health Policy Studies

Lee Sechrest

There are, obviously, several ways in which psychologists interested in and knowledgeable about health might have an impact on the health of the nation and its people. Researchers can produce information critical to decisions about how best to improve health, some by research on specific health problems and services and some by research on organization and delivery of services. Health services providers can assist in ameliorating the distress of those individuals with health problems. Prevention specialists can help to develop programs in communities to forestall the development of health problems. But some psychologists may want to get more directly involved in defining and influencing policy decisions. Some psychologists are likely to be able to insinuate themselves directly into the processes that result in establishing of policy, e.g., by possession of some special expertise or by dint of position. Other psychologists will, however, find it efficient or even necessary to seek training specifically in the processes by which policies—local, state, or federal—are shaped. Training in policy processes is usually called either policy studies or policy science.

For many years the scientific tradition of objectivity and noninvolvement prevailed in psychology, and neither the discipline nor many of its practitioners were much involved in the analysis and setting of public policy. That is not to say that individual psychologists, let alone the American Psychological Association, did not attempt to influence public policy. The attempts were, however, sporadic and unsystematic and, more often than not, were directed toward issues of direct interest to psychology and psychologists, e.g., professional licensure or funding of scientific research. More recently,

I wish to thank Dr. Judith Meyers, a former APA Congressional Fellow and Director of the Bush Program in Child Development and Social Policy for very helpful comments on an earlier draft of this paper.

though, psychology and psychologists have begun to take an active and direct interest in public policy across a broad range of issues, with many activities more in the nature of *pro bono* efforts rather than narrow self-interests. A notable manifestation of the interest of psychology as a whole in public policy is the *American Psychologist,* which not only added a section on "Psychology in the Public Forum" in 1982, but which began to feature articles written by public figures such as senators. A question that naturally began to arise was whether psychologists were really prepared for a role in the policy arena.

An influential treatise of only a few years back advanced the notion that academicians and policymakers represent "two communities" (Caplan, Morrison, and Stambaugh 1975) that are destined never to meet. Academically trained persons without experience "in the real world" were alleged to be naive. Certainly friends and acquaintances of mine who were psychologists who happened to have reached positions in which their decisions could bear on policy warned me and others that the policy arena was different from academia, that it required special understanding and skills in order to permit effective operation within it (e.g., Patrick DeLeon of Senator Inouye's office; James Kaple of the Social Security Administration and later Health Care Financing; John Marshall of the Bureau of Community Health Services and later the National Center for Health Services Research). Psychology was not prepared with an obvious mechanism for educating itself about the rigors of policy setting.

To some extent, of course, if only slightly, we are educated about the setting of public policy when we take "civics" courses in school, when we study political science, when we discuss legislative issues, and so on. But this informal training is haphazard, usually superficial, and of dubious effectiveness. Therefore, specific training programs in policy studies have been proposed and developed in various universities and other institutions. The American Psychological Association annually sponsors two younger members as Congressional Fellows for one year of in-service training in the offices of U.S. legislators. Rand Corporation gives a Ph.D. in policy studies and recently, with support from the Pew Memorial Trust, established the Rand-UCLA Center for Health Policy Study which will support five predoctoral fellows each year as well as offer midcareer training for persons already involved in health employment.

In general, it seems agreed that policy studies refers to a broad, interdisciplinary program with a strong emphasis on economics, but with political science, law, and management science ranking just behind economics in importance. Policy studies is essentially analytic in approach; hence, traditional research methods receive somewhat less emphasis than in most discipline-oriented programs. In general, however, quantitative methods are much emphasized.

As Masters (1983) has noted, training programs in the area of policy studies, at least in psychology, are as yet quite new. They are evolving and changing with experience and the development of more and better knowledge about the policy setting process. The Bush Programs in Child Development and Social Policy at UCLA, the University of Michigan, the University of North Carolina, and Yale are examples of such training efforts. Funded by the Bush Foundation since 1978, the programs aim to train predoctoral and postdoctoral students in areas relevant to the applications of child development research to social policy. Each of the programs has developed its own curriculum and model of training over time. No national training conference along the lines of the Boulder conference on clinical training has as yet been envisioned for policy studies training. Consequently, there is probably relatively little uniformity in training programs. Moreover, it might not be especially safe to predict what they might be like ten or fifteen years from now. No great uniformity may ever develop.

Terminology

As is so often true of a new enterprise, terminology and taxonomy are as yet variable and imprecise. *Policy studies* seems the better generic term to refer to a range of interests and roles in relation to the interface between research and policy-making. *Policy analysis* seems most often used to describe attempts to forecast the effects of policies being considered in relation to a specific problem. *Policy research* seems most often used to refer to the activities that policy analysts engage in in the course of their attempts to forecast effects. In this paper I will use the term policy studies generically.

Part of the problem stems from lack of agreement about just what it is we want a person "trained in policy" to do. The policy person could serve as an adviser to policymakers (probably the policy analyst's role), could be an activist trying to bring about changes in public policy, could try to be a catalyst to improve connections at the interface of research and policy, e.g., by improving the policy-relevance of research, or the policy person could try in some manner or other to become a policymaker. Obviously these roles are quite different in their requirements and so, presumably, would be the training needed for them. Rather the opposite of Pirandello, it seems that we may have six roles in search of an actor.

The Case for Postdoctoral Training

Two options to bring the influence of psychology to bear on public policy present themselves. One is to train policy scientists (and public administrators, which is where many policy scientists end up) and try to persuade some of them to specialize in psychology and include a heavy concentration of work in psychology in their programs. Thus, in programs such as at Rand or at the University of Michigan in which it is possible to get a Ph.D. in policy studies, some graduates would, one hopes, be well informed about psychology and its implications for public policy. One would, however, have to rely on the haphazard processes of selection and the vagaries of individual interests to ensure that psychology would ultimately be represented among those with policy studies training. The other option is to identify psychologists (Ph.D. level) with an interest in public policy and provide them with the requisite training for a career related to the making of public policy.

For several reasons, I very much favor the latter option, i.e., for postdoctoral training in policy studies. Probably I favor that option even more for health psychology policy studies than for psychology policy studies in general. First, although it may be possible to produce a technocrat's knowledge of psychology in the course of public policy training, it is not likely that that training would result in the depth of knowledge required as a base for informed decision making about the diverse issues for which psychology is relevant. Second, psychology and its views need advocates in the course of establishing policy. Dispassionate presentations by those without personal commitments to the field are not likely to be persuasive, especially in the face of arguments that may be made by persons committed to other points of view.

Some writers (e.g., Takanishi 1981) have argued quite strongly for the necessity of training within a discipline as a prerequisite for policy studies training. The argument is not particularly relevant in relation to proposals for postdoctoral training since, by definition, persons with doctorates would have been trained in some discipline.

Health psychology is, I think, particularly likely to suffer from superficial approaches to it and from a relative lack of commitment to the psychological approach to health. Those persons with inadequate background in psychology may be apt either to exaggerate the potential of psychology out of an uncritical attitude or to underestimate it out of excessive narrowness. Sweeping claims of efficacy are often made on behalf of psychology, and it sometimes requires a fair degree of sophistication to be able to evaluate those claims and put them in an appropriate perspective. On the other hand, many less than completely informed persons equate psychology with psychoanalysis, psychotherapy, mental testing, or some other circumscribed view or activity. Such persons are unlikely to comprehend the value that psychology may have in community interventions, increasing compliance with medical regimens, altering habitual behavior, and so on. Psychology must be viewed as a rather broad analytic perspective and not simply as a small bag of tricks. Health is a problem area that easily generates heat, and there are many different points of view vying for attention. Some of these points of view are likely to have powerful or vociferous proponents or both, and if psychology is to receive attention, it is likely to need the persistence and vigor in its champions that characterizes only the fully committed.

Postdoctoral training in policy studies, coming as it does after extensive training in the content and methods of psychology, can concentrate on the additional knowledge and skills and on the point of view characteristic of good quality analysts. The psychologist wishing to become an effective policy analyst will have to acquire new knowledge, new methods, and a new way of looking at things: knowledge of the political system, new ways of analyzing data, and a pragmatic view.

As Masters (1983) notes, policy studies training programs are essentially remedial in their nature. They are required because ordinary doctoral training in a discipline does not prepare one for working in the policy arena. A postdoctoral training program has, or ought to have, the aim of ameliorating the naivete alleged, almost certainly quite correctly, by Caplan, Morrison, and Stambaugh (1975). The "remedial" should, however, be advanced as a qualification only with caution and without contempt. Disciplinary training is not ordinarily meant to be policy oriented, nor should it be. Only a handful of the doctorates in any discipline are likely ever to become involved in policy setting, and there is no reason that the vast majority should be trained to become policy analysts. And, on the other hand, politicians and bureaucrats are mostly quite naive about the various academic disciplines and what they have to offer. Advancing the case for training in policy studies is not at all disrespectful to the discipline. On the contrary, it is highly respectful since, if the discipline had nothing to offer, neither would there be any case to be made for policy studies training.

Reference was made earlier to the lack of any accepted prescriptions for training of psychologists for policy roles. Indeed, it may be that no substantial uniformity will ever be desirable, especially at the postdoctoral level. By its very nature, postdoctoral training probably needs to be largely ad hoc, addressing itself to the particular needs and interests of individual trainees. Postdoctoral trainees are likely to bring to policy studies training very diverse interests and skills arising out of similarly diverse backgrounds and experiences. Some may already be in midcareer stages and desire further fairly specific training to enable them to enhance effectiveness in particular jobs (Masters 1983). Others may be new Ph.D.s concerned with enlarging their employment opportunities. Some postdoctoral trainees, even if new Ph.D.s, may have had extensive work experience in policy relevant settings; others will have had little work experience at all. Postdoctoral policy studies training will not lend itself to lockstep programs.

The Breadth of Policy Studies Training

The University of Michigan has an Institute of Public Policy Studies (IPPS) that offers various training programs, including one leading to a doctorate in public policy. Although the IPPS program is but one of many, it serves to illustrate both the orientation of such programs and the uncertainties about just what is entailed by them. The prologue to the description of the Institute and its programs states rather well the case for policy studies and the nature of the training entailed:

> In a society such as ours, with multiple, vague and conflicting goals, and unequal, but widely shared power, institutions must meet a dual test of political acceptability and operational feasibility. Institutions, therefore, need to be managed by individuals who understand the great complexity of the policy environment itself and possess the skills necessary to grasp and develop solutions. . . . The challenge is to prepare unusually able individuals for a career in public service in a profession requiring analytic skill and sound judgment. These persons must be at once sensitive, conscientious, and tough-minded. They must, as a matter of habit, keep broadly informed and communicate widely. They must tackle problems with imagination and creativity.
>
> In order to accomplish this, the curriculum must provide students with a set of attitudes and skills that are best described as being analytical or having a problem-solving orientation. Because no single scholarly discipline is broad enough to provide feasible solutions across the spectrum of policy issues, a familiarity with the basic principles of economics, law, political science, psychology, industrial engineering, and management science is necessary, as well as an ability to apply those principles to particular problems.
>
> This must be coupled with an understanding of the decision-

making environment; an ability to work effectively as a member of a decision-making team; and an ability to communicate effectively in stating problems and proposing solutions.

(Institute of Public Policy Studies, University of Michigan 1984, 3)

The assertion in the IPPS prologue that "familiarity with the basic principles of economics, law, political science, psychology, industrial engineering, and management science *is necessary*" could be startling, to say the least. Six diverse fields are specified (and one wonders how members of other disciplines, such as sociology or statistics, might feel at being left out). Even if one takes a restrictive view of what is meant by "basic principles," learning them in six fields is a tall order. In fact, however, the actual program of the IPPS requires demonstrated doctoral level proficiency in only two fields, with demonstrated competence required in three concentrations, one usually being quantitative methods. It is not clear how seriously the "is necessary" is taken with respect to the six disciplines named, but the program description contains no specific provisions for either obtaining or demonstrating familiarity with basic principles in all six fields. Whether the failure to follow through explicitly on the stated requirement represents a compromise with reality or is merely a reflection of a very low standard for familiarity is not clear. The important point is that an extraordinary diversity of background knowledge is regarded as at least highly relevant, if not absolutely necessary, for a career in the policy arena.

A Plea for Training in Research Methods

I would make a special case for the very best training possible in research methodology for any psychologist intending to become involved in policy analysis or policy setting. It seems to me to be professionally and ethically imperative that when a psychologist evaluates the scientific evidence for a potential policy action, that that evaluation be truly informed and expert. There is no place in policy-making for the casual or noncompetent analyst.

Methodological training is best obtained at the predoctoral level. I do not believe that all Ph.D. psychologists are well trained in research methodology, particularly in the type likely to be required for sophisticated policy analysis. Standard research methodology such as is customarily taught in connection with psychology laboratory courses is not a sufficient background for the kind of research analysis that is necessary in the much messier "real world." Data available in most policy areas is likely to come in the form of nonexperimental findings, quasi-experiments, epidemiological studies, and so on. Unless psychologists aiming to establish policy are truly sophisticated in analysis and interpretation of these kinds of data, their recommendations may be well off the mark.

As indicated, my belief is that methodological training of the kind needed ought to be acquired at the predoctoral level. Postdoctoral training programs ought to develop specific mechanisms for diagnosing the methodological sophistication of trainees and for remediating identified deficiencies.

Internships and Field Training

It would seem evident that academic training is not, itself, sufficient for the development of even entry-level skills for a policy-oriented job. Quite some time ago, Matarazzo (1965) made the case for postdoctoral residency training in clinical psychology, and those arguments would seem to apply readily to policy training. A major part of the argument concerns the need for actual experience in the complex, "hot" atmosphere of practice. Kubie (1948) had previously noted that, "This atmosphere is so important in training for therapy of any kind, that without it all intellectual and technical equipment is of little value" (p. 49). That observation applies acutely to training for the practice of (ameliorative) policy analysis and policy formation. Takanishi (1981) has made a particularly strong case for the necessity of internship or equivalent training in policy studies.

In a later paper, Matarazzo (1971) suggested quite strongly that the apprenticeship is probably the only reasonably dependable way of training practitioners in areas lacking a strong scientific data base. Certainly that describes the field of policy studies. Although there may be a reasonably good scientific data base involved in the development of some policies, there is no such data base to guide the processes required to absorb and evaluate all the information and concepts relevant to a policy and then to derive inferentially the best recommendations for action. Matarazzo, writing of psychotherapy, insisted that it is far more art than science and that it is best learned by doing in the presence of an experienced and accomplished mentor. The same position with respect to policy analysis and policy-making could easily be defended.

There is an apocryphal story about a psychoanalyst who claimed to have had a thousand hours of training from an analyst who had had three hundred hours of training from someone who had had none at all. Policy studies is a new field, and trainees are really in very much the position of a psychoanalyst being trained by someone with at best minimal personal training. A central question is whether training for policy studies is necessary—or even possible. Most policymakers have had no specific training, and in recommending apprenticeships, one must keep in mind that trainees will of necessity be mentored by persons whose outlook may be distinctly non-academic. It is at least conceivable that the best preparation for policy studies is simply doing it—being in the trenches month after month.

One of the uncertainties that raises the possibility that the best preparation for policy-making may be doing it is the seemingly extraordinary variability in policy problems and settings. If every issue and every setting are different from others in important ways, development of a training program is, at best, a haphazard enterprise. The very existence of special centers for child development and social policy suggest that policy training may have to be very diverse, that separate training may be needed for different areas of interest. The paper by Masters (1983) entitled "Models for Training and Research in Child Development and Social Policy" presupposes that models might have to be separately developed for every field. The point made previously about the possibility that training in policy studies for psychologists may never be highly uniform is reinforced.

Analyst or Activist?

Should the health psychologist interested in policy be trained for the relatively passive role of analyst or the active role as policymaker? The distinction is akin to that often made between staff and line positions in organizations. I am dubious of the prospects for deliberately training psychologists for policy-making roles. Policy-making, when it is of any consequence, is fundamentally political. Some persons are good at politics, and some are not. Candidates get elected to office, and other persons get appointed to policy-making positions based on their skills in navigating through the rocks and shoals of the political seas. Whether those navigational skills can be deliberately trained and fostered rather than simply being allowed to develop naturally, remains to be demonstrated. We have no examples of schools to follow. We are on sounder footing (I think) in our efforts to train psychologists to be careful and knowledgeable analysts of policy. What they are then able to do with their analyses may depend much more on abilities that are beyond our own capacity to engender.

Many of us have an abiding faith in "planned change," that is, in the likelihood that society can be improved by deliberately stimulated or fostered changes. That faith may or may not be warranted (see Bennis, Benne, and Chin 1969 for a still provocative discussion). Many social changes have proven extraordinarily difficult to bring about, such as altering our system of medical care, and other changes when successfully negotiated prove to have unanticipated negative effects that may well outweigh the intended positive ones—screening populations for health problems may result in "labeling" people in quite undesirable ways. Still other changes, although desirable in principle, may be beyond our capacity to manage and, hence, result in effects that are a shambles: the deinstitutionalization of mentally disturbed persons is an example. Perhaps psychology should be reticent to move in the direction of any program to train its policy analysts to be change agents. When we *train* psychologists to do something, we become, perforce, responsible for their doing it.

Kelly[1] (1969) has provided a particularly cogent discussion of the role of the expert in society, pointing both to the advantages and the dangers of the expert role. These advantages and dangers pertain both to the expert and to society. Kelly makes what appears to me to be an important distinction, quite relevant to training in policy studies, between *macroexpertise* and *microexpertise*. The macroexpert function occurs when a society or one of its organs is in a state of perturbation or crisis. The macroexpert is asked to give advice on how to resolve the problem, how to restore equilibrium. The advice given by the macroexpert is not presumed to be universal or timeless; it is specific to extant conditions. Microexpertise is directed toward the improvement of society. It is guided by some vision of what society ought to be, i.e., it is *utopian*. For example, we currently have experts telling us how to save the nuclear family, how to deal with the crisis in our schools, what to do about unemployment. As Kelly sees it, these are macroexperts, or at least persons trying to function as such. Presumably they require a broad knowledge and a capacity to foresee consequences of various societal or governmental actions. But they need not be, perhaps should not be, guided by any particular ideology. And when equilibrium has been restored, the macroexpert is no longer needed and, in theory at least, retreats to the venue from which he or she came. By contrast, we also have experts telling us how the family may be restructured so as to permit women to achieve personal fulfillment. We have experts telling us how schools may be reorganized so that all children may receive an optimal education. These experts, microexperts, have a vision of the perfect society, or some segment of it, and provide advice on a continuing basis in an attempt to move society along the path to that perfection (utopia). Kelly suggests that few experts really want to *become* the power, that their temperament and inclination are otherwise engaged. But they do naturally wish that their ideas will prevail.

1. This is not George A. Kelly, the psychologist, although the first name and middle initial are the same.

These two potential expert roles, macroexpert and microexpert, are important to distinguish. Obviously, the same person may occupy either role on different occasions, but one needs to be aware of which role it is when. The role of the microexpert is partisan and may involve a long-range view that is inappropriate in a situation of organizational or societal disequilibrium. Training programs might well pay explicit attention to the characteristics and needs of these two roles and to the possible differences in policy analyses required for each.

Mead (1983) has been severely critical of policy studies for the nearly exclusive emphasis he believes the approach places on economic factors in decision-making as opposed to political and ethical factors. As Mead sees it, the role of policy analysts tends strongly to consist of determining whether a proposed means to reach an end is cost-effective. Policy analysts are too little inclined to question whether the end is worthwhile or whether the proposed means are politically feasible, legally sustainable, and morally acceptable. Mead concedes the improvements that have come about in policy-making from being sure of "the numbers," but he notes that policy scientists are often overruled by politicians because the former neglect the critical political elements in the decision process. Policy scientists may lack good knowledge of the law governing the decision areas in which they work, and moral positions are often explicitly eschewed. Without sound legal underpinnings and in the absence of any moral considerations, what is left of policy analysis? Perhaps, precisely as Mead asserts, nothing much more than costs in relation to gain.

Should training programs attempt to deal with problems of values and morality? It is difficult to see how such problems can be ignored. Whether they can be resolved is another matter. But at the very least, postdoctoral training programs for policy studies involving psychologists should illustrate value problems in policy contexts. It is neither possible nor fair for experts working in the intense political arenas surrounding social problems to claim truly to be neutral with respect to values and morals.

Training for Administrative Positions

Since one can expect that at least some proportion of postdoctoral trainees in policy studies will end up in administrative/managerial positions, the question arises whether part of postdoctoral training time ought to be devoted to training for administration. I would argue not. First, the time available for postdoctoral training is likely to be quite limited, and there is enough to be done to absorb the material that is required for astute policy analysis. Second, it is not entirely clear that we know very much about how to train people for administrative positions, especially positions for which requirements are unknown at the time of training. Third, training everyone in a policy studies program for administrative positions is wasteful unless most persons end up in such positions. And, fourth, administration may well be something that is best learned by doing it, albeit best with gradual exposure.

There is a tradition in many fields and many jobs for persons needing specialized training to enter degree programs designed to provide that training. The M.P.H. and the M.B.A. are degree programs designed specifically for such purposes. Both programs may afford psychologists the kind of training that would be desirable for pursuing careers as administrators. They seem, therefore, to be appropriate recommendations for psychologists who would be administrators and are likely to be more satisfactory than training that might be devised and tacked onto an already demanding program in policy studies.

Support for Postdoctoral Training

Support for postdoctoral training will not come easily. Still, support for postdoctoral training may be more likely these days than support for predoctoral training. For one thing, postdoctoral training is likely to be considerably briefer than predoctoral training. In general, however, federal agencies have shown reduced sympathy in recent years for support of training at the predoctoral level for persons who are expected to move into well-paying jobs.

Masters (1983) notes that the three most important sources of funding for policy studies in child development have been three private foundations. That seems likely to continue, but psychology is going to have to be imaginative in its search for funds generally. If it is important to psychology as a whole to have more psychologists involved in policy, then perhaps the discipline as a whole should give consideration to supporting a modest number of trainees each year, a step that could be taken either by the American Psychological Association or the Association for Advancement of Psychology, or both. It should be noted that the APA already funds two Congressional Fellows each year, and the Society for the Psychological Study of Social Issues, Division 9 of APA, funds one Public Policy Fellow each year to work at APA.

Evaluation of Training

Unfortunately, we do not yet know much about how to evaluate training programs at the professional level. An American Psychological task force

(Task Force on Evaluation of Education, Training, and Practice 1983) could do little more than recommend initiating a program of research in order to learn how to evaluate training programs. Nonetheless, at least some evaluation of postdoctoral training in policy studies seems mandatory. The beginning step in an evaluation will be to specify with care the goals of the training program, preferably in terms of knowledge and skills to be acquired.

Postdoctoral training in policy studies might benefit from an explicitly product-oriented approach. That is, one of the requirements of postdoctoral training might be that each trainee should produce a usable study of some policy. Not only would such a product demonstrate the competence of the trainee, and therefore be helpful in evaluating the training program, but the attempts to produce the study, along with the processes involved in it, could help generally to illuminate the nature of policy studies by psychologists. I think that, in truth, we as yet know very little. Moreover, the emanation of a series of quality policy studies from a training program might do a great deal of elicit support for it. On the other hand, the difficulty of producing usable policy papers should not be underestimated, and the usefulness of a product-oriented training effort is not assured.

In the long run, of course, we would like to think that our training programs are evaluated by the quality of the work done by their graduates. That evidence may, unfortunately, be long in coming and uncertain in meaning. More immediately, we ought to learn to ask ourselves whether it makes sense to have training programs that we cannot evaluate. If, as I believe, the answer is no, then we ought to get on with the development of an evaluation. We are presumably at some advantage in the case of postdoctoral programs in policy studies since they are new. It ought to be easier to build in evaluations of programs starting from scratch.

Reforms as Experiments and Experimenting Societies

Donald T. Campbell (1969) made a cogent and persuasive (to many social scientists) case for proposing social reforms as experiments to be undertaken and evaluated. Social reforms should not be presented as panaceas or even as mere solutions for problems, but rather as ideas to be tested empirically. Social reforms should consist of the potential changes surviving the crucible of evaluation.

Obviously Campbell's proposals have not come to pass, and we are still not an experimenting society. In my view, however, his arguments are still cogent and persuasive. The experimenting society is, itself, an idea that ought to be tried. At the very least, programs to train psychologists for roles in the making of public policy ought to strive mightily to avoid the traps fostering unwarranted certainty about policy and its basis in empirical fact. Hubris does not become the psychologist who is a student of policy. A good way to avoid this is to consider carefully the case for social experiments and to encourage and actively promote the systematic testing of proposed solutions to social problems. Policy studies programs that do not foster such views are, in my estimation, derelict.

REFERENCES

Bennis, W. G., K. D. Benne, and R. Chin. 1969. *The planning of change.* New York: Holt, Rinehart, and Winston.

Campbell, D. T. 1969. Reforms as experiments. *American Psychologist* 24:409–29.

Caplan, N., A. Morrison, and R. J. Stambaugh. 1975. *The use of social science knowledge in policy decisions at the national level.* Ann Arbor: University of Michigan, Institute for Social Research.

Institute of Policy Studies. 1984. Institute brochure. Ann Arbor, MI: University of Michigan.

Kelly, G. A. 1969. The expert as historical actor. In *The planning of change,* edited by W. G. Bennis, K. D. Benne, and R. Chin. New York: Holt, Rinehart, and Winston.

Kubie, L. S. 1948. Elements in the medical curriculum which are essential in the training for psychotherapy. *Journal of Clinical Psychology* 4(Monograph Supplement no. 3): 46–51.

Masters, J. C. 1983. Models for training and research in child development and social policy. *Annals of Child Development,* vol. 1, edited by G. Whitehurst. Greenwich, CT: JAI Press.

Matarazzo, J. D. 1965. A postdoctoral residency program in clinical psychology. *American Psychologist* 20:432–39.

———. 1971. The practice of psychotherapy is art and not science. In *Creative developments in psychotherapy,* edited by A. R. Mahrer and L. Pearson, 364–92. Cleveland, OH: Case Western Reserve Press.

Mead, L. M. 1983. Policy science today. *The Public Interest,* no. 73:165–70.

Takanishi, R. 1981. Graduate education for roles in child development and social policy. *UCLA Educator* 23:33–37.

Task Force on Evaluation of Education, Training, and Practice. 1983. Final Report. American Psychological Association.

28

Respecialization and Continuing Education for Health Psychology

Wilbert E. Fordyce and Manfred J. Meier

This chapter concerns two separate but related issues: respecialization and continuing education. They share a number of important objectives and methods but require separate treatment.

Respecialization has special importance to health psychology. In the formal and titular sense, there are no health psychologists. There are many psychologists who are functioning professionally as health psychologists. Yet others now in the training pipeline are being prepared for such roles. Many of those now filling the role of health psychologist, or who will soon do so and have appropriate credentialing in background, training, and experience, will undoubtedly in due course be "grandfathered in" as health psychologists. It seems reasonable to expect that many psychologists presently identifying themselves in other fields of the profession will seek to become health psychologists. Economic and vocational or professional opportunity in the rapidly expanding health care/behavioral science area will attract some. Some will come because of the opportunity to study and explore an exciting frontier of human service. Perhaps some will come because they see the field of health psychology as a way of seeking to credential activities heretofore perceived as on or beyond the fringe of scientific legitimacy. Respecialization must cope with these diverse issues. It must provide ample opportunity while maintaining rigorous quality control.

Just as with respecialization, continuing education also presents special challenges to a new field. It is important first to clearly distinguish between them. Respecialization can be seen as preparation added on to earlier completed training for entering a field and continuing education as keeping up with a field once entered.

Special note should be made of the contributions of the Respecialization and Continuing Education Working Group: Timothy Baker, Roy Grzesiak, William Johnson, and Charles Swencionis.

The particular need for top-quality continuing education resources in health psychology derives from the rapid emergence of new concepts, new problems, new methods. It is of paramount importance that there exist mechanisms for fostering maintenance and advancement of knowledge and competence in this rapidly moving field.

Respecialization

A new field faces many and diverse challenges. One of the more important challenges is to generate an identity—an articulation of who we are and who we aren't. In the domain of health/behavioral science, that becomes particularly important. There is a long and not always meritorious history of pronouncements concerning relationships between sickness/health and human behavior. Clearly, a simple disease model of sickness/health is insufficient. However, the concepts and methods which have been brought forth either as alternatives to disease models or as management strategies to be used with them often have been insufficiently grounded in empirical data or in the conceptual bases of behavioral science. These often shaky bases for highly touted movements alleging to apply psychological principles to problems of sickness/health have led to innumerable fads and, all too often, to black marks on the credibility of behavioral science. It is particularly important at this initial phase of a new field to recognize our responsibility to proceed with caution and to articulate our identity in ways that enhance credibility. Here, of course, "credibility" is to be defined in terms of intellectual and professional excellence.

Respecialization inevitably will play a significant role in providing the basis for credentialing health psychologists. It is incumbent on us that respecialization be implemented in ways which strike the right balance between providing opportunity for those with doctorates in other areas of psychology (who thus are appropriately prepared to enter training via respecialization in health psychology) and preserving scientific and professional credibility.

Scientific and professional credibility will be accorded first as a consequence of demonstrated competence in their endeavors by the health psychologists now in place. Secondly, credibility will be assigned by the reputations of training facilities. That kind of anticipatory credibility dictates that respecialization have eminently respectable academic roots. Respecialization should be the mission of academic institutions. Respecialization is not a simple matter of accrual of credits by whatever mechanism. It requires the resources of the academic setting and the institutionalized quality-control mechanisms characteristic of established academic programs.

In light of the foregoing considerations, the Working Group on Respecialization and Continuing Education formulated a series of recommendations as to the proper structure and format for respecialization.

1. Respecialization into health psychology of professionals holding doctorates in other areas of psychology should occur exclusively within APA-approved programs in academic settings. As a corollary, academic institutions must make provision for respecialization tracks within their doctoral programs in psychology.
2. Academic institutions should develop training track alternatives to full-time course work which combine academic study with paid (if possible) practicum experiences and training. That will permit greater accessibility to respecialization by psychologists not able to enter a full-time academic program.
3. The academic program must provide the respecialist with training equivalent to that required in predoctoral, postdoctoral, and apprenticeship training.
4. The academic program should grant approval, on a carefully controlled basis, for transfer of academic credit and professional experience for prior training equivalent to health psychology requirements.
5. As possible, the respecialization academic training model should be an extension of the one currently in place in that institution.

Continuing Education

The first mission of continuing education is, of course, to assist in the development of the newly required skills and the maintenance of competence. A related mission is to assist in meeting the requirements of state-mandated licensure and the professional organizations' requirements for continued upgrading and updating of knowledge and skills.

Given the new and rapidly expanding nature of health psychology, there is a particular need for continuing education resources sufficient to disseminate emerging knowledge and skills. The distinction between knowledge and skills should be kept clear. Knowledge is not something over which a professional field should seek proprietary control. Efforts to constrain access to knowledge are inappropriate. The situation is different with respect to skill training. There is a professional responsibility to be concerned about the proper preparation of the persons who would use those skills and about the monitoring of competency in the exercise of skills.

The very nature of the field of health psychology is to interface with numerous other professional fields and specialities. It follows that continuing education offerings from within health psychology will attract members of other professions. Where the topics and training format focus on dissemination of knowledge, there is no problem. Where, however, skill training is involved, it is essential that there be appropriate safeguards against permitting access by those who have the potential for misuse of those skills. It follows that continuing education courses which teach assessment or intervention skills must be carefully considered by the purveyors. The level and type of training of applicants who come from within psychology and the training and professional qualifications of people from other fields must be reviewed and appropriate screening exercised before entry into the skill-training programs is permitted.

Health psychology's multiple linkages to other fields and professions dictates that the continuing education process draw on the working relationships with those fields and professions. It is essential that liaisons with other fields be pursued. To do so is to enrich the continuing education process for health psychology by appropriate offerings developed elsewhere. At the same time it promotes infusion of the continuing education offerings of other fields by health psychology and the related behavioral science into other fields. These liaison relationships should help avoid redundancy in continuing education offerings across disciplinary boundaries and aid the exercise of more effective quality control over what is offered and who may enroll.

The continuing education process presents a number of additional issues. Continuing education is not presently confined to academic settings. That, in turn, has necessitated often elaborate and complex procedures for attempting to maintain appropriate quality control when the mechanisms and related quality control resources of the academic setting are not present. This burden generally has been undertaken by professional organizations such as the APA. The importance of continuing that effort is ever greater until such time as academic settings may fulfill this mission. This is so because the pace of advances in knowledge and skills threatens to outrun effectively controlled dissemination resources. But as the burden grows so also does the opportunity for it to be shared. Development and greater use of liaison relationships within APA, between divisions and the central office, and between divisions should occur.

In line with the preceding discussion, a series of recommendations regarding continuing education were formulated at the May 1983 National Conference on Graduate Education and Training in Health Psychology:

1. The American Psychological Association must continue to accept responsibility for review and approval of continuing education offerings.

2. The American Psychological Association should maintain and strengthen its present continuing education evaluation mechanism by drawing on the expertise of its divisions. This can be accomplished by: (a) each division identifying one or more persons to serve coordinator and liaison functions with the American Psychological Association regarding evaluation of the continuing education mechanisms available to its division members; and (b) the American Psychological Association drawing on those people in the review and approval process.
3. Continuing education credit in health psychology should be contingent upon the American Psychological Association approval of the continuing education offering.
4. Continuing education offerings which include skill training must specify the prerequisites for attendance/participation; and the American Psychological Association approval must be contingent upon doing so.
5. The American Psychological Association should develop liaisons between divisions and with other appropriate professional groups with regard to continuing education policies and requirements.

Two additional issues remain to be considered: the continuing education strategy of competency-based training and the resource development of the Assessment Center concept.

Competency-based Training

The issue of the strategy for evaluation of continuing education must be addressed. We endorse a competency-based training model as a desirable heuristic for the design and implementation of continuing education programs. The competency-based training concept draws the distinction between demonstrating the mastery of a knowledge set or a skill by performance and documenting exposure to a training period in regard to the knowledge or skill. The student *performs* to the satisfaction of the teacher. In the case of a knowledge issue, performance may, for example, be by generating an outline or description of some course of action dictated by the knowledge. In the case of a skill issue, the learner demonstrates the level of mastery attained. We believe that a competency-based model will permit and, in fact, foster: (a) the identification of core knowledge and skills; (b) the accurate evaluation of skills acquisition in the learner; and (c) the accurate evaluation of continuing education programs, per se.

We realize that in some areas of service delivery and health psychology, the definition and assessment of competence constitute measurement challenges of profound proportions. We advocate that the American Psychological Association investigate multiple avenues through which basic core competencies may be identified and characterized and that measurement strategies be developed to assess individuals' levels of competence. Procedures could then be instituted to provide appropriate individuals (i.e., those with appropriate professional certification and academic degrees) the information and skills considered seminal to a particular competence. Such training modules should be self-contained and should necessarily incorporate assessments that reflect the acquisition of the competence information and skills.

Assessment Centers

The traditional postdoctoral continuing education model for professional psychology has emphasized didactic workshops and conferences rather than a competency-based or competency-determined approach. Workshops and conferences are certainly appropriate vehicles for transmitting knowledge in an existing or evolving area of practice. However, the goals of these traditional continuing education activities are characteristically limited to the transmission of new knowledge with little if any opportunity for practical experience directed toward expanding skills or establishing new competencies. As more predoctoral apprenticeship and postdoctoral programs develop competency-determined training modules, their utilization in an externship through continuing education should become feasible. With appropriate adjustments, externship activities could provide a step-wise opportunity to acquire verifiable new competencies through the export of the competency component of apprenticeship and postdoctoral programs. A key methodological approach for achieving this goal on a continuing education basis is the Assessment Center approach.

In this country, the concept of an Assessment Center originated in the Office of Strategic Services (OSS) during World War II and subsequent applications have been extended in management selection and placement programs in large multinational corporations (Bray 1983). Assessment Centers can be designed to include learning components and, thereby, facilitate the acquisition of new knowledge and the incorporation of knowledge into new proficiencies and competencies in a given specialty area such as health psychology. An example of a specific learning component would be acquisition of the skills required in cardiac pulmonary resuscitation (CPR), while another would involve learning the skill of systematic desensitization. This approach does not necessarily imply a single physical resource or location. Rather it is characterized as a multimethod resource for transmitting, collecting, reviewing, and integrating information in the development, evaluation, and deployment of competencies in particular settings (Cyrs 1976). For purposes of continuing education, such resources can collectively be designated as Learning and Assessment Centers in which the necessary materials for learning are identified and made available to the professional in the field as part of a larger continuing education strategy.

The Learning and Assessment Center concept has the potential for extending competency-determined training modules into practice settings where the professional in the field can maintain or expand proficiencies and competencies without extended periods in residence at an educational institution (McClelland 1973). In fully developed form, the center could provide the foundation for an open-ended postdoctoral program without extended absence from professional practice. Short of such an elaborate goal, the approach appears to have considerable merit for complementing traditional conference and workshop activities as a means of pursuing continuing education.

A difficult but not insurmountable obstacle to the effective implementation of the Learning and Assessment Center concept is the as yet incomplete identification of core and specialized competencies in health psychology. As these competencies are identified, they will need to be defined in operational terms to specify how the cognitive, affective, and psychomotor components of a competency relate to the desired behavioral outcomes in professional practice. The elements of a given professional role are approximated in such centers by work sample simulations and exercises, test-item banks, and the entire range of possible tests and autotutorial procedures necessary for acquiring the knowledge, attitudes, and skills for subsequent integration in competent performance.

Such elaborate exercises in instructional methodology have been introduced in other professions (MacKinnon 1975). This advanced technology, developed by educational psychologists and instructional design personnel, is available for application in continuing education as well as for the pre- and postdoctoral professional education. As competencies become defined in the field, the terminal performance objectives necessary for effective professional practice can be translated into modules or self-contained instructional packages. The learner can then be subjected to direct tests and be given the necessary supervision for refining the competency in accord with accepted standards of practice. In addition, the professional may be assisted to qualify for a new practice area in which he/she may not have received primary training. Division 38 can be seen as the central guiding force for defining health psychology competencies and for assisting professional organizations, credentialing bodies, and educational institutions in the design of training modules.

The timeliness of this approach is underscored by the recent decision of the American Board of Professional Psychology to award the diploma in new areas of practice in addition to the traditional areas of clinical, counseling, school, and industrial/organizational psychology. Thus, clinical neuropsychology and, soon, forensic psychology will be recognized as discriminable and valid new areas of practice. In light of a variety of competencies that are emerging, health psychology appears to be in a strong position to build a structure for a seventh such specialty. Criteria for the identification and continued recognition of proficiencies and new specialties are being defined by the Subcommittee on Specialization of the Board of Professional Affairs of the American Psychological Association. It appears likely that a policy statement and decision regarding new specialties may soon reach the floor of the American Psychological Association Council of Representatives. These developments are rapidly converging and call for appropriate innovation in continuing education. A performance analysis of the roles of health psychologists will be needed to identify the cluster of competencies that qualify health psychology as a new specialty. The relatively broad definition of health that prevailed at the Arden House Conference suggests that from a proficiency/competency perspective, health psychology will become differentiated into many proficiencies if not, later, also into one or another subspecialty.

Although psychologists have generated much of the technology that underlies the Center concept, the necessary analyses of competencies and the self-contained training modules remain to be developed. This is an extremely large undertaking that requires the cooperation and active participation of the American Psychological Association, state associations, state licensing boards, and national credentialing agencies such as ABPP and the National Register of Health Service Providers in Psychology. The effectiveness of the process toward encouraging lifelong commitment to maintaining and expanding professional competencies will depend on the strengthening of the secondary reinforcement to be derived from pursuing continuing education opportunities on a regular basis. While there are intrinsic rewards in competency validation, other reinforcements will be needed to ensure this commitment. In this direction, a number of developments are noteworthy. Introduction of continuing education requirements on the part of the state licensing boards beyond the twelve that now mandate it by statute should facilitate commitment to continuing education. Also, increased competition in the health services marketplace will require a higher and more effective level of professional competence for survival in the future.

The Learning and Assessment Center concept has considerable potential for serving individuals in the field who are faced with contraints relative to releasing the large blocks of time necessary for the pursuit of a formal postdoctoral program. Such an extension of the Center concept to serve as a vehicle for respecialization, however, may be (but not necessarily is) more remote than the immediate goal of providing more systematic continuing education opportunities for the practicing health psychologist in the field. Such centers could become a powerful resource for the growth and effectiveness of existing as well as evolving psychological specialties.

Summary

The need for special attention to respecialization and continuing education resource development for health psychology is discussed. The major points can be summarized by indicating the twelve recommendations made.

1. Respecialization into health psychology should occur exclusively within APA-approved programs in academic settings.
2. Academic institutions should develop training track alternatives to full-time course work to permit greater accessibility for respecialization by psychologists not able to enter a full-time academic program.
3. The respecialization academic program must provide training equivalent to that required in predoctoral, postdoctoral, and apprenticeship training.
4. Transfer of academic and professional experience credit should be approved but on a basis carefully controlled to ensure equivalency to health psychology requirements.
5. As possible, the respecialization academic training model should be an extension of the one currently in place in the institution.
6. APA must continue to accept responsibility for review and approval of continuing education offerings.
7. APA should maintain and strengthen its continuing education evaluation mechanism by identifying and drawing on members from each division to assist.
8. Health psychology continuing education credit should be contingent upon APA approval of the continuing education offering.
9. Continuing education offerings that include skill training must specify the prerequisites for attendance and participation; APA approval must be contingent upon doing so.

10. APA should develop liaison mechanisms between divisions and with other appropriate professional groups in regard to continuing education policies and requirements.
11. A competency-based training model is recommended.
12. Assessment Centers, characterized as a multimethod resource for transmitting, collecting, reviewing, and integrating information in the development, evaluation, and deployment of competencies, should be developed to facilitate continuing education.

REFERENCES

Bray, D. W. 1983. ABPP Conference on Competence Evaluation. Washington, D.C., 12 October.

Cyrs, T. E. 1976. Modular approach to curriculum design using the systems approach. In *Instructional media and technology*, edited by P. Sleeman and D. M. Rockwell, 117–38. New York: Halsted Press.

MacKinnon, D. W., 1975. *An overview of assessment centers.* Greensboro, NC: Center for Creative Leadership.

McClelland, D. C. 1973. Testing for competence rather than intelligence. *American Psychologist* 28 : 1–14.

29

Accreditation of Training Programs

Paul D. Nelson

The history of accreditation, as that of psychology, is one of controversy and change, as well as consensus, on fundamental issues of higher education. The thesis to be advanced in this chapter is that developments in the field of health psychology are as likely to influence the future course of accreditation in psychology as are training programs in health psychology to be shaped by the criteria and practices of accreditation.

In a recent publication summarizing the history, current practices, and future challenges of accreditation, Kenneth Young, founding president of the Council on Postsecondary Accreditation, entitles his prologue "The Changing Scope of Accreditation," thus establishing a frame of reference for the treatise which follows. Reflecting on the post–Civil War period of social and technological change in our society, and the concomitant changes effected in education, Young sets the stage for the advent of what we know today as accreditation, "born," as Young states (Young 1983a, 5), "during a time of ferment and hope."

That same spirit, one might add, has characterized all of psychology during the past thirty-five years, as it does, in particular, those who today make the case for and debate the issues of health psychology as a discipline and profession. Moreover, one might reason, resolution of these issues will have an effect on the future of professional psychology in general, and therefore, as well, on accreditation as practiced by the American Psychological Association. To make that point, it seems appropriate to briefly review certain aspects of the philosophy and practices of accreditation, the history of accreditation in American psychology, and to summarize by addressing the issues which appear central to the future accreditation of professional psychology training programs, including those in health psychology.

Unless otherwise indicated, the opinions expressed in this chapter are those of the author and should not be construed as necessarily reflecting policy of the American Psychological Association or the endorsement of its governance.

Philosophy and Practices of Accreditation: An Overview

What is accreditation? It is both a status of public recognition and a process of evaluation. It is voluntary, self-regulatory, and nongovernmental in nature, initiated by educational institutions or specialized programs thereof. The Council on Postsecondary Accreditation defines accreditation as "a system for recognizing educational institutions and professional programs affiliated with those institutions for a level of performance, integrity, and quality which entitles them to the confidence of the educational community and the public they serve" (COPA 1983, 1). Young defines accreditation as "a process by which an institution of postsecondary education evaluates its educational activities, in whole or in part, and seeks an independent judgment to confirm that it substantially achieves its objectives and is generally equal in quality to comparable institutions or specialized units" (Young 1983b, 21). In referring to accreditation as the "conscience" of the educational community, Millard suggests that "accreditation as a process has two fundamental purposes: to certify to the quality of an institution or program and to assist in the further improvement or enhancement of such quality." He adds: "Basically, what accreditation attests to is that an institution or program has both clearly defined and educationally appropriate objectives, that it maintains conditions under which such achievement reasonably can be expected, that it appears in fact to be accomplishing them substantially, and that it can be expected to continue to do so" (Millard 1983a, 11).

As a system to assess and enhance quality in education, accreditation rests on three basic processes: (1) self-study by the educational institution or program, (2) on-site evaluation by a selected group of peers, followed by (3) review and decision of an independent accrediting body, by which accreditation is sought in accordance with published standards or criteria of educational quality set forth by that accrediting body. Without all three of these processes, the cycle of accreditation activities is incomplete.

It was early in this century that specialized accreditation of professional training programs got its start, notably in the fields of medicine and law (Glidden 1983). Those efforts to standardize and review professional education were to be followed in subsequent decades by other professions, among them psychology. The evolution of accreditation practices suggests that while standards were prescriptive at first, a point of view was developed eventually to evaluate institutions and programs in the context of their setting, their goals, and the processes by which they achieve those goals (Millard 1983b). Beyond that, moreover, specialized accreditation standards typically denoted a sensitivity to national norms or standards of practice in the specialized field of interest. Thus, Millard argues, specialized accreditation standards are related not only to improvement of the professional training program, but also to the profession itself, an orientation to quality of outcome as well as resources and processes of education and training.

Brief History of Accreditation in Psychology

The accreditation of doctoral training programs in psychology did not begin until after the Second World War. The demand at that time for clinical psychologists was especially acute, prompted by the numbers of neuropsychiatric casualties among military service personnel and the need to provide psychological assistance to veterans upon their return to civilian life. The Veterans Administration, followed by the U.S. Public Health Service, recognized that need and requested from the American Psychological Association "a list of institutions that possessed adequate facilities for providing training to the doctoral level in clinical psychology" (Sears 1947, 199).

The task of evaluating programs was assigned to the Association's Committee on Graduate and Professional Training, chaired at that time by Robert Sears. Following a study of those institutions that gave public notice of their intent to offer doctoral training in clinical psychology, the committee published an account of its work in 1947. It included the first public listing of institutions within which doctoral programs in clinical psychology had been evaluated in terms of criteria established on a national basis by a body of the American Psychological Association. Essentially, those criteria had to do with characteristics of the faculty, the curriculum, and the practicum facilities. With a prophetic tone, moreover, the committee concluded: "If accreditation continues to be desirable for the profession, new criteria will gradually develop. . . . The present criteria must be viewed only as steps along the way; they are useful for measuring one stage in a type of professional training that is changing and growing every year" (Sears 1947, 204).

To advance those first efforts, a new Committee on Training in Clinical Psychology was appointed under the leadership of David Shakow. Although Shakow and his colleagues, guided in part by the earlier Flexner Report on medical education and training, attempted to develop a more formal set of standards for training in clinical psychology, the orientation of the committee was not entirely prescriptive. The following was written as the preface to its work:

> The general principles which underlie the graduate program appear to us of primary importance—in fact much more important than

the details of the program. If clarity in the formulation of goals exists, there should be relatively little difficulty about agreeing on the means for implementing them. As has already been indicated, it is the opinion of the committee that the setting up of a detailed program is undesirable. Such a step, if accepted generally, would go far in settling clinical psychology at a time when it should have great lability. Considerable experimentation with respect to the personality and background of students as well as the content and methods of courses will for a long time be essential if we are to develop the most adequate program. Our aims are rather to achieve general agreement on the goals of training and encourage experimentation on methods of achieving these goals and to suggest ways of establishing high standards in a setting of flexibility and reasonable freedom. We also hold that the goals should not be determined by special situations and special demands, but should be oriented toward the question of what is the best training for the clinical psychologist. (APA Committee on Training in Clinical Psychology 1947, 543)

That statement, intended by the committee for the benefit of psychology, is woven with a number of threads essential to the fabric of accreditation. Among those essentials are the clear statements of program goals, the emphasis on allowing programs flexibility to develop and innovate, the inference that programs should be evaluated in terms of the model of training they set forth, and a generic orientation to the profession and its training requirements. Two years later the committee summarized its efforts by stating:

We are convinced of the importance of setting standards and evaluating performance in clinical training—in fact we see this process as inevitable if clinical psychology is to establish itself soundly and be a credit to psychology as a whole. We have set up criteria and administered procedures in ways that seemed best; we are neither satisfied that they are perfect nor persuaded that they are dangerous or ineffective. It is natural that there should be differences of opinion in the Association regarding the goals and the techniques we have accepted. Both these differences and our own convictions are still matters of opinion rather than demonstrated fact. The real answer to the question "Shall we evaluate?" lies somewhere in the future— a future which must include among other considerations, a systematic appraisal of the effects of the committee's work, not only on the clinical psychological products which the universities turn out, but on other psychological products, and university staffs and administrations as a whole.

(APA Committee on Training in Clinical Psychology 1949, 340–41).

In other words, does accreditation make a difference? That question remains central to issues of accreditation philosophy and practice.

Accreditation Standards and Criteria in Psychology

Throughout the history of accreditation by the American Psychological Association a few principles have governed the development of standards or criteria against which training programs in professional psychology have been evaluated. In the course of its work, the committee chaired by Shakow (APA Committee on Training in Clinical Psychology 1947) articulated the following principles of doctoral training in clinical psychology: (1) that a clinical psychologist must first and foremost be a *psychologist,* having a point of view and core of knowledge common to all psychologists; (2) that the program of education for the doctorate in clinical psychology should be as rigorous and extensive as that for the traditional doctorate; (3) that preparation should be broad, directed to research and professional goals, not to technical goals; (4) that programs should be organized around careful integration of theory and practice, of academic and field work, by persons representing both aspects; (5) that research and an inquiring attitude be an essential aspect of the orientation and training for the practice of psychology; and, (6) that students develop an early identification with the profession and a sense of professional responsibility at the level of society as well as that of the individual patient or client.

Reviews by Goodstein and Ross (1966), Shakow (1978), and most recently Matarazzo (1983), provide summaries of how professional psychology training programs have developed during the past three decades. Despite the changes which have occurred in the field of psychology, including the development of professional schools and alternative philosophies of training, the principles set forth in 1947 remain basic to the accreditation criteria for professional psychology programs today.

In translating those principles into standards or criteria for accreditation, an effort has been made over the years to achieve balance between that which prescribes and that which guides, between that which requires uniformity and that which encourages innovation, between that which is specific and that which is general. The construct that perhaps best embodies the spirit of these principles is that referred to as the program's "training model." The following text, for example, is embedded in the American Psychological Association's current accreditation criteria:

> Various models of training exist. A diversity of philosophies, goals and practices from program to program and from individual student to individual student must be permitted. Each program must specify its training model and goal in writing. The responsibility for definition of its model and goals rests with the faculty of the training program. . . . Programs are evaluated in terms of the model endorsed, the goals stated and the success in meeting these goals. The training model and goals are evaluated in terms of their relevance to available resources and to local, regional and national needs. The goals of professional training may be achieved through a variety of formal and informal curricula. A primary emphasis should be on helping the student acquire proficiency in the broad area of professional practice at a high level of skill. A commitment to lifelong professional development should be incorporated as a basic value to be adopted by faculty and students.[1]

Evaluating programs in the context of their training models, yet also within the framework of national standards deemed valid by professional colleagues for the purpose of preparing students at the entry level of the profession, is a practice consonant with principles of specialized accreditation. That process also serves as a potential source of tension between professional and academic needs or values, between the accrediting association and the program or institution being accredited, and between training practices that are normative or traditional and those that are idiosyncratic or innovative. Psychologists responsible through the years for developing accreditation criteria seemed mindful of these matters, as are those engaged in the development of standards for evaluation practices in general (see Rossi 1982).

Another issue germane to discussion of training models and program emphases is that of specialization within the profession. For most professions accreditation applies to the generic field of training and academic degree level appropriate for entry into the profession (Glidden 1983). For psychology that has been, and remains, at the doctoral level of education and training. In terms of the professional field of focus, however, accreditation of psy-

---

1. American Psychological Association, *Accreditation Handbook,* March 1983 edition, Appendix B, pp. 9–10.

chology programs has developed with "one foot in the generic bucket" and "one foot in the professional specialty bucket." That is, the scope of accreditation in psychology has been limited to programs publicly identified by what the American Psychological Association recognizes as professional specialties, notably those of clinical, counseling, and school psychology. Yet, the accreditation criteria employed in evaluating those programs have been decidedly more generic in nature than attentive to the uniqueness of each specialty. Aspects of training that are unique to a specialty can be incorporated in a particular program's training model. One might expect, therefore, somewhat greater similarity of training models among programs that purport to prepare students for the same specialty area of professional psychology than among those that prepare students for different specialty areas.

Attention to issues of uniqueness and overlap among specialty fields of professional psychology was an issue thirty years ago, as it is today. In 1951, the Committee on Intraprofessional Relationships in Psychology, chaired by Carroll Shartle, published several statements on this matter. One was that a common core of theory, concepts, and research seemed to have become a part of the basic training of all doctoral students in psychology. The committee encouraged that practice as a way of providing professional unity to psychology. In addition, the committee noted overlap in professional functions of the specialties of clinical psychology, counseling and guidance, and school psychology. It recommended, therefore, that "Ph.D.-level training in school psychology and counseling and guidance be evaluated along with clinical training programs" (APA Committee on Intraprofessional Relationships in Psychology 1951, 93).

During the following year, a group charged with developing guidelines for the accreditation of doctoral training programs in counseling psychology reported:

> The training program for counseling psychologists overlaps with training for other psychological fields. The delineation of similarities and differences in either practice or training is not, however, an appropriate problem for unilateral action by representatives of one area. This collaborative effort lies in the future.
> (APA Committee on Counseling Training, Division of Counseling and Guidance 1952, 180)

Thus, by 1953, the criteria initially established for use in review of clinical psychology programs were applied to counseling psychology programs and, in 1971, to doctoral programs preparing students for the specialty of school psychology, as well. Public recognition of accredited programs was specific to the professional specialty area in which the program offered training. The criteria for accreditation, however, were essentially generic, as they have remained.

Accreditation Issues Related to Health Psychology

As new fields or emphases of professional service in psychology emerge, inevitably the question of whether or not such fields or emphases represent new specialties of professional psychology is raised. Health psychology is not an exception. Whether health psychology is or is not a specialty, in the sense defined by the American Psychological Association Committee on Standards for Providers of Psychological Services (1981), or whether it meets the general criteria of a profession noted earlier by Sanford (1951) and more recently by Peterson (1976), is not the central issue of this chapter. These are relevant questions simply in the context of current accrediting practices of the American Psychological Association, the scope of which is defined in terms of the professional specialty designation of doctoral programs, even though generic criteria are employed in their evaluation. More fundamental a question is the extent to which doctoral programs in health psychology have the goal of preparing students for professional services in psychology. For if they do, based on the history of accreditation in psychology and the nature of the accreditation criteria, one might argue with good reason that those criteria are as applicable to health psychology as they were thirty years ago when applied to counseling psychology and school psychology programs.

In a survey of graduate programs in psychology, Belar, Wilson, and Hughes (1982) sought to determine where, how, and for what purposes doctoral training is afforded in the field of health psychology. By coincidence, the number of doctoral programs responding that they provide training in health psychology ($n=53$) is not appreciably different from the number of clinical psychology programs initially listed thirty-five years ago by the APA Committee on Training in Clinical Psychology (1949). Health psychology is carried typically as a track or emphasis within another psychological discipline or professional specialty area (e.g., social, clinical, experimental psychology), the most commonly reported one being clinical psychology. Some programs seem focused predominantly on research, while others are principally concerned with preparing students for professional practice. In most instances, regardless of theoretical orientation or program goals, formal coursework and laboratory experience is combined with experience in applied settings (reinforcing the value of apprenticeships in psychology, a topic reviewed by Strickland in chapter 24). Belar discusses those issues further in her chapter (chapter 22) on current training practices in health psychology.

Most important for purposes of accreditation is the extent to which a program makes its purpose and goals clear, how it plans to achieve those ends, and how well it does in that endeavor. Such is the point from which the program self-study begins, the cornerstone of the accreditation process. It is the basis on which the program is evaluated and offers the essential characteristics of the program's training model. In that vein, Levy (1984) argues that all psychology training programs focused on human services should be eligible for accreditation. Offering a three-dimensional matrix of human services psychology, he recommends that programs "be required to identify the specialties for which they provide training and those cells within the human services psychology matrix upon which they focus, and they should be evaluated in terms of how well they accomplish their goals" (p. 491). Others, similarly, have offered multidimensional models of training for professional services in psychology, such as the cube model on dimensions of intervention for student development advanced by Morrill and Hurst (1980).

To be clear about one's purpose in training is especially important in a new field of study, let alone one as broad in scope as health psychology (see Belar et al. 1982; Matarazzo 1982 and 1983; and Stone 1983). Once a training program declares its intent to prepare psychologists to render professional services to the public, it assumes certain obligations. Specifically, it assumes the obligation to train students in accordance with broadly accepted professional standards of practice and a body of ethics appropriate to the profession. With that knowledge, as well, the student is expected to develop a set of attitudes, if not always skills, by which to challenge in a scholarly, exploratory, and professional manner the traditions and habits of professional practice, continually seeking new knowledge and more effective methods by which to render those professional services for benefit of the public.

These latter aspects of program development seem to be acknowledged already, if not altogether resolved, among health psychology doctoral training programs. Indeed, from proceedings of the National Working Conference on Education and Training in Health Psychology (Stone 1983) and the expanding scientific literature in health psychology, there is a strong sense of a commitment among health psychologists to the development of professional practices based on empirical evidence of effect. The methods of scientific inquiry and verification, program evaluation research, and epidemiology are almost without exception central to the thinking of health psychologists. Among the leaders in the field, there is insistence on rigor but at the same time tolerance of alternative methodological models. There is likewise an interdisciplinary emphasis among health psychologists, reminding one of the position advocated by Shakow and his colleagues more than three decades ago, namely that students learn to value and participate in a multidisciplinary team approach in rendering professional services, as well as in research, on problems as complex in nature as those pertaining to health of people (APA Committee on Training in Clinical Psychology 1949, 545).

In the final analysis, one might suggest that the prevalent and increasing interest of so many psychologists in the relation of psychology to health and fitness in the most general sense affords professional psychology an opportunity to revisit once again the fundamental issues of "who and what psychologists are, and what they do," addressed at least some forty years ago and periodically by national forums since that time. The interest in health psychology comes at a time during which essential questions are being raised about psychology as a profession (Peterson 1976), the quality of professional training (Strupp 1976), and the nature of professional specialties in general and clinical psychology in particular (Fox 1982; Shakow 1976). Moreover, Fox (1982) and Matarazzo (1982) frame the challenge to psychology in terms of the prevalence of general health and fitness problems, associated with which are behavioral or psychological conditions of significance for those who plan the strategies and public policies, develop methods and implement programs of prevention, treatment, and rehabilitation. Indeed, the questions raised and the tenor of the times bear some resemblance, at that, to the post–World War II era during which the roles of psychologists and psychology in mental health services became matters of public discussion and debate.

It was in that context, of course, that accreditation in psychology took root. In much the same sense, the future of accreditation in psychology may be influenced significantly by the discussions held at this time about health psychology and its relation to all of psychology. The questions raised about the professional functions for which psychologists need to be trained to render or participate in a broad range of health services, and how well our training programs do in preparing students for those roles, are the very issues of public accountability in education and training that are central to accreditation. Indeed, the articulation of training goals that are deemed professionally valid, and the process of evaluating how well those goals are achieved, became priority matters for accredited programs.

Thus, in this period of ferment and hope, the impact of health psychology is likely to be registered not only on professional services rendered by psychologists or in the substance of graduate training programs, but even in the evolving process of accreditation as practiced in psychology. Those charged with the task, in time ahead, with a look at the future of accreditation in professional psychology might benefit as well from the wisdom of our earlier generation of colleagues who, in 1947, first worked on issues of accreditation in psychology and stated:

> If clarity in the formulation of goals exists, there should be relatively little difficulty about agreeing on the means for implementing them. . . . Our aims are . . . to achieve general agreement on the goals of training and encourage experimentation on methods of achieving these goals and to suggest ways of establishing high standards in a setting of flexibility and reasonable freedom.
> (APA Committee on Training in Clinical Psychology 1947, 543)

REFERENCES

APA Committee on Counseling Training, Division of Counseling and Guidance. 1952. Recommended standards for training counseling psychologists at the doctorate level. *American Psychologist* 7:175–81.

APA Committee on Intraprofessional Relationships in Psychology. 1951. Fields of psychology and their implications for practice and training. *American Psychologist* 6:90–93.

APA Committee on Standards for Providers of Psychological Services. 1981. Specialty guidelines for the delivery of services by clinical psychologists. *American Psychologist* 36:640–81.

APA Committee on Training in Clinical Psychology. 1947. Recommended graduate training program in clinical psychology. *American Psychologist* 2:539–58.

———. 1949. Doctoral training programs in clinical psychology. *American Psychologist* 4:331–41.

Belar, C. D., E. Wilson, and H. Hughes. 1982. Health psychology training in doctoral psychology programs. *Health Psychology* 1:289–99.

Council on Postsecondary Accreditation (COPA). 1983. *The balance wheel for accreditation.* Washington, D.C.: Council on Postsecondary Accreditation.

Fox, R. E. 1982. The need for a reorientation of clinical psychology. *American Psychologist* 37:1051–57.

Glidden, R. 1983. Specialized accreditation. In *Understanding accreditation,* edited by K. E. Young, C. M. Chambers, H. R. Kells, and Associates. San Francisco: Jossey-Bass Publishers.

Goodstein, L. D., and S. Ross. 1966. Accreditation of graduate programs in psychology: An analysis. *American Psychologist* 21:218–23.

Levy, L. H. 1984. The metamorphosis of clinical psychology: Toward a new charter as human services psychology. *American Psychologist* 39:486–94.

Matarazzo, J. D. 1982. Behavioral health's challenge to academic, scientific, and professional psychology. *American Psychologist* 37:1–14.

———. 1983. Education and training in health psychology: Boulder or bolder. *Health Psychology* 2:73–113.

Millard, R. M. 1983a. Accreditation serves as a 'conscience' of the educational community. *Proceedings, Southern Association of Colleges and Schools* 35: 11–14.

———. 1983b. Evolution of accrediting standards. *Accreditation, Council on Postsecondary Accreditation Newsletter* 8, 2.

Morrill, W. H., and J. C. Hurst. 1980. *Dimensions of intervention for student development.* New York: John Wiley & Sons.

Peterson, D. R. 1976. Is psychology a profession? *American Psychologist* 31: 148–58.

Rossi, P. H., ed. 1982. *Standards for evaluation practice.* San Francisco: Jossey-Bass, Inc.

Sanford, F. H. 1951. Annual report of the Executive Secretary: 1951. *American Psychologist* 6:664–70.

Sears, R. R. 1947. Clinical training facilities: 1947. A report from the Committee on Graduate and Professional Training. *American Psychologist* 2:199–205.

Shakow, D. 1976. What is clinical psychology? *American Psychologist* 31:553–60.

———. 1978. Clinical psychology seen some 50 years later. *American Psychologist* 33:148–58.

Stone, G. C., ed. 1983. Proceedings of the National Working Conference on Education and Training in Health Psychology. *Health Psychology* 2(5): 1–153, supplement section.

Strupp, H. H. 1976. Clinical psychology, irrationalism, and the erosion of excellence. *American Psychologist* 31:561–71.

Young, K. E. 1983a. Prologue: The changing scope of accreditation. In *Understanding accreditation,* edited by K. E. Young, C. M. Chambers, H. R. Kells, and Associates. San Francisco: Jossey-Bass.

———. 1983b. Accreditation: Complex evaluative tool. In *Understanding accreditation,* edited by K. E. Young, C. M. Chambers, H. R. Kells, and Associates. San Francisco: Jossey-Bass.

30

Curricula of Graduate Training Programs in Health Psychology

Joseph Istvan and Daniel C. Hatton

Since the publication of Matarazzo's (1980) article as charter president of the Division of Health Psychology of the APA in which he presented an overview of some of the interests and content areas of health psychology, doctoral programs offering either core training in health psychology or a health psychology emphasis within an allied specialty area have grown at a rapid rate. Without a history of prior specific models upon which to base their decisions concerning an appropriate course of study, program directors and faculty curriculum committees have had to rely largely on their own notions concerning both the *content* and *context* of education and training in health psychology at their respective institutions. Discussion of issues surrounding appropriate research/practicum experiences and academic coursework for those seeking graduate training in health psychology was, of course, one of the primary objectives of the 1983 National Conference on Graduate Education and Training in Health Psychology. We felt that it would be useful to examine how the first graduate programs responsible for producing the upcoming generation of health psychologists have structured their training experiences.

Although useful information concerning the characteristics of graduate programs that provide training in health psychology either as a specialty area or as a track within a health-related specialty area has been published by Belar, Wilson, and Hughes (1982), there is presently little specific information available concerning the actual coursework in such curricula. Toward the end of rectifying that deficiency, Matarazzo (1983) recently described *four* such programs. In this chapter, we present a more extensive sample of such doctoral programs. In addition to documenting the nature of a set of existing programs, we hope that these curricula might provide at least a partial perspective for faculty interested in developing similar programs and a useful beginning guide for informed choices by prospective graduate students considering health psychology as an area of advanced study.

To gather the data for the present analyses, in February and March of 1983 we sent letters to the department heads or program directors of each of the 42 graduate departments listed in the article by Belar et al. (1982) as a provider of graduate training in health psychology, requesting both a brief written overview of the program and a sample outline of both recommended and required courses for an individual receiving training in health psychology. Responses were obtained from twenty-one of these institutions. Eight of the twenty-one respondents indicated that the faculty was unable at present to describe a specific curriculum for training in health psychology. Generally, these program or department heads stated that their departments did not offer administratively acknowledged graduate training in health psychology at either the minor or major concentration level, although some courses which focused primarily on health-relevant issues were at least occasionally offered, and practicum or research experience could involve populations drawn from university or community health-care settings. Two departments provided information we considered too incomplete to be included in the present chapter. Nine responding departments offered either a minor or major concentration in health psychology and sent curriculum information complete enough for inclusion. During the summer of 1985 these nine departments, as well as the four programs reported in Matarazzo (1983), were given the opportunity to update and revise their curriculum descriptions. Two of the responding departments indicated that they had terminated their health psychology programs during the intervening two years and were dropped from the final sample.

Thus, responses were obtained from slightly more than half of the departments which indicated that they offered graduate training in health psychology. Although a higher response rate would have been desirable, this proportion of returns is comparable to that found in the Belar et al. (1982) survey. Overall, however, the following descriptions and sample courseloads, modeled after the format in Matarazzo (1983), should be regarded as illustrative examples of the manner in which education in health psychology has been structured at a variety of institutions and not as an exhaustive guide for those seeking training at, or information about, a specific institution. The courses offered in each program and the written description of each curriculum are presented below exactly as provided to us by the psychology faculty of each university except for very minor editing.

Ph.D. Program at the University of Alabama in Birmingham: A Medical Psychology Emphasis within the Clinical Psychology Track

The University of Alabama in Birmingham (UAB) offers a jointly sponsored doctoral program in Clinical Psychology with an emphasis on Medical Psychology. This program was begun in 1981 and is directed by a Medical Psychology Committee made up of psychologists from the Department of Psychology in University College and psychologists employed in nine different schools, departments, or institutes within the medical center complex of UAB. This is a five-year program with four years in residence and a fifth involving a full-time clinical internship. The emphasis of the program is on developing research-based, theoretically competent psychologists with basic clinical skills who have spent the last two years of their program emphasizing coursework, research, and clinical activities directed toward behavioral problems in a health-care setting. The program of study is highly structured in the first two years which includes an array of didactic courses in basic psychology, clinical psychology, and health psychology and also involves completion of a Masters degree. Comprehensive examinations are taken in the third year and the dissertation must be essentially completed prior to leaving for internship. Basic and clinical scientists from the neuroscience program, the Center for Development and Learning Disorders, and the departments of anatomy, physical therapy, neurology, neurological surgery, pediatrics, and the schools of optometry, public health, medicine, and allied health provide instruction, research facilities, and practicum opportunities under the sponsorship of psychologists working in those several settings. The individualized curriculum of the last two years includes advanced training in related areas and specialization in basic and clinical psychology as they apply to human health.

Ph.D. Program at the Louisiana State University: A Medical Psychology Emphasis within the Clinical Psychology Track

A Ph.D. specialty track in medical psychology is offered by the Louisiana State University Department of Psychology within its clinical training program. This track was designed to prepare students to work effectively as clinical psychologists in medical settings such as medical schools, family practice clinics, VA hospitals. Along with general clinical courses (e.g., assessment, psychopathology, interventions), students are required to take a number of specialty courses including behavior therapy, behavioral medi-

TABLE 30.1 The Ph.D. Program at the University of Alabama in Birmingham: A Medical Psychology Emphasis within the Clinical Psychology Track

Fall Quarter	Winter Quarter	Spring Quarter	Summer Quarter
		FIRST YEAR	
Statistics and Computer Tech (4)	Research Design and Computer Tech (4)	Statistics (4)	Psychopathology
Psychophysiology (4)	Learning/Cognitive	Psychopharmacology	Psychotherapeutic Methods
Professional Issues (1)			
	One-year Clinical Assessment		
	Sequence of Segments, Each 5–8 Weeks in Length		
	(1) Interviewing, Behavioral Observation	(4) Projective Personality Assessment	
	(2) Cognitive Adult Assessment	(5) Objective Personality Assessment	
	(3) Cognitive Child Assessment		
Research (1)	Research (1)	Research (1)	Research (1)
		SECOND YEAR	
Interpersonal Psychotherapy (2)	Behavioral Therapy (2)	Health Psychology I (3)	Health Psychology II (3)
Social Psychology (3)	Developmental Psychology (3)	Personality (3)	Neuropsychology I (4)
Research (1)	Research (3)	Neural & Humoral Bases of Behavior (4)	Research (2)
Clinical Practicum (2)	Clinical Practicum (2)	Research (2)	Clinical Practicum (2)
		Clinical Practicum	
		THIRD YEAR	
Psychotherapy elective (2)	History and Systems (3)	Public Health I (3)	Public Health II (3)
Health Psychology III (3)	Neuropsychology II (3)	Electives (3–6)	Electives (3–6)
Research (2)	Research (2)	Research (2)	Research (2)
Clinical Practicum (2)	Clinical Practicum (2)	Clinical Practicum (2)	Clinical Practicum (12)
		FOURTH YEAR	
Research (2)	Research (2)	Research (2)	Research (2)
Clinical Practicum (2)	Clinical Practicum (2)	Clinical Practicum (2)	Clinical Practicum (2)
Electives (3–6)	Electives (3–6)	Electives (3–6)	Electives (3–6)
		FIFTH YEAR	
		Clinical Internship	

cine, biological basis of psychopathology, behavior neurology, and psychopharmacology. The integration of psychological and bio/medical coursework is designed to provide medical psychology students with a foundation of knowledge necessary to perform the appropriate assessments and provide effective interventions for medical patients with both psychological and physical disorders.

Medical psychology students at LSU receive supervised clinical practicum experience in two settings, the Psychological Services Center of the Psychology Department and Earl K. Long Memorial Hospital. Practicum at the Psychological Services Center offers the opportunity for students to develop their clinical skills in working with a community population on an outpatient basis. Earl K. Long Memorial Hospital is part of the LSU School of Medicine Residency Training Program and offers medical psychology students a number of practicum alternatives including placements in pediatrics, family practice clinic, or general consultation and liaison. Medical psychology students participate in practica in this hospital setting during their first and third years. These placements provide students with a broad experience in managing medical patients with a diversity of physical and psychological problems. Along with developing skills in dealing with medical patients, students gain experience in working in a hospital setting and become knowledgeable in hospital procedure. Lastly, medical psychology students are required to conduct at least three research projects in fulfillment of their doctorate requirements. These include a masters thesis, an intermediate project, and a doctoral dissertation concerning issues in the areas of behavioral medicine or medical psychology.

Ph.D. Program at the University of California in Los Angeles: A Health Psychology Emphasis within a Social or Clinical Psychology Track

The Department of Psychology at UCLA has had a Health Psychology Program since 1979. Initially developed within the social psychology area, health psychology is now an interarea program between social psychology and clinical psychology, at both the predoctoral and postdoctoral levels. Students from areas in addition to social and clinical also participate in the program, which at present leads to a minor concentration in health psychology. Offerings include basic coursework in health psychology, field placements, and advanced statistical and methodological training. Participation from faculty and liaisons with the School of Public Health, the Department of Psychiatry, the Jonsson Cancer Center, and the Neuropsychiatric Institute round out the program's offerings. In addition, the Los Angeles area affords a wide variety of health settings for field placements and research.

TABLE 30.2 The Ph.D. Program at Louisiana State University: A Medical Psychology Emphasis within the Clinical Psychology Track

Fall Semester	Spring Semester
FIRST YEAR	
Statistics (3)	Methodology (3)
Physiological Psychology (3)	Learning (3)
Assessment, Part I (3)	Assessment, Part II (3)
Practicum (1)	Practicum (1)
SECOND YEAR	
Psychopathology (3)	Behavior Therapy (3)
Intervention (3)	Practicum (2)
Practicum (2)	Thesis (3)
Thesis (3)	Biological Basis of Psycho-pathology (3)
THIRD YEAR	
Behavioral Medicine (3)	Psychopharmacology (3)
Measurement of Behavior (3)	Professional Considerations (3)
Practicum (3)	Practicum (3)
Intermediate Project (1)	Intermediate Project (1)
FOURTH YEAR	
Behavioral Neurology (3)	Dissertation (6)
Dissertation (3)	Practicum/Research (1)
Practicum/Research (1)	Elective (3)
Elective (3)	
FIFTH YEAR	
Internship	Internship

Examples of illustrative programs of study for social and clinical students are provided in tables 30.3 and 30.4. Health psychology offerings can also be integrated into other areas within psychology, including physiological, learning and behavior, developmental, etc. As can be seen in the sample programs, students are required to take a number of introductory and advanced courses in their major area of concentration (e.g., social) and to include a variety of advanced statistical and methodological training courses as well. Health psychology typically constitutes one of the two minors that must be completed to obtain the degree.

The Health Psychology Program is supported, in part, through an NIMH Training Grant, which is held jointly by the programs of Social Psychology and Clinical Psychology.

TABLE 30.3 The Ph.D. Program at UCLA: A Health Psychology Emphasis within the Social Psychology Track

Fall Quarter	Winter Quarter	Spring Quarter
	FIRST YEAR	
Social Psychology A	Social Seminar of Choice	Social Psychology B
Statistics A	Statistics B	Introduction to Health
Research Methods A	Research Methods B	Psychology
Psychology Core Course	Psychology Core Course	Research Methods C
Lecture Series in Health	Lecture Series in Health	Behavioral Medicine A
Psychology A	Psychology B	
	SECOND YEAR	
Interpersonal Influence and	Social Epidemiology A	Behavioral Medicine B
Health	Practicum in Health	Social Epidemiology B
Practicum in Health	Psychology	Social and Interactional
Psychology	Advanced Statistics	Aspects of Stress
Research Methods in Social	Research	Social Seminar of Choice
Psychology	Lecture Series in Health	Research
Research	Psychology B	
Lecture Series in Health		
Psychology A		
	THIRD YEAR	
Advanced Statistics	Personality and Behavioral	Social Seminar of Choice
Health Promotion in	Factors in Cardiovascular	Research
Minority Populations	Disorders	
Lecture Series in Health	Research	
Psychology A	Lecture Series in Health	
	Psychology B	
	FOURTH YEAR	
Dissertation	Dissertation	Dissertation
Lecture Series in Health	Lecture Series in Health	
Psychology A	Psychology B	

Ph.D. Program at the University of Georgia: A Behavioral Medicine Emphasis within the Clinical Psychology Track

The purpose of the doctoral program in clinical psychology with a specialization in behavioral medicine is: (a) to give students a knowledge of the field of psychology as a method of inquiry into human behavior and variations from psychological and physiological norms; (b) to train students in the techniques and procedures of clinical psychology with special emphasis on health psychology, neuropsychology, and behavioral medicine; (c) to develop research and clinical competence in behavioral medicine; (d) to give

TABLE 30.4 The Ph.D. Program at UCLA: A Health Psychology Emphasis within the Clinical Psychology Track

Fall Quarter	Winter Quarter	Spring Quarter
	FIRST YEAR	
Foundations of Clinical Psychology A	Foundations of Clinical Psychology B	Foundations of Clinical Psychology C
Clinical Psychology Methods A	Clinical Psychology Methods B	Clinical Psychology Methods C
Research Methods A	Research Methods B	Psychology Core Course
Statistics A	Statistics B	Introduction to Health Psychology
Lecture Series in Health Psychology A	Lecture Series in Health Psychology B	
	SECOND YEAR	
Clinical Assessment A	Clinical Assessment B	Clinical Field Placement C
Clinical Field Placement A	Clinical Field Placement B	Advanced Clinical Methods B
Research Methods C	Advanced Clinical Methods A	Behavioral Medicine A
Interpersonal Influence and Health	Psychology Core Course	Research
Lecture Series in Health Psychology A	Lecture Series in Health Psychology B	
	THIRD YEAR	
Field Work in Clinical Psychology (Health Setting)	Field Work in Clinical Psychology (Health Setting)	Advanced Clinical Seminar
Psychology Core Course	Psychology Core Course	Social and Interactional Aspects of Stress
Research	Research	Advanced Statistics
Lecture Series in Health Psychology A	Lecture Series in Health Psychology B	Research
	FOURTH YEAR	
(Clinical student would not be supported on training grant during this year)		
Health Promotion in Minorities	Personality and Behavioral Factors in Cardiovascular Disorders	Internship
Internship	Internship	
Lecture Series in Health Psychology A	Lecture Series in Health Psychology B	
	FIFTH YEAR	
Dissertation	Dissertation	Dissertation
Lecture Series in Health Psychology A	Lecture Series in Health Psychology B	

students an identification with clinical psychology and behavioral medicine; (e) to provide the student with knowledge of the professional standards and ethical values of psychology and medicine; and (f) to train students with professional competence to function in various medical and health settings including general hospitals, rural medical situations involving behavioral medicine, and medical schools and universities which emphasize health psychology and behavioral medicine.

The program employs an apprenticeship model with continuous activities in coursework, clinical practicum or internship, and research. Clinical teams in both research and clinical activity are utilized with the final year of the doctoral program emphasizing the acquisition of supervisory skills. While the program normally takes five years to complete, in special circumstances it can be finished in four years.

Ph.D. Program at the State University of New York at Buffalo: A Behavioral Medicine Emphasis within the Clinical Psychology Track

The specialization in behavioral medicine within the Clinical Psychology Training Program trains clinical psychologists at the predoctoral level to work in the provision of psychological services as they relate to general health. This includes the applications of research and therapy with "psychosomatic" disorders, as well as areas of general medical practice in which behavioral or psychological phenomena may have impact (e.g., compliance, preparation for hospitalization, counseling of terminally ill, bioethics). Students in this APA-approved, clinical program take work in psychophysiology, behavioral medicine research and practica, biofeedback, prevention, and intervention and assessment methods. In addition to their dissertations, students are expected to produce several professional works reflecting intensive study of subjects related to health and behavior. Students receive didactic and practicum training in the Psychology Department and its Psychological Services Center; in addition, arrangements have been made for a variety of placements in the community, including Erie County Medical Center, Children's Hospital, etc. Students are expected to complete a full-year internship in a medical setting in addition to practicum requirements. Upon completion of training, students are eligible to work in medical schools, hospitals, outpatient clinics, and research and training institutes emphasizing the study and treatment of health disorders and the promotion of health.

TABLE 30.5 The Ph.D. Program at the University of Georgia: A Behavioral Medicine Emphasis within the Clinical Psychology Track

Fall Quarter	Winter Quarter	Spring Quarter	Summer Quarter
		FIRST YEAR	
Adult Psychopathology (5)[a]	Child Psychopathology (5)[a]	Methods of Practice in Clinical Psychology (5)[a]	Psychological Testing (5)[a]
Biological Foundations of Behavior (5)[ac]	Statistics I (5)[a]	Statistics II (5)[a]	Developmental Psychology or Individual Differences or
Clinical Practicum (2)[a]	Clinical Practicum (2)[a]	Clinical Practicum (2)[a]	Theories of Personality (5)[b]
			Neuroanatomy (5)[c]
		SECOND YEAR	
Behavioral Assessment (5)[ac]	Behavior Therapy (5)[ac]	Thesis (5)[b]	Neuropsychological Assessment (5)[ac]
Learning and Motivation (5)[b]	Social Psychology (5)[b]	Behavioral Medicine/Health Psychology (5)[b]	Psychophysiology (5)[c]
Clinical Practicum (2)[a]	Clinical Practicum (2)[a]	Clinical Practicum (2)[a]	
		THIRD YEAR	
Physiology I (5)[c]	Physiology II (5)[c]	Advanced Research Design (5)[b]	
Pharmacology (5)	Physiologic Dysfunctions (5)[c]	Elective in Behavioral Medicine (5)[c]	
		FOURTH YEAR	
	Clinical Psychology Internship with Behavioral Medicine Emphasis (20, four quarters)[a]		
		FIFTH YEAR	
Dissertation (5)	Dissertation (5)	Dissertation (5)	
Electives (5)[d]	Electives (5)[d]	Electives (5)[d]	
Clinical Supervision Practicum (2)	Clinical Supervision Practicum (2)	Clinical Supervision Practicum (2)	

[a]Clinical Psychology Requirement
[b]Basic Psychology Requirement
[c]Behavioral Medicine Requirement
[d]Elective

TABLE 30.6 The Ph.D. Program at the State University of New York at Buffalo: A Behavioral Medicine Emphasis within the Clinical Psychology Track

Fall Semester	Spring Semester
FIRST YEAR	
Statistics	Statistics
Personality Assessment	Research Methods
Behavioral Medicine course	Clinical Theories of Personality or
Distribution Requirement	Modification of Behavior Systems
	Distribution Requirement
SECOND YEAR	
Psychopathology	Behavioral Medicine course
Introduction to Psychotherapy	Distribution Requirement
Research	Free elective
Behavioral Medicine	Behavioral Medicine Practicum
Practicum	
THIRD YEAR	
Psychotherapy elective	History and Systems of Psychology
Behavioral Medicine	Behavioral Medicine Practicum
Practicum	Electives
Psychotherapy elective	
Elective	
FOURTH YEAR	
Dissertation	Dissertation
FIFTH YEAR	
Internship	Internship

NOTE: Behavioral medicine electives include Behavioral Medicine Seminar, Biofeedback Theory and Practice, Human Psychophysiology, Behavior Genetics, Aging, Behavioral Pharmacology, Biopsychology of Stress, Prevention, Epidemiology.

Distribution courses are selected from Biopsychology, Cognitive, and Social Areas, and additional work is available in Developmental Psychology; clinical practica are offered in child therapy, family therapy, cognitive behavior therapy, and community therapy.

Ph.D. Program at the Uniformed Services University of the Health Sciences: A Medical Psychology Specialization

The Ph.D. program in medical psychology at USUHS was conceived as a research training program capitalizing on the resources of a medical school and associated hospitals. The program emphasizes social, environmental, endocrinological, and psychophysiological aspects of health and illness and incorporates rigorous exposure to biomedical sciences as part of the curriculum. Students complete coursework in medical school courses in physiology and pharmacology as well as completing a series of courses in psychology. Clinical topics are included, but practica are not part of the program. The program is designed to be completed in four years. Research is a continuing requirement throughout these years. Each student is required to work with at least two faculty members each year and is expected to develop individual research programs or to assume major responsibility for implementing research as part of an ongoing project.

The department is now almost six years old, and the first group of students (accepted in 1979) has completed their dissertation research. Almost all of the advanced students have worked on projects with patient populations and medical collaboration, and all except the first-year students have participated in scientific presentations at national and regional meetings.

Ph.D. Program at the University of California—Irvine: Health Psychology Emphasis within a Social Ecology Program

The program in social ecology provides the intellectual and organizational context of graduate studies in health psychology at the University of California, Irvine. Graduate training emphasizes the scientific analysis of contemporary problems in the social and physical environment; problems are studied from the diversified viewpoints of a multidisciplinary faculty including specialists in health, community, environmental, developmental, and social psychology; urban sociology; and public health. In August, 1981, the Program in Social Ecology was awarded a five-year, predoctoral and postdoctoral training grant from the National Institute of Mental Health in Environment, Development and Health. The training program provides a structured context in which students focus intensively on the relationships among health, environmental conditions, and life span developmental processes. The interdisciplinary nature of the program prepares graduates for research and teaching positions in health psychology and related academic fields as well as for research-administrative positions such as jobs within public health agencies.

The specific objectives of the graduate curriculum in health studies at Irvine are: (1) to expose pre- and postdoctoral students to conceptual issues concerning the sociophysical environment, life span developmental processes, and mental and physical health; and (2) to foster the development of multidisciplinary research skills for examining these issues. In addition to completing all prerequisites for the Ph.D. in social ecology, students specializing in health psychology take a minimum of six elective courses, com-

TABLE 30.7 The Ph.D. Program at the Uniformed Services University of the Health Sciences: A Medical Psychology Specialization

Fall Quarter	Winter Quarter	Spring Quarter	Summer Quarter
FIRST YEAR			
Statistics I Research Methods & Complex Human Experimentation History & Systems Medical Psychology Seminar Research	Statistics II Introduction to Medical Psychology Medical Psychology Seminar Research	Statistics III Introduction to Medical Psychology Medical Physiology Medical Psychology Seminar Research	Research
SECOND YEAR			
Learning (Behavioral Factors in Chronic Illness) (Analysis in Psychology) (Human Sexuality) Medical Psychology Seminar Research	Pharmacology (Social Psychology) (Social Psychology & Health) (Psychology of Gender) Medical Psychology Seminar Research	Pharmacology (Psychopharmacology) (Interventions) Medical Psychology Seminar Research	Research
THIRD YEAR			
(Psychophysiology) (Analysis in Psychology) (Appetitive Behaviors) Medical Psychology Seminar Research	(Developmental Psychology) (Behavioral Assessment) Medical Psychology Seminar Research	(Advanced Social Psychology) Medical Psychology Seminar Research	Research
FOURTH YEAR			
Medical Psychology Seminar Research	Medical Psychology Seminar Research	Medical Psychology Seminar Research	

NOTE: Courses listed in parentheses are elective courses. All other courses are required.

plete a research practicum over three to four quarters under the supervision of one or more faculty, participate in a biweekly research seminar, and pass a written comprehensive examination during the third year of graduate study. Table 30.8 provides a model program of study.

The social ecology program is part of a University of California Health Psychology Consortium including all nine University of California campuses. This intercampus cooperation allows students greater opportunities to be exposed to other health psychology perspectives through taking a course (or even spending a term) at another campus and through participating in an annual intercampus conference on health psychology.

Ph.D. Program at the Chicago Medical School: A Health Psychology Emphasis within the Clinical Psychology Track

The University of Health Sciences/The Chicago Medical School is located forty miles north of Chicago on ground leased from the North Chicago Veterans Administration Hospital. The School of Graduate and Postdoctoral Studies was established in 1968 in response to the need for more highly qualified biomedical researchers and teachers in the rapidly expanding health sciences, and the first masters and doctoral-level graduate programs were offered in the basic medical sciences. In keeping with the University's mission, new programs in health related disciplines were added in 1977. One of these was a doctoral program (Ph.D.) with a specialization in clinical psychology. In the 1984–85 graduate handbook available from the school's Department of Psychology is the statement that:

> Our goal is to graduate psychologists who are well trained in clinical and scientific skills with emphasis in Health Care Psychology. The overall emphasis in health care is represented in the general course requirements and the two general elective areas: Clinical Neuropsychology, Clinical/Health Psychology. A Child-Clinical emphasis is available within the health or neuropsychology area. The health care psychology orientation provided by the program prepares students for clinical service and research in medical, mental health, and academic settings. Our graduates receive training in a variety of assessment methods and goal-oriented psychotherapy. The graduates are well prepared to enter academic fields because of their solid grounding in scientific, data-oriented disciplines and an emphasis on developing strong theoretical and research skills. The training assures the development of broad-based clinical skills and an emphasis area which encourages close cooperative work with other health care specialists such as pediatricians, internists, neurologists, neurosurgeons, and psychiatrists.

TABLE 30.8 The Ph.D. Program at the University of California—Irvine: A Health Psychology Emphasis within a Social Ecology Track

Fall Quarter	Winter Quarter	Spring Quarter
	FIRST YEAR	
SE 200 Principles of Social Ecology	SE 213 Issues in Social Intervention	SE 268 Environmental Psychology
SE 201 Research Methods	SE 264 Statistics	SE 265 Statistics
Elective*	Social Psychology	Elective
	SECOND YEAR	
SE 291 Program Evaluation or	SE 258 Health Psychology	SE 267 Human Stress
SE 224 Behavioral Epidemiology	Elective	Elective
Human Development (Child, Adolescent or Adult)	SE 241B Seminar in Environment, Development, and Health	SE 271 Research Tutorial in Environment, Development, and Health
SE 241A Seminar in Environment, Development, and Health		
	THIRD YEAR	
SE 299 Research Practicum	SE 299 Research Practicum	SE 299 Research Practicum
Elective	Elective	Elective
Written Comprehensive Examination	Develop Dissertation Proposal	Develop Dissertation Proposal
	FOURTH YEAR	
Dissertation Research	Dissertation Research	Dissertation Research

*Electives include the following: Community Psychology, Seminar in Social Gerontology, Family and Illness, Medical Sociology, Mental Health and Social Policy, Management of Health Care Systems, Atypical Child Development, Introduction to Survey Research.

The summary description of an illustrative program of study is reproduced here in table 30.9. Students are required to take clinical and research practica as well as eighteen to twenty-two hours of electives. Electives have included aphasiology, advanced neuropsychology, child clinical neuropsychology, advanced behavioral medicine, behavioral psychopharmacology, biofeedback, child psychopathology, and family and child therapy.

Ph.D. Program at the University of California—San Francisco: A Health Psychology Specialization

In 1961 an independent graduate division was added to the schools of medicine, dentistry, nursing and pharmacy, which then comprised the University of California—San Francisco. Stone (1979, 1981) has described how, in the short period of only four years, a Ph.D. program in psychology with an emphasis on biopsychology, personality, and psychopathology was added in 1965 to the nineteen doctoral programs in the basic sciences already in place and how this program in psychology was augmented by a new research training track in "health psychology" that admitted its first students in 1977. The aim of this newer program was to develop psychologists trained in social and personality areas of psychology who are prepared for a career of research in the health care process; specifically, for research, teaching, and consulting careers dealing with the cognitive, personality, and social psychological issues that affect the outcomes of health transactions. Recently the biological component of the original program was incorporated into the health psychology curriculum. Students in this program thus may emphasize their studies in social, personality, organizational, or biobehavioral areas.

The four-year curriculum is reproduced in table 30.10. As is shown, the required courses are heavily concentrated in the first two years of the four-year program, and the "basic psychology courses of the first year are taught much as they might be taught in any academic program, although they make more use of the literature of health psychology than would usually be the case. However, there is not yet much material available that links health problems to the central theoretical issues of psychology" (Stone 1981, 228).

Ph.D. Program at the University of Maryland: A Health Behavior Specialization within a Department of Health Education

The brochure description of this program suggests it might fit into one of the models described by Dwore and Matarazzo (1981) which could be developed by the cooperative effort of faculties within the college of education

TABLE 30.9 The Ph.D. Program at the Chicago Medical School: A Health Psychology Emphasis within the Clinical Psychology Track

First Quarter	Second Quarter	Third Quarter	Summer Quarter
FIRST YEAR			
Learning Interview & Behavior Observation Psychopathology I Professional Issues I Physiological Psychology	Behavioral Therapy Tests & Measures/Cognitive Assessment Statistics I Neuropsychological Theory Practicum	Infant & Child Assessment Psychopathology II Statistics II Computer Science Practicum	Practica
SECOND YEAR			
Social Psychology Health Psychology I Neuropsychological Assessment Electives/Practica	Research Design Projective Assessment Electives/Practica	Structured Personality Assessment Research Seminar Electives/Practica	Practica
THIRD YEAR			
Personality & Theories of Psychotherapy Electives/Practica Dissertation Research	History & Systems Professional Issues II Electives/Practica Dissertation Research	Electives/Practica Dissertation Research	
FOURTH YEAR			
Internship/Dissertation	Internship/Dissertation	Internship/Dissertation	Internship/Dissertation

TABLE 30.10 The Ph.D. Program at the University of California—San Francisco: A Health Psychology Specialization

First Quarter	Second Quarter	Third Quarter
	FIRST YEAR	
Social Psychology (4)*	Learning and Cognition (4)	Proseminar in Health Psychology (4)
Personality Psychology (4)*	Research Methods (3)	Statistics of Rates and Proportions (3)
Introduction to Biopsychology (3)*	Applied Regression Analysis and Analysis of Variance B (4)	Introduction to Health Psychology (1)
Applied Regression Analysis and Analysis of Variance A (4)	Introduction to Health Psychology (1)	Electives include:
Introduction to Health Psychology (1)	Electives include:	Research Methods B (3)
Electives include:	Neurophysiological Mechanisms of EEG and Event-Related Potential (3)	Program Evaluation in Health and Other Human Service Organizations (2)
Introduction to the Computer (3)		Cerebral Hemispheric Specialization and Integration (2)
Psychophysiology (2)		Health Transactions (2)
	SECOND YEAR	
Physiological Basis of Health Psychology (4)	The Health System	Research Project and Seminar C (4)
Research Project and Seminar A (4)	Research Project and Seminar B (4)	Electives include:
Electives include:	Electives include:	Communication Skills C (2)
Psychology of Pain (2)	Communication Skills B (2)	Reproductive Behavior (3)
Health Status and Behavior (3)	Psychological Stress and Coping (4)	Stress and Bodily Disease (4)
		Developmental Psychology (3)
	THIRD YEAR	
Individual and tutorial study plus elective courses in preparation for Qualifying Examination and Dissertation Proposal (total 8–12 units per quarter)		
	FOURTH YEAR	
Dissertation	Dissertation	Dissertation

*Students take two of these three courses.

NOTE: Other requirements include: (a) five approved elective courses; (b) students must pass an examination in History and Systems of Psychology by Winter Quarter of the second year.

and the college of arts and sciences. The doctoral degree programs developed at the University of Maryland in College Park leads to a masters or doctor of philosophy degree specializing in "health behavior." The health behavior program was launched in 1980 by psychologists and health educators under the direction of Robert H. L. Feldman, a social psychologist whose postdoctoral training was in health psychology. As summarized in the brochure available to prospective students the Ph.D. program in health behavior reproduced in table 30.11 consists of four components and is offered by the Department of Health Education, an autonomous department within the College of Physical Education, Recreation and Health, which is one of the colleges in the Division of Human and Community Resources of the University of Maryland.

The first component presents a survey of the field of health behavior, including the theories, empirical research findings, and methodologies of psychology, social psychology, sociology, and anthropology as applied to health care. The second component is concerned with training competent researchers in health education—those who can understand, evaluate, and carry out research. The third component emphasizes the professional health educator's role as a provider of service. Finally, the fourth and last component is related to the practical application of these skills and emphasizes the need for supervised practice as a health practitioner.

Ph.D. Degree Program Emphasis in Behavioral Cardiology Research within an Experimental-Physiological Psychology Track at the Oregon Health Sciences University

The psychology faculty in Oregon had been offering since 1958 a masters degree with a track in experimental-physiological psychology to a highly selective group of medical students who added two extra years of study to their curriculum to earn combined M.D.-M.S. degrees in one of the basic sciences. When an autonomous departmental status was established in 1961, the psychology faculty built on this experience and established a Ph.D. program in psychology in 1962 for graduate students with an interest in a research career in general experimental-physiological psychology.

From the inception of this Ph.D. program one of its areas of emphasis within this experimental-physiological psychology track has involved research at the interface between behavior and cardiovascular function. The graduate students in this research area (as well as other graduate students whose track of training emphasized the brain-behavior area or the learning-motivation area) have been supported from 1962 to the present time by fed-

TABLE 30.11 The Ph.D. Program at the University of Maryland: A Health Behavior Specialization within a Department of Health Education

Fall Semester	Spring Semester
FIRST YEAR	
Hlth 665 Health Behavior I (3)	Hlth 666 Health Behavior II (3)
Hlth 720 Scientific Foundations of Health (3)	Hlth 688S Writing for Communication in Health Education (3)
Edms 645 Quantitative Research Methods I (3)	Edms Quantitative Research Methods II (3)
SECOND YEAR	
Hlth 650 Foundations of Health Counseling (3)	Hlth 780 Applied Principles of Health Education (3)
Hlth 775 Health Education Program Planning and Evaluation (3)	Hlth 710 Methods and Techniques of Research (3)
Elective in Advanced Statistics and Computer Usage (3)	Elective (3)
THIRD YEAR	
Hlth 785 Externship in Health Education (3)	Hlth 740 Modern Theories of Health (3)
Electives—6 hours from courses such as:	Electives—6 hours from courses such as:
Hlth 688T Stress and Stress Control (3)	Hlth 688 Biofeedback in the Health Professions (3)
Hlth 750 Stress and Disease (3)	Hlth 688 Research Assistance (3)
Hlth 688 Relaxation Theory and Practice (3)	Hlth 688 Reaching Practicum: "Controlling Stress and Tension" (3)
Hlth 688 Psychological Aspects of Coping with Stress and Tension (3)	Hlth 688 Field Work or Independent Study (1–6)
FOURTH YEAR	
Dissertation Research (6)	Dissertation Research (6)

eral training grants provided variously by NIMH, NIAAA, and NIH. When the present one of these training grants was applied for and received in 1977 this earlier emphasis within our Ph.D. program was labeled a training program in "psychology" with a track of study which emphasized animal models for research in "behavioral cardiology," a term we coined from the zeitgeist. The research Ph.D. program in psychology which the department has offered with this emphasis has evolved considerably, and a summary of its current curricular content is provided in table 30.12.

Most of the graduates of this program either have gone on for further postdoctoral training, joined the faculty of a medical school or university, or became students in medical school to further their educational preparation for a career of clinical research. It is the hope of the faculty providing this training that, after further postdoctoral training, most of the graduates of this program will initiate lines of research on some processes involved in the mechanisms by which physiological, biochemical, and behavioral processes interact to produce normal and pathological functioning in animals and humans.

Discussion

Although *de facto* standardization of curricula may someday occur in health psychology, much as has happened in clinical psychology, this state of affairs is likely far in the future, if one is to judge from the curricula in the tables above. The major specialty-area training of half of these eleven "health psychology" programs described was clinical psychology, while health or medical psychology *per se* accounted for only three of these programs. Among the remaining curricula, health or medical psychology appeared as a minor concentration within the areas of social psychology, biopsychology, and social ecology, respectively.[1] Clearly, there is the potential for as many health psychology "emphasis-within-a-track" programs as there are special areas of training in psychology, since issues of health and illness are potentially germane to any of the traditional content areas of psychology. However, it would seem important for the half of the faculties offering nonclinical health psychology as either a primary area of training or as a minor emphasis within a nonclinical area of psychology to describe clearly the skills their graduates will have upon completion of their programs.

Although there are differences in the "home" specialty of health psychology programs, there do appear to be some basic consistencies among these programs. For instance, it seems clear that in common with other graduate programs in psychology, most of these curricula offer coursework in areas that characterize the foundations of psychology as a scientific and scholarly discipline. Thus, students in these programs generally will experience exposure to coursework and/or practical experience in accord with the 1977 APA Accreditation Guidelines (see chapter 23 by Boll). Also, with differing emphases on specific content areas, most curricula seem to include coursework in the four "core" content areas of biological, cognitive/affective, social, and individual difference foundations of behavior.

---

1. Although these respondents might not be typical of all programs offering training in health psychology, the proportion of clinical and nonclinical respondents is similar to that reported by Belar et al. (1982).

TABLE 30.12 The Ph.D. Program of the Oregon Health Sciences University: An Emphasis on Research Training in Behavioral Cardiology

Fall Quarter	Winter Quarter	Spring Quarter
	FIRST YEAR	
MPs 511 Statistics (3)	MPs 512 Research Design (3)	Phy 410 Human Physiology (7)
MPs 515 Learning & Conditioning (3)	MPs 517 History of Psychology (3)	MPs 518 Physiological Psychology (3)
MPs 514 Sensory Processes (3)	MPs 507 Laboratory Instrumentation	MPs 521 Theories of Learning (3)
MPs 501 Research (3)	Techniques (3)	MPs 501 Research (1)
	MPs 501 Research (3)	
	SECOND YEAR	
MPs 507 Behavior Genetics (3)	Con 412 Cardiovascular	An 412 Neuroanatomy (4)
Phy 517 Advanced Cardiovascular	Pathophysiology (6)	MPs 507 Endocrine & Hemodynamic
Physiology (4)	Phc 607 Pharmacology of Autonomic	Consequences of Stress (3)
MPs 507 Laboratory Computer	Activity (3)	Elective Medical Psychology or Basic
Methods (3)	Elective Medical Psychology or Basic	Sciences (3)
MPs 507 Research (3)	Sciences (3)	MPs 503 Thesis Research (3)
	MPs 503 Thesis Research (3)	
	THIRD YEAR	
MPs 507 Cardiovascular Function &	MPs 507 Cardiovascular	Electives in Medical Psychology or Basic
Disease (3)	Psychophysiology (3)	Sciences (6)
Med 691 Electrocardiography (2)	MPs 507 Behavioral Cardiology	MPs 501 Research
MPs 501 Research (3)	Seminar (3)	
	MPs 501 Research (3)	
	FOURTH YEAR	
Advanced Electives (3–6)	Advanced Electives (3–6)	Advanced Electives (3–6)
MPs 503 Dissertation Research (6)	MPs 503 Dissertation Research	MPs 503 Dissertation Research (6)

Exposure to this common core of psychological knowledge during a student's graduate career would seem to be particularly important for those seeking a career in health psychology. If past trends continue, many of these students will not be employed in a traditional college or university-based department of psychology upon receiving their doctoral degree. Rather, the employment settings of some of these graduates will more likely be at community hospitals, medical schools or health science universities, or any of the broad array of institutions dedicated to research and/or service delivery in behavioral health and behavioral medicine. Psychologists employed in such settings will frequently find themselves one of a small handful of behavioral scientists in their department or institution, and in exceptional cases, may be the sole representative of the profession of psychology. As such, they will lack the reciprocal reinforcement of professional identity that continually occurs in a traditional department of psychology. Thus, an important—and clearly not superficial—function of coursework and professional experience in the content areas that define psychology as an independent scientific discipline is to foster students' identification with psychology in contrast to other scientific or professional disciplines. Also, we should not ignore the fact that the feature of health psychology that unites us—a concern with the applications of psychology to health and illness—rests upon a base of shared knowledge. If we, as health psychologists, are to claim the possession of competencies in either research or clinical practice more directly applicable to health-related issues than those of other psychologists our knowledge of the process of atherosclerosis must be greater than what we might have read in area-specific journals such as *Health Psychology* or *Journal of Behavioral Medicine*. The eleven doctoral programs described in this chapter generally do make an effort to acquaint their students with the academic subject matter in relevant areas of biomedical science and in a broad range of medically-related content areas of psychology (e.g., psychopharmacology, neuropsychology) as well.

Of corresponding importance to the value of any training experience in health psychology is access to appropriate medical care settings and subject/client populations. This point is made in several of the chapters of this volume. In this respect, there are undoubted advantages to being affiliated with schools of medicine, and indeed, four of the eleven programs described above are located exclusively at medical schools (Uniformed Services University of the Health Sciences, Chicago Medical School, University of California—San Francisco, Oregon Health Sciences University). Of the remainder, most apparently have ties with nearby medical schools and other private or public medical institutions. Future reviewers of the history of health psychology no doubt would seriously question the value of any graduate program in health psychology that does *not* maintain such ongoing liaisons.

As is clear from both the content of this chapter and previous discussions of graduate training in health psychology (e.g., Belar, et al. 1982; Matarazzo 1980, 1982, 1983), health psychology curricular offerings remain, in most institutions, a hybrid offshoot of one or another traditional content areas of graduate training. Perhaps this is, at present, a "healthy" state of affairs. We feel that until the job availability for primary interest area training in health psychology is well defined, it would not be useful for our graduate programs nationwide to churn out more Ph.D.s in this nontraditional area than the job market might possibly be able to absorb. Students presently in those few programs currently offering primary interest area training in health psychology will, like it or not, be experimental subjects in a test of the viability of health psychology as a discrete content area of psychology. We wish them well.

References

Belar, C. D., E. Wilson, H. Hughes. 1982. Health psychology training in doctoral psychology programs. *Health Psychology* 1:289–99.

Dwore, R. B., and J. D. Matarazzo. 1981. The behavioral sciences and health education: Disciplines with a compatible interest? *Health Education* 12:4–7.

Matarazzo, J. D. 1980. Behavioral health and behavioral medicine: Frontiers for a new health psychology. *American Psychologist* 82:807–17.

———. 1982. Behavioral health's challenge to academic, scientific, and professional psychology. *American Psychologist* 37:1–14.

———. 1983. Education and training in health psychology: Boulder or bolder? *Health Psychology* 2:73–113.

Stone, G. C. 1979. A specialized doctoral program in health psychology: Considerations in its evolution. *Professional Psychology* 10:596–604.

———. 1981. Training for health systems research and consultation. In *Linking health and mental health*, edited by A. Broskowski, E. Marks, and S. Budman. Beverly Hills, CA: Sage.

Part Seven

Sites for Training Health Psychologists

Editor: Jerome E. Singer

As some of the earlier chapters have indicated, health psychology first took shape in medical settings and in centers of health research. Likewise, the first efforts to establish programs for training health psychologists occurred at these sites. During the first decade of rapid growth, however, psychologists in a variety of settings recognized the potential of this new area of concentration, and training programs began to develop in many different contexts. In this section, those who have played an active role in the programs consider the strengths, weaknesses, and special features of each as a place to train students and fellows in health psychology.

Throughout this book the message that there is no single model of health psychologist against which all trainees should be gauged is reiterated. Correspondingly, there is no single setting that is necessarily best for training all of the different kinds of health psychologists who will be needed. Chapter authors have been asked, therefore, to consider whether their own setting is a place where sound psychological training of some kind can be carried out. Not too surprisingly, each of them gives an affirmative answer to this question. They then consider what special kinds of training within the broader field are well suited to each location and what special pitfalls have to be avoided.

Part 7 begins with a chapter by Judith Rodin and Johanna Freedman that deals with the traditional site of psychological training, the university department of psychology. These authors provide a good framework for the evaluation of any training site and then use it to examine the capabilities of conventional departments. Such departments have usually had many years to develop a resource base, a stable faculty, and tested educational approaches. The first departments venturing into the area of health psychology were limited by the very small number of academic psychologists who recognized the opportunities available in the health system and by the limited access of psychologists to the health system. The authors discuss how such limitations can be overcome.

Levin and Swencionis describe the academic medical center, a complex organizational structure which, they believe, is understood by few persons who are not a part of one. They characterize the differences between the climate of work in this environment and that encountered by students in colleges of letters and science. The pervasiveness of rapidly progressing, richly funded biomedical research and of the urgent problems of patients and others engaged with the health care system can be stimulating and challenging, and it can also tempt students into premature, overly technical specialization. The authors argue that these hazards are best avoided by maintaining strong links with academic colleagues.

An unusual setting in which a strong, clinically oriented health psychology program has developed is described by Nathan Perry. He provides an explanation of the term "allied health professions" and gives an overview of the kinds of educational activities that occur in schools of the allied professions. He outlines the opportunity for autonomous provision of health services that such schools can offer psychology, although he recognizes that relatively few of them enjoy the particular combination of circumstances that has fostered the development of the successful program at the University of Florida.

Some of the most significant impetus to the development of health psychology was provided by a group of psychologists working for the U.S. Public Health Service in the 1950s and 1960s. A number of those psychologists have moved on to positions in schools of public health, from which they have continued to publish the results of their work. When health psychology became more visible, other schools of public health added psychologists to their faculties, and they naturally began to think of training opportunities. Matthews and Siegel exemplify this new generation of public health psychologists. There are, as yet, no predoctoral health psychology training programs based in schools of public health, and these authors do not anticipate that there soon will be. They do believe that their schools can make important contributions to training both pre- and postdoctoral students in public health approaches to health problems.

Another unique program is described by Eagleston and Thoresen. A health psychology curriculum is being established within a seasoned counseling psychology program located in the School of Education at Stanford University. These authors present the argument that one of the major ways of improving health is through counseling that will lead to more adaptive health behaviors and that counseling is essentially an educational activity. Thus they see their program as one that could be widely emulated.

The final chapter in this section discusses a training site that has been the subject of much controversy. The "professional schools of psychology" have been viewed skeptically by many established academic departments of psychology for various reasons. Perhaps the most important of these is that a number of professional schools have been established as freestanding enterprises without affiliation to any other academic organization. But this is not true of all of them. Another source of controversy is that many of the professional schools have abandoned the "Boulder model" of the scientist-practitioner, which continues to be the approved approach for the training of clinicians in the view of much of the psychological establishment. Nelson Jones discusses these issues and describes a number of variations on the basic pattern of the professional school. He argues that professional schools must be acknowledged as a significant component of training in psychology and that they can provide excellent training, including training in health psychology, under appropriate circumstances. The psychological establishment should judge them in terms of the quality of the education they provide individually rather than trying to wish them out of existence.

31

Health Psychology Training in University Departments

Judith Rodin and Johanna Freedman

What constitute the appropriate venues for the training of future health psychologists? The simple fact of posing such a question is noteworthy since traditionally, doctoral training in the field of psychology has taken place in schools of liberal arts and sciences. A relatively recent phenomenon, associated with the growth of more applied fields of psychology, e.g., clinical practice or health care, is the development of alternative training sites such as professional schools or programs in schools for the biomedical science disciplines (e.g., medicine, dentistry, nursing). Now that multiple options for training settings have become available to health psychology, it becomes important to examine the strengths and weaknesses of each, in part so that we provide the best training possible within each particular context. Attempts to evaluate critically these various settings and make recommendations, however, must be done at present without the type of comparative outcome data among alternative venues that we would demand in our research inquiries (Hogan 1979; Koocher 1979; Peterson and Bry 1980; Stern 1984). Let us be clear then at the outset that the views in this chapter are based more on general principles than on specific data and admittedly reflect the biases and values of someone who was trained and trains others in a traditional, university-based department of psychology. The specific task of this chapter will be to comment on the strengths and weaknesses of university-based health psychology training within departments of psychology.

Implicit in the choice of venue are values concerning the identity, function, and responsibilities of health psychologists. A university site for training, and specifically one in a psychology department, emphasizes the field's historic identification with psychology, perhaps to a greater extent than other settings. In other words, it emphasizes the "psychologist" as much or even more than the "health." Health psychology training programs in departments of psychology are tied strongly to the view that the broad knowledge base of psychology is requisite to the training and function of a health psychologist and that such knowledge is best conveyed by experts in each of the major subdisciplines of psychology, e.g., clinical, developmental, social. Most such programs also hold a commitment to the scientist-practitioner model when training clinicians, either in general or in health psychology in particular. Finally, research training within psychology departments aspires to making scientific contributions to the knowledge base of psychology in general, as well as to fields more directly related to physical health and illness (Stone 1979).

The Requirements of a Training Program in Health Psychology

Numerous goals for predoctoral training were articulated at the Arden House Conference (Boll et al. 1983). Many represent requirements for any good psychology program; others are unique to training in health psychology in particular. Since virtually all aspects of psychology are relevant to health psychologists, a broad foundation of training is essential (Ebert-Flatteau 1981; Matarazzo 1983b; Miller 1983; Olbrisch and Sechrest 1979; Peterson 1976a, 1976b). Of utmost importance for any setting wishing to establish a predoctoral training program in health psychology are classroom and experimental training in biopsychosocial aspects of health care and the integration of theory and practice ensured by access to an adequate range of patients, research subjects, and teaching opportunities relevant to health psychology (Asken 1975; APA Task Force on Health Research 1976; Matarazzo 1983a; Schneiderman et al. 1983; Sechrest 1974; Stone 1979).

Because the field is so broad and varied, structured introductory courses in health psychology should be provided which cover the field's intellectual roots, present areas of work, and appropriate research and clinical methods. Such training should provide a strong background in research, both psychological and biostatistical (McNamara 1981), and in application. Training for the health psychology provider should share grounding in the basics of psychology and biostatistics with the researcher and should enable those intending to do clinical work to be sophisticated in evaluating and utilizing research findings (cf. Gentry, Street, Masur, and Asken 1981). The training model assumes that there is synergy between care and research, with research supplying answers to the questions raised by clinical practice and clinical work being informed by research activity (Miller 1983). Because of the goals of health psychology, training should also emphasize and make available, for those who intend to provide service to patients, assessment and intervention skills to promote performance within health care settings, both through interdisciplinary collaboration and through effective care of clients, patients, and their families.

Access to health care settings and study of the special issues relevant to these settings is vital to good training; scientific theory and technique are useless without an adequate understanding of the conditions in which they must be applied (Miller 1983; Stone 1979, 1983). Training should be provided in health care organization and health care policy since health practitioners must be capable of identifying a problem in a given population, deriving its probable cause, and positing solutions to maladaptive behavioral contingencies in the form of preventive interventions (Runyan et al. 1982; McNamara 1981). Students must be made aware of the numerous ethical legal and professional issues involved in the care of medical patients and in the extensive remediation in client life-style that health practitioners must often urge.

The final requirement is a purely pragmatic one—but nonetheless vital—namely, all this must be accomplished within a feasible time limit and courseload, or health psychology may suffer the same break between the real and the ideal as has occurred too often in clinical psychology (Matarazzo 1983b). If the scientist/practitioner model set forth as an ideal at the Arden House meeting is to be realized for health psychology, predoctoral training in both research and praxis must be made more coherent.

It also seems reasonable to specify that a health psychology training program should be administered by a psychologist, including supervision of curriculum development, recruiting and selection of faculty, admission of students, and allocation of the budget. In each program there must be a sufficient number of psychologists with skills and interests in the field of health to represent the profession and implement the curriculum. Ideally the core faculty providing most of the training should be health psychologists who, if they are service providers, represent the scientist/practitioner model and can provide students with a close mentor relationship and adequate practical experience in research, and health-care services when appropriate, under supportive supervision (Schwarz et al. 1983; Stone 1979).

University-based Psychology Programs?

Can the traditional, university-based psychology program, as it stands or in some modified form, fulfill the needs specified above? As long as the doctorate is seen as the entry-level degree of choice for tomorrow's health psychologist, the university-based psychology program remains well suited to provide the training required. Universities are at present the most common sites for the training of the health psychologist and seem likely to remain so in the future (Olbrisch and Sechrest 1979). Ideally such settings are characterized by the autonomy, stability, and resources necessary to establish and maintain a training program (Schwartz et al. 1983).

The advantages of the "multiversity" with its wealth of academic departments and ready access to public and private financial and educational resources seem clear. Still, there are a number of present and potential problems inherent in the university setting that must be identified and ameliorated if universities are to offer optimal training in health psychology and educate scientists and practitioners capable of fulfilling the demands of the profession, i.e., contributing educationally, scientifically, and professionally to the promotion and maintenance of health; the prevention of illness; the identification of etiologic and diagnostic correlates of health, illness, and related dysfunctions; and the analysis and improvement of the health care system and health policy formation (Matarazzo 1980; Schwartz et al. 1983; Schneiderman et al. 1983).

Advantages of University-based Psychology Programs

The advantages of a university-based psychology program seem readily identifiable. These will be discussed briefly below. Since the university-based training program is currently the most common training site for health psychologists, more extensive attention will be paid to the disadvantages of this venue in the section that follows. By specifying the benefits and costs of the traditional department of psychology as a training site, we may make more informed comparative judgments among settings and point to conditions that merit change within university-based programs.

CURRICULUM

Students learning to be health psychologists in traditional university-based psychology programs are viewed as, and therefore trained to be, psychologists. Thus their graduate-level training typically includes comprehensive introductory and advanced coursework in all subspecialties of psychology. They receive extensive training in research methods and data analysis and are supervised by psychologists in their research and clinical activities. Because they are in psychology departments they are exposed to opportunities for continuous cross-fertilization between health psychology and other areas of psychological knowledge and inquiry. Since developmental, social, clinical, and biological psychology all relate to health psychology in numerous important ways, interactions with students and faculty in these areas enlarge and fundamentally inform the training experience of health psychologists. Students interested in health ask questions and frame concepts in ways that reciprocally expand the horizons of their colleagues in psychology's more traditional subspecialties.

Another extremely valuable resource within many psychology departments is the clinical psychology teaching-research clinic. Though not all departments have such clinics, in those that do the clinic can be an excellent setting for health students to gain necessary clinical experience. In addition, as Olbrisch and Sechrest (1979) have pointed out, research-oriented health psychologists often can be helpful in assisting such clinics to plan long-range research programs and data collection procedures.

While adequate support for students' interest in health must come from within the psychology department if they are to maintain their primary identity as psychologists, additional resources provided by a university enrich and insure the inter- and intradisciplinary nature of health psychology training. Medical schools associated with many universities are potential resources which could afford health psychology students in-depth courses in basic and clinical medical sciences, as well as familiarize them with a major health setting and likely future work sites. In addition, medical schools are likely to be able to extend students' ties beyond the school to local private practices and community and public health clinics. The student health services facilities, if available to students, are of enormous value for pilot work in health psychology projects. Anthropology departments might offer a useful cross-cultural perspective since students may be dealing with clients with a variety of ethnic backgrounds; economics courses could extend to the interested student an insight into the burgeoning costs of health care and possible courses of remediation (Schwartz and Weiss 1978). A law school affords the student an understanding of the legal and ethical issues inherent in health care delivery, an area of vital importance to health psychologists since they are more likely than other psychologists to deal with people at a high medical risk (Miller 1983).

STABILITY OF FUNDING

While no schools or programs enjoy the type of resources and financial security that was experienced in the 1960s and early 1970s, university-based psychology programs have typically had a more certain and stable funding base—the university itself—than programs in other training settings. Even medical schools within the same institution have typically relied more on "soft" money, funding more of their programs and faculty salaries as well as research by grant support, compared to psychology departments. This stable funding base in the arts and sciences typically allows for more prospective planning efforts regarding resource allocation, which impacts directly on training.

MOBILITY

When all psychology students are trained together, in a single department with uniform criteria and eligibility requirements, significant latitude is possible for changing one's area of subspecialization within psychology. This might occur while one is still a student or as a reflection of a change in interest or focus later in one's career. Not only does this give a person being trained as a health psychologist increased options and career flexibility, but it provides options to switch fields more readily for students and colleagues from other subspecialties who become interested in health. With adequate additional training, such people, who have extensive knowledge in another area of psychology, will bring important fresh perspectives to the field of health psychology, potentially enriching and expanding the discipline (Matarazzo and Carmody 1983).

Disadvantages of University-based Psychology Programs

DEPARTMENTAL SYSTEM

Departments have been criticized since their inception in American higher education for what Dean Andrew F. West called "the break-up of knowledge into pieces" and what Irving Babbitt put in stronger terms as "the maiming and mutilation of the mind that comes from over-absorption in one subject" (Veysey 1965). Surprisingly few health psychologists are aware of their debt to the fields of medical sociology or psychosocial epidemiology, for example. The theories and methods of both fields have, from the beginning, defined human beings as bio-psycho-social entities, and health psychologists trained in ignorance of this as a consequence of "departmentalism" may be condemned to repeat unknowingly the "discovery" of old findings. As universities grew in size, psychology split from its roots in philosophy and, isolated from departments such as anthropology, sociology, education, and biostatistics (Schwartz and Weiss 1978) with which it shared common interests, became increasingly insular (Matarazzo 1983c). This obviated the sharing of perspectives, a chief value of the university, and increased the possibility that students' choices of research problems would lack perspective and relevance (Smith 1981).

Though set up in part to facilitate teaching and education, departments can act as a constraint on cross-disciplinary work. While psychology departments were useful in developing the discipline, they have too often ossified, demanding that students fulfill irrelevant or obsolete requirements and emphasizing specialization at the expense of generalization and multidisciplinary studies. This situation is especially dangerous for future health psychologists. Their necessarily interdisciplinary training needs will vary widely depending on a number of factors, including their choice of the scientist or professional role, their special area of interest, the environment they will eventually practice in, and the changing requirements of the profession as health psychology evaluates and modifies its goals (Belar, Wilson, and Hughes 1982).

There are many other hazards of the traditional psychology department. In their own research activities members of departments may keep up with scientific change, yet show a tendency toward safe conservatism in pedagogy in the form of opposition to curricular changes, to the introduction of new subspecialties, and to experimentation with new teaching methods. Too often the untenured avoid controversy, and those who are given tenure are either selected in the tenured faculty's own image or are faced with an impermeable network of departmental politics and red tape. Initially departments increased faculty power against administrators, governing boards and forces beyond the campus, but now that it is time to take other initiatives, it is possible that departmentalism may stand in the way (McHenry 1977). Moreover, departmental influence over degree requirements often can have more to do with protecting departmental enrollment than with educational theory. In consequence the reification of departmental boundaries can prevent students from achieving the integrated understanding of their subject so vital for health psychologists.

Location in Colleges of Arts and Sciences

Not all universities include or are near health care settings such as hospitals or dental and medical schools in which students can gain vital training in the various epistemologies and methods used by medicine, epidemiology, public health, and dentistry and become familiar with the social mores, codes, and norms of the various health settings in which they will have to function effectively. Even psychology departments that are geographically proximate to health care settings may not be able to utilize them as training sites, given local competition, lack of appreciation for the potential contribution of the behavioral sciences within medicine, or insufficient funding for training opportunities for health professionals other than physicians, to name only a few reasons. With the limited access to relevant populations provided by many university-based psychology programs, the student may gain insufficient understanding of the populations most relevant to health psychology theory and practice. Such a student might be wholly incapable of either working as an effective clinician in a health care setting or of planning truly fundamental health research outside the immediate university setting.

SOURCES OF FUNDING

Concerns about funding are undoubtedly threatening the autonomy of the academy, despite its relatively more stable funding base. The ideal of the autonomous university cannot be realized without complete financial independence (Hetherington 1965; Cowley 1980) since industry and governmental funding of academic work can create pressure to choose potentially remunerative research, to rush research, to produce "appropriate" results, and can create problems of ownership of resultant data. Society will not let higher education function entirely free of government direction if there is a prospect that its work will affect political, economic, or health-relevant decisions of the day (cf. Price 1971).

At present the locus of power seems to be shifting from inside to outside the university, from the community of scholars to the public domain (Kerr 1964; Dressel and Faricy 1972), from the university's historic position of privilege and immunity to one of responsibility and accountability (Woodward 1974). Since at least 1964 when President Lyndon Johnson first managed to coerce American health scientists and professionals into pursuing fewer theoretical and more applied research and training activities through a shift in financial support, it has been clear that the supposedly value-free objectivity of the research university could all too easily be undermined. Presidents Nixon, Ford, Carter, and Reagan enforced this demand that scientific and teaching institutions refocus their priorities and pay attention to the human and financial cost of health care (Matarazzo 1982). What may be gained in the short term for government in this form of control is initially lost only to the university; subsequent losses may well be to the community as a whole as more and more basic research is left undone.

Fifty years ago, researchers rarely received federal research grants or consulted with businesses. Though their research may have been relatively limited, professors were largely free of extra-academic restraints. Today, most faculty members in the social and health sciences rely heavily on outside funding from government and industry and may adapt their views to official policies, replacing critical analysis with pragmatism. If faculty members depend on outside funds to carry out their research, the subjects they choose to investigate will be influenced by the opportunities available to obtain the necessary resources (Bok 1982). For example, the extensive financing for cardiovascular research and training may have determined the course of more than a few careers (Matarazzo 1980, 1983a; Rothenberg and Matulef 1969; Weiss 1978). What is more, the time spent on monitoring the use of funds and filling out forms to prove they were neither misallocated nor used in violation of federal regulations is virtually incalculable (Bok 1982; Giamatti 1981).

The corporate world is becoming increasingly concerned about maintaining the health of its employees to improve the quality of life and increase productivity and profit (Matarazzo 1980). With the current economic climate of the country, reflected in the federal mandate for reduced federal spending, it seems likely that health psychologists will be forced to turn to the private sector (business and industry) for financial support (Matarazzo and Carmody 1983; Matarazzo 1980). Such support may in some instances force health psychologists to turn from certain areas of interest to those that are more pragmatic and immediately applicable.

While the problems just discussed are not unique to university-based psychology departments, they represent the weakness of a training structure based in any part on funding by sources outside the university. Such funding strategies can also injure students. Restrictions tied to funds may tendentiously affect admissions. Affirmative action programs for the population of the funder's choice could replace other presumably more objective and fair reasons for acceptance. Less obviously, large grants need large staffs, and it is possible that too many students could be accepted with a view to their use as research assistants but no thought as to their future if too many Ph.D.'s glut the market. Finally, students could be pushed to work on problems of little intrinsic interest to them, simply to fulfill the faculty's research obligations.

Conclusions

There are many difficulties with the university-based psychology department as a training site. Some are simply inherent in the structure of a university and would be discounted as the fixed cost of education. Yet these flaws may have more serious ramifications for health-oriented psychologists and are potentially more evitable, since health training programs are not entrenched at present. Can this multiplicity of problems be alleviated? Can the utility of university-based programs be adequately enhanced? We believe that the answer to both questions is yes. Clearly, universities are not ideal. Yet many of the disadvantages are shared by other training sites. Regardless of setting, now that health psychology has defined a shared training agenda at the Arden House meeting (Boll et al. 1983), it will be essential for all training sites to streamline their requirements to achieve these goals, giving students more coherent, less global programs which are better suited to appropriate training and more feasible in the long run.

One problem that must be resolved to enhance the effectiveness of university-based training in psychology departments is that of communication across disciplinary boundaries. It seems commonly recognized to the point of cliche that such communication is vital to the survival and expansion of understanding and practical skills among all areas touched on by health psychology. While only slightly more than half the programs offering health psychology training in psychology doctoral training programs at present have interdisciplinary faculty, many more offer such contact as an option should the student choose it (Belar 1979; Belar and Tavel 1982; Belar, Wilson, and Hughes 1982; Stone 1979). In addition, if channels of communication are opened interdepartmentally through shared students, it seems plausible that faculty will discover shared interests and goals, thereby forwarding the present cause of health psychology as well as the training of its future scientist/practitioners (Matarazzo and Carmody 1983; Matarazzo, Carmody, and Gentry 1981). Dwore and Matarazzo (1981) have suggested health educators can benefit from interchanges of perspective through visiting faculty exchanges, team-taught classes and seminars on the same campus, and interdisciplinary research and service projects.

Sources of funding are a deeper problem, but again, not one limited to university-based psychology programs. Funding agencies will continue to finance whom and what they choose, and while universities may try to set aside money for "unsalable" research and training, it is unlikely they will be able to do so in sufficient quantity. In short, to quote Bok (1982) "we must reluctantly accept the fact that as the research university has grown in influence, a measure of scholarly independence has been lost." Of all of the possible training settings, however, the university-based psychology department may be the one most likely to nurture and promote basic research and scholarly activity, a background that is essential for training both research scientists and practitioners of health psychology. It is this commitment to psychology as both an academic and clinical science that has been a fundamental characteristic of the large number of psychology programs that train health psychologists.

REFERENCES

APA Task Force on Health Research. 1976. Contributions of psychology to health research: Patterns, problems, potentials. *American Psychologist* 31:263–74.

Asken, M. 1975. Medical psychology: Psychology's neglected child. *Professional Psychology* 6:155–60.

Belar, C. D. 1979. Training the clinical psychology student in behavioral medicine. *Professional Psychology* 10:596–604.

Belar, C. D., and E. Tavel. 1982. Health psychology training in psychology doctoral programs. Surveyed by the Education and Training Committee, Division 38, American Psychological Association.

Belar, C. D., E. Wilson, and H. Hughes. 1982. Health psychology training in doctoral psychology programs. 1(3): 289–301.

Bok, D. 1982. *Beyond the ivory tower.* Cambridge: Harvard University Press.

Boll, T., C. Thoreson, N. Adler, J. Hall, T. Millon, D. Moore, M. E. Olbrisch, N. Perry, L. Weiss, J. Woodring, and C. Wortman. 1983. Working group on predoctoral education/doctoral training. *Health Psychology* 2(5): 123–30.

Cowley, W. H. 1980. *Presidents, professors, and trustees: The evolution of American academic government.* San Francisco: Jossey-Bass.

Dressel, P. L., and W. H. Faricy. 1972. *Return to responsibility: Constraints on autonomy in higher education.* San Francisco: Jossey-Bass.

Dwore, R. B., and J. D. Matarazzo. 1981. The behavioral sciences and health education: Disciplines with a compatible interest? *Health Education* 12:4–7.

Ebert-Flatteau, P. ed. 1981. The workshop of establishing research training programs in behavior and health. Proceedings of the Workshop Establishing Research Training Programs in Behavior and Health. National Research Council, Commission on Human Resources, Washington, D. C.

Gentry, W. D., W. J. Street, F. T. Masur, and M. J. Asken. 1981. Training in medical psychology: A survey of graduate and internship training programs. *Professional Psychology* 12(2): 224–28.

Giamatti, A. B. 1981. *The university and the public interest.* New York: Atheneum.

Hetherington, H. 1965. *University autonomy: Its meaning today.* Paper no. 4. Paris: International Association of Universities.

Hogan, D. B. 1979. *The regulation of psychotherapists.* Vol. 1 of *A study in the philosophy and practice of professional regulation.* Cambridge, MA: Ballinger.

Kerr, C. 1964. *The uses of the university.* Cambridge: Harvard University Press.

Koocher, G. P. 1979. Credentialling in psychology: Close encounters with competence. *American Psychologist* 34:696–702.

Matarazzo, J. D. 1980. Behavioral health and behavioral medicine: *Frontiers for a new health psychology. American Psychologist* 35(9): 807–17.

———. 1982. Behavioral health's challenge to academic, scientific and professional psychology. *American Psychologist* 37(1): 1–14.

———. 1983a. Biobehavioral resources, manpower, and training programs. In *Behavior and arteriosclerosis,* edited by A. J. Herd. New York: Plenum.

———. 1983b. Education and training in health psychology: Boulder or bolder? *Health Psychology* 2(1): 73–113.

———. 1983c. Behavioral immunogens and pathogens: Psychology's newest challenge. *Professional Psychology: Research and Practice* 14:414–16.

Matarazzo, J. D., and T. P. Carmody. 1983. Health psychology. In *The clinical psychology handbook,* edited by M. Hersen, A. E. Kazdin, and A. S. Bellack, 657–82. New York: Pergamon Press.

Matarazzo, J. D., T. P. Carmody, and W. D. Gentry. 1981. Psychologists on the faculties of the United States schools of medicine: Past, present, and possible future. *Clinical Psychology Review* 1:293–317.

McHenry, D. E. 1977. *Academic Departments.* San Francisco: Jossey-Bass.

McNamara, J. R. 1981. Some unresolved challenges facing psychology's entrance into the health care field. *Professional Psychology* 12(3): 391–99.

Meltzoff, J. 1984. Research training for clinical psychologists: Point-counterpoint. *Professional Psychology* 15(2): 203–9.

Miller, N. E. 1983. Some main themes and highlights of the conference. *Health Psychology* 2(5): 11–14.

Olbrisch, M. E., and L. Sechrest. 1979. Educating health psychologists in traditional graduate training programs. *Professional Psychology* 10:589–95.

Peterson, D. R. 1976a. Is psychology a profession? *American Psychologist* 31: 572–81.

———. 1976b. Need for the Doctor of Psychology degree in professional psychologists. *American Psychologist* 31:792–93.

Peterson, D. R., and B. H. Bry. 1980. Dimensions of perceived competence in professional psychology. *Professional Psychology* 11:965–71.

Price, D. K. 1971. Purists and politicians. In *In defense of academic freedom,* edited by S. Hook. Indianapolis: Pegasus, Bobbs-Merrill.

Rothenberg, P. J., and N. J. Matulef. 1969. Toward professional training: A special report from the national council on graduate education in psychology. *Professional Psychology* 1(1): 32–37.

Runyan, C. W., R. F. DeVellis, B. M. DeVellis, and G. M. Hochbaum. 1982. Health psychology and the public health perspective: In search of the pump handle. *Health Psychology* 1(2): 169–80.

Schneiderman, T., T. Baker, J. Borysenko, J. Matarazzo, B. Strickland, and C. Wortman. 1983. Task group on basic research. *Health Psychology* 2(5): 67–71, supplement section.

Schofield, W. 1979. The clinical psychologist as a health professional. In *Health psychology,* edited by G. C. Stone, F. Cohen, and N. E. Adler. San Francisco: Jossey-Bass.

Schwartz, G. E., and S. M. Weiss. 1978. Yale conference on behavioral medicine: A proposed definition and statement of goals. *Journal of Behavioral Medicine* 1:3–12.

Schwartz, G., C. Wortman, J. A. Best, J. Polascovicovich, J. Borysenko, R. Faden, M. Follick, W. Fordyce, N. Jones, N. Perry, D. Russo, N. Schneiderman, J. Singer, C. Swencionis, C. Thoresen, L. Temoshok, and J. Woodring. 1983. Task group on training venues. *Health Psychology* 2(5): 110–13, supplement section.

Sechrest, L. 1974. Training psychologists for health research. *APA Task Force on Health Research Newsletter* 1:1–6.

Smith, A. F. 1981. Graduate education and law. Unpublished manuscript. State University of New York, Binghamton.

Stern, S. 1984. Professional training and professional competence: A critique of current thinking. *Professional Psychology: Research and Practice* 2:230–43.

Stone, G. C. 1979. A specialized doctoral program in health psychology: Considerations in its evolution. *Professional Psychology* 10:596–604.

———. 1983. Summary of recommendations. *Health Psychology* 2(5): 15–18, supplement section.

Veysey, L. R. 1965. *The emergence of the American university*. Chicago: University of Chicago Press.

Weiss, S. M. 1978. News and developments in behavioral medicine. *Journal of Behavioral Medicine* 1:135–39.

Wiens, A. N. 1979. Dentist professional: The appropriate training model for the mainstream of clinical psychology. *Professional Psychology* 1(1): 38–42.

Woodward, C. V. 1974. Erosion of academic privileges and immunities. *Daedalus* 103:33–37.

32
Training Health Psychologists in the Academic Medical Center

Gilbert Levin and Charles Swencionis

The academic medical center provides a dynamic setting for graduate education in health psychology, one rich in both opportunities and hazards. Because of its unusual nature and history the academic medical center is not
widely understood. This stems from the fact that the majority of the centers
do not have a formal independent corporate identity. Most do not have a
strong chief executive officer. Many have hyphenated names. They are really
coalitions of apparently separate medical schools and hospitals that have
evolved into a genuinely, and by all odds permanent, symbiotic relationship.
Many people who work in the centers, including psychologists, are only
faintly aware that they are part of a center since their personal identification
may not extend beyond that of the school or the hospital or even a department or still smaller unit. This myopic condition was probably harmless
during the recent extended period of expansion in the health care world. Today's circumstances require a broader vision. Several recent publications
provide a vivid picture of this institution and its current crisis, the outcome
of which is certain to affect the development of health psychology training
(Rogers 1978; Association of Academic Health Centers 1980; Lewis and
Sheps 1983).

There are today more than one hundred academic medical centers spread
throughout the country, many of them concentrated in major metropolitan
centers. There are seven in New York and five in Philadelphia. Some of the
centers spend as much as a quarter of a billion dollars annually. Many are
the largest employers in their communities. Taken together, the centers spent
a total of $43 billion in 1979, fully twenty percent of all public and private
health expenditures for that year (Lewis and Sheps 1983, chap. 5). Even
these impressive statistics do not tell the whole story of the centers' power
and influence as it is exerted through secondary hospital affiliates and as a
result of the centers' role as pace setter and model in the development and
dissemination of technological innovation.

An academic medical center consists of a medical school, its principal teaching hospital or hospitals, and often other affiliated hospitals as well. These medical centers evolved from the need for clinical teaching sites for medical students, a requirement of the reforms set in motion by Abraham Flexner's watershed 1910 critique of American medical education (Flexner 1925). The bond between medical school and hospital gave society better trained physicians and had the added benefit of providing quality health services for citizens who could not afford private health care. Fostered by various societal developments over the years, the medical center has broadened considerably; its size, its complexity, and its influence have all increased. Its period of greatest expansion occurred in the 1950s and 1960s largely as a consequence of the generous infusion of federal funds to support biomedical research, medical education, and hospital construction. Research funds also helped to defray the cost of medical education. Medical education, research, and patient care have traditionally been regarded as the three goals of the academic medical center and are often seen as inextricably intertwined. Delivery of health services to the local community, in many cases a disadvantaged local community, would be added to the trinity by some advocates. The academic medical center is an American invention and it has been a productive one, especially as regards the development of biomedical knowledge and its translation into technologically sophisticated specialty practice.

In some fashion and to some degree virtually every health psychology training program relates to an academic medical center. A program that is solidly grounded in a school of arts and sciences may limit its involvement to the informal placement of individual students around a specific project, which may have been initiated by the student. Programs located in public health schools or schools of allied health are likely to have a deeper involvement. A few programs are fully integrated into the medical center, as is the case with the Einstein/Ferkauf program, which is a formal collaboration between a graduate psychology department and a medical school department of epidemiology and social medicine. Programs with the greatest level of involvement are positioned to make maximum use of the centers' extraordinarily rich resources. They are also maximally subject to influence from a variety of desired and undesired forces within the medical center and from its organizational culture.

Professional Socialization in the Academic Medical Center

Those of us who are responsible for graduate training programs devote a lot of time and effort to planning and carrying out the formal curriculum. At the same time we are aware that the informal curriculum, that is the opportunities and constraints inherent in the training environment, play a large, perhaps decisive role in shaping our students' identities and careers.

A graduate student trained primarily in a medical center automatically learns the language of the medical center and assimilates elements of its culture into his or her professional identity. This occurs spontaneously as the student attends classes together with medical students or other health care trainees, sits in at case conferences, or participates in ward and clinic life in different medical specialties. A student socialized in this way develops an understanding of and a feel for the politics, the ideals, and the manners and mores of the medical center that can be acquired only with great difficulty by one who grew up professionally outside of this setting.

The socialization process continues as the student assumes the role of apprentice by entering into an internship or fellowship. The trainee then may find generous offers of resources in support of the shared goals of the health team into which the trainee has become integrated. But in dreams begin responsibilities and the trainees may be expected to help bring in funds to support their own efforts as well. The atmosphere of the medical center differs sharply from that of the academic psychology department or other applied settings. There is more money in the medical center, most often soft money and therefore great uncertainty and an air of speed and urgency, of rapid accomplishment, a sense that the next grant is just around the corner.

The professional identity of the next generation of health psychologists will include elements that mirror the aspirations, tensions, achievements, and failures of today's academic medical center. The medical center will provide a context for large contributions and satisfactions, but at the price of strenuous effort, more than a little stress, and some disappointment.

Research and Service Opportunities

The academic medical center offers the trainee a wide variety of research opportunities and improved chances to apply such areas as social, personality, and physiological psychology than was the case previously when psychologists concentrated on problems of mental health and illness. With a wealth of patients, equipment, laboratories, skilled colleagues and other resources, the potential to help patients and discover better ways of helping them clearly exists. This is not the "psychology of the college sophomore." It is an opportunity to use psychological knowledge and skills to better understand and to help solve some of society's problems.

The prevailing values in the academic medical center favor research and encourage faculty in all specialties and at all levels to engage in it. However, medical education does not usually prepare physicians to conduct research, especially research involving human subjects. The health psychology graduate student and his or her psychologist mentor is thus likely to encounter no shortage of physicians interested in research collaboration and able to bring important intellectual and practical resources to the venture. This potential for collaboration is one of the factors that make the center so attractive as a setting for health psychology research and research training.

The medical center is equally rich in opportunities for learning about the process of providing personal health services to patients and the vast majority of trainees—medical students, resident physicians, nursing students, social work students, clinical psychology interns and others—are in the medical center to do just that.

The presence of patients in need together with trainees and professionals in various disciplines striving to meet these needs can create pressures on health psychology students to participate in the treatment process beyond the level that their graduate program has prepared them for. This challenges those responsible for health psychology training programs to carefully define the extent and the limits of the service role of the health psychology graduate student, to provide close supervision, and to communicate with their colleagues in other disciplines. The other members of the health team are unlikely to be able to make fine distinctions between types and kinds of psychologists without guidance from psychologists themselves. Obviously no consensus now exists in the profession as to the proper extent and limits of graduate training in patient service skills—this is a tension that we are likely to have to endure for some time to come.

Academic Standards

Training in service skills is only an aspect of the larger issue of the maintenance of academic standards. How, in the high-pressured, somewhat opportunistic world we have described with all of its uncertainty and its emphasis on solving problems immediately, is it possible to assure that students will acquire the skills and attitudes required to conduct research that measures up to the highest scientific standards?

This is a valid source of concern and only time will tell if it can be addressed adequately. The means available to assure quality are to apply the same standards in evaluating graduate student research in the medical center that are applied to research conducted in other settings and to make sure that the right psychologists are involved in the right components of the curriculum.

Psychologists working in the academic medical center are the right people to teach the specifics of psychological factors in aging, heart disease, cancer, or other specific and technical topics. They are often the wrong people to teach basic psychological topics. Students frequently learn by imitation and tend to focus prematurely on the technical aspects of a disease, avoiding consideration of the psychological processes and theoretical issues involved. This difficulty can be ameliorated if a graduate psychology department is involved in the training. Without some ties to a graduate school or another part of a university where academic values are represented, a program based at a medical center would be vulnerable to pressures to produce technicians rather than applied scientists.

The Current Scene

The academic medical centers are now going through a period of severe criticism from many quarters, including health consumer interests, local communities, the general public, their own faculties, their parent universities and, most importantly, the federal government. David Rogers, president of the Johnson Foundation and a former academic medical center director, describes the center as "a stressed American institution" and calls attention to a growing confrontation between the centers and the government, one that will benefit neither side (Rogers and Blendon 1978; Rogers 1978). The government sees the centers as spending too much money and failing to provide, and to train medical students to provide, the primary care services that today's health care needs require. Medical center faculty and administration resent governmental meddling in the centers' affairs and the progressive tightening of the flow of funds upon which the centers have grown dependent.

Whatever the outcome of the confrontation, the relationship between the government and the medical centers has transformed the health care world, and the influence of both parties is such that they are now the two dominant organized forces within the health system and are likely to remain so in the future (Lewis and Sheps 1983). The current pressures of government are almost entirely aimed at cost containment, leading the centers to provide ever increasing amounts of fee-for-service medical practice in what they see as the best means available for their financial survival. Unfortunately, the actual effects of the government's actions are proving to be quite different from those intended. The government's actions greatly hinder the centers in their efforts to govern themselves effectively, to teach, to do research, and to perform community service. At the same time the government's actions actually *increase* the nation's total health care bill. This is so because the cost of rendering service at an academic medical center inevitably far exceeds the cost of service provided through any other mechanism.

Health psychology is taking shape as a discipline and a profession at a crucial moment in the history of the academic medical center. Its role in the centers' evolution is in the process of being defined. The nature of that role will ultimately be determined by forces both within and outside of psychology. What the public and the government want from the health care system and its medical centers is a kind and quality of care that psychologists seem increasingly willing and able to help provide. Psychologists have only recently joined the ongoing public dialogue on national health policy and, like other interested parties, could affect the outcome of the debate. At the very least, such participation improves the prospects that the potential contributions of psychology will be heard in future rounds of health legislation. This appears to be one of those happy occasions when a set of narrow discipline interests are in simple harmony with those of the nation. However, any influence that psychology exerts is sure to be met by pressures to modify its own priorities to better meet national needs.

REFERENCES

Association of Academic Health Centers. 1980. *Organization and governance of academic health centers,* vols. 1–4. Washington, D.C.

Flexner, Abraham. 1925. *Medical education: A comparative study.* New York: Macmillan.

Lewis, Irving J., and Cecil G. Sheps. 1983. *The sick citadel: The American academic medical center and the public interest.* Cambridge, MA: Oelgeschlager, Gunn & Hain.

Rogers, David E. 1978. *American medicine.* Cambridge: Ballinger.

Rogers, David E., and Robert Blendon. 1978. The academic medical center: A stressed American institution. *New England Journal of Medicine* 298 : 940–50.

33
Schools of the Allied Health Professions

Nathan Perry

There is currently only one academic department of psychology located within a college or school of allied health. The Department of Clinical Psychology which awards the Ph.D. in clinical psychology at the University of Florida is one of ten departments in the College of Health Related Professions. The college in turn is one of six in an academic health center. There are many advantages in being located in the college and in an academic health center for training in clinical psychology with a major focus in health. A primary one, other than proximity to academic medicine and access to medical patients is that the basic purpose of the department is to produce psychologists. Before discussing the advantages and implications of such a location for a psychology department, and particularly a psychology department with a major emphasis in training in health psychology, it will be helpful to first discuss education and training in allied health in general. The term "allied health" ordinarily refers to those occupations and professions which either provide health services or promote health. The list of such occupations and professions is very large (more than 150), and the levels or ranges of training required for the different occupations are great.

There are currently more than sixty schools or colleges of allied health, with medical technology representing the largest single profession being trained. The programs offered vary greatly. Colleges with six or seven programs are among the largest. Virtually all of the allied health professions have been created since the turn of the century and, in fact, the majority within the last three decades. Most originated as training programs within hospitals and medical departments and such venues are still common for many.

There are two major organizations which represent allied health. The Committee on Allied Health Education and Accreditation (CAHEA) is a joint program with the American Medical Association and helps formulate standards for the accreditation of professionals in occupational therapy, medical technology, physical therapy, medical record administration, along with radiology technologists, cytotechnologists, respiratory therapists, among others. CAHEA was formed in the 1930s. The other association is the American Society of Allied Health Professions (ASAHP). The latter association was formed in 1958 to concentrate primarily on collegiate higher education. Most psychologists, and I suspect even most health psychologists, are unaware of either of these associations, and the APA has no liaison with either.

In 1977, the Kellogg Foundation sponsored the National Commission on Allied Health Education which was charged with the task of making recommendations for the next decade in allied health education. Chapter four of the commission report, "Scope and Diversity of Allied Health Education" (Dickey 1980, 66–128), does not once mention psychology. Elsewhere the commission does briefly acknowledge the possibility of including clinical psychology as an allied health profession since it is recognized as such in federal legislation. In another place, however, the report also locates psychology with those professions that are related to allied health. "In developing the questionnaire for the survey mentioned previously, the staff compiled a list of all the occupational titles included in the ASHAP Glossary—adding physicians, dentists, psychologists, nurses, and other occupations . . ." (p. 27). The professions or occupations ordinarily considered "allied health" have varied some with the times but have never been as inclusive as the label implies. For example, nursing has at times been characterized as part of allied health and at other times not. Currently, nursing is not. Medicine and other advanced degree professions have never been associated with or considered part of "allied health." The inclusion of psychology with primarily bachelor-level programs creates a minor disadvantage which will be discussed later.

Between 1965 and 1974, the federal government was extremely active in promoting an increase in absolute numbers of all health occupations and professions. The first such legislation specifically recognizing allied health was the Allied Health Professional Personnel Training Act which was passed in 1966. The definitions of what constituted allied health personnel changed with subsequent acts, apparently depending on what group Congress was trying to provide funds for. The initial legislative intent to increase numbers of health and allied health personnel has shifted to concerns with specific target populations and problems of maldistribution and cost containment. The shift in support goals did not produce any substantial change in the definitions of fields.

Section 787 of the Public Health Act authorizes the Secretary of Health Resources and Services to make grants to schools of medicine, osteopathy, public health, dentistry, veterinary medicine, optometry, pharmacy, podiatry, and allied health. Twenty-seven occupations/professions are listed in that act under allied health professions. Psychologists may be surprised to learn that one of these is clinical psychology. In fact, clinical psychology is the only field listed at the doctoral level. At the masters level are speech pathologists and audiologists. At the associate degree level are clinical dietetic technicians, cytotechnologists, and dental assistants. The remaining twenty-two occupations are at the baccalaureate level of training. Thomas D. Hatch of the Bureau of Health Professions recently stated that "I am not sure that clinical psychologists have always been particularly happy about being identified as an 'allied health' profession" (VandenBos and Batchelor 1983, 1363). I would suspect that very few psychologists are even aware of such a possible identity. Awareness aside, it would seem desirable for psychology to be recognized legislatively as an allied health profession, particularly when the intent is to support manpower needs.

However, it might be more sound from an educational viewpoint to consider issues raised by such an identity independent of federal or other funding sources. If psychology (and health psychology in particular) were an allied health profession in terms of training venue and practice, what kinds of consequences would result? As noted earlier, there is currently only one doctoral degree program in psychology at an allied health school, but the history and present status of that program does allow some rough generalizations or speculations.

In 1958, the College of Health Related Professions joined the colleges of medicine, nursing, and pharmacy in the J. Hillis Miller Health Center at the University of Florida. Colleges of veterinary medicine and dentistry have since been added. The health center was designed and started so that multiple fields could share common resources and engage in interdisciplinary collaboration and this was the basis for forming the new college. At the time, such an academic health center *was not common* and of those that existed, none had a school or college of health related professions. Subsequently established schools or colleges adopted the title of "allied health" rather than "health related" but were very similar in structure to the first one at Florida.

However, the College of Health Related Professions at Florida included a component that was not included in any of the subsequently developed colleges—a psychology service. The psychology service resulted from the collaboration of the Deans of Medicine and Health Related Professions (George Harrel and Darrel Mase, respectively) and Chairs of Psychiatry and Psychology in the College of Arts and Sciences (Peter Regan and Wilse Webb, respectively). The unit was to provide a service to psychiatry and a training setting for clinical psychology students. The psychology service became the psychology clinic within the Department of Clinical Psychology in Health Related Professions which was created in 1961, and the first department chair (Louis Cohen) was simultaneously the Director of Clinical Training in Psychology in Arts and Sciences. Since 1977, the Ph.D. in clinical psychology has been awarded from the Department of Clinical Psychology rather than from the Department of Psychology in Arts and Sciences. In retrospect, the location of a psychology service system outside of a department of psychiatry or a college of medicine within a large academic health center was much more significant than its specific location within a college of health related professions.

Independence from medicine in the health center meant that the department had all of the advantages for health psychology of proximity to other health disciplines and patients of those departments and divisions of psychology within medicine. More importantly, psychology could set its own educational goals and had control of the programs and resources leading to those goals. Thus, budgets were (and are) developed and defended solely on the basis of what was needed to educate and train psychologists. While such budgets are common in traditional academic psychology departments, they are unheard of in medical settings, even academic medical settings. Colleges of medicine may have many departments with Ph.D. programs, but the primary mission of those departments is to serve the educational needs of the medical students and residents. Similarly, a psychiatry department may have a division of psychology which engages in the training of psychologists, but the higher priority of the department for training by that division would be for psychiatry residents and fellows if there were any problems in obtaining or allocating resources. Of course, a secondary priority, while less desirable does not necessarily mean inadequate training for psychologists.

At the university, the primacy of psychology training in an academic health center and its hospitals has continued and broadened through the addition of the department's Ph.D., internship, and postdoctoral programs. The Ph.D. program in clinical psychology was accredited by the APA in 1953 and the general clinical psychology internship program was accredited in 1963. Training in health psychology (both applied and research) in all of the department programs evolved over the past twenty years based on faculty interests and philosophies, available resources, and societal needs. Health psychology training has become more programmatic or structured with the addition of tracks or minors within the Ph.D. and internship programs in clinical psychology with adult and child emphases. The tracks are medical psychology, pediatric psychology, and neuropsychology. Postdoctoral fellows are in their respective areas full-time.

Thus, all basic educational goals of the department involve training psychologists only and its resources are devoted to this goal. There are no requirements, other than those expected from simple courtesy or collegiality and mutual interests, for the department and its faculty to participate in the educational goals of the College of Medicine or other colleges in the center. There are a wide variety of relationships between students, residents, fellows, and faculty of the department with other health center units, but because all of these must meet a need of psychologists or psychology, they are reciprocal and truly collaborative. For example, there are fourteen physicians who are jointly appointed in the department in recognition of their much more than courtesy contribution to the department. In terms of psychology, it should be noted that only four of the fourteen physicians are psychiatrists.

The formal or administrative independence of the Department of Clinical Psychology, while designed to facilitate training clinical psychologists, also led directly to the development of health psychology within the department and in its various programs. The department and its clinics served initially (and today) as a "mental health" resource to the clinical medicine departments and particularly to psychiatry. From the beginning, however, the department also served as what has now come to be called a health psychology resource. That is, consultations and referrals were received from throughout medicine for problems that would not then or now be defined as "mental health" and there was collaborative research involving medical patients and psychological variables. Originally, the majority of the requests did involve applied or research questions regarding mental health, but today such requests are few relative to health psychology requests.

The shift has been marked and steady. It could be argued that it was greatly facilitated by the independence of the clinical psychology program from psychiatry. Then and now, a typical pediatrician is likely to think of psychiatry when confronted with a psychotic child but not when a child with cancer becomes upset and resistant to repeated spinal taps. Now, a large, visible, and directly accessible psychology clinic is likely to be thought of by that typical pediatrician with the latter patient. This perception has resulted from the offering of consultation, direct patient treatment, and support and education of staff and faculty for over twenty-five years. The educational advantages for health psychology, cited for administrative independence of the training programs from medicine and psychiatry, are not specific to locations within allied health but are specific to location in an academic health center. A psychology department with a primary goal of educating psychologists could theoretically be established in any college, including medicine, within an academic health center. In fact, given the breadth of psychology, a school or college of psychology within an academic health center is feasible.

What are the disadvantages or problems of psychology training with allied health? The problems created within the college are the most visible but also perhaps the greatest. Whereas, the term allied health is indeed broad, a doctoral psychology program will be extremely unusual in a college of allied health, even if the college is considered to have a wide or heterogenous range of programs. As a consequence, a disadvantage is the need for greater education about psychology within the college, and particularly for research at the doctoral level, than within a traditional arts and science college. The clinical psychology Ph.D. program at Florida is a strong advocate of the scientist-practitioner model and the combination of professional training with graduate school matriculation under that model of training is unique. It is poorly understood by many outside of psychology (or even perhaps some within it). For many programs in allied health, the bachelor's degree is the terminal and entry-level degree, so research is not a component that allied health schools in general must consider. This means that acceptance of the research demands and requirements of a doctoral program and graduate faculty must be taught to the college. Conversely, unlike the situation of clinical programs in traditional colleges of liberal arts and/or science, the necessity and requirements for clinical training is well understood and accepted. The anomalous nature of a psychology program will be even greater if, as is true at Florida, the program has no undergraduate programs or responsibilities, which is the training level of most of the other departments in the college. The Florida program does have undergraduate psychology honors students engaged in health-related research projects with the faculty.

The perceptions of psychology by colleges in the academic health center and the university outside of allied health are, of course, difficult to determine, as are problems created by those perceptions. Those who view applied psychologists as technically skilled people carrying out physicians' orders or as subordinate members of a "team" would presumably have those views reinforced by seeing psychology located within allied health. This has not happened to an apparent extent at Florida, in part because of the wide confusion over what "allied health" means. Thus, a complex and rapidly changing discipline and profession like ours within allied health apparently has fewer rather than more stereotypes to correct. A large part of what a faculty member must do when pursuing "health psychology" is to educate physicians and others about the presence of a health psychology resource and the nature and limits of that resource. This type of education seems to be relatively independent of the administrative location of psychology.

Also, regardless of location, a clinical psychology Ph.D. program in an academic health center must have, either within the program or available to the program, a broad resource in the general content of psychology, comparable to a large graduate department, and broad content in statistics. At Florida we have been fortunate to have the basic psychology and statistics needs met by the Departments of Psychology and of Statistics in the College of Arts and Sciences. It is unlikely that these resources could be made available or developed within a psychology department in a school of allied health.

I believe that success of the clinical psychology program at the University of Florida clearly demonstrates that a location in allied health can work well indeed. It is assumed that this successful outcome cannot be attributed solely to the administrative structure, and the uniqueness of the structure at Florida makes isolation of the effect of the structure *per se* even more difficult. It does seem that the structure has helped in attracting very able faculty and facilitated their many and varied contributions to health psychology. Also, despite the apparent success of psychology training in allied health at Florida, there are apparently no plans to establish a similar program in any of the more than sixty other colleges or schools of allied health.

A presumptive speculation is that the administrative structure that would offer the greatest advantages to training in health psychology would be a college of psychology as one of several in an academic health center. Such a college would encompass all of the substantive experimental and applied areas of psychology as departments or as divisions of departments. A college would have all of the advantages cited earlier for an independent department and more, but would also allow all of psychology's strengths to be brought to bear on health in an integrated and programmatic manner. This extensive emphasis of a college could be expressed whether there were a separate department of health psychology or not. I personally believe that health psychology is too young for such a designation. It should also be noted that while such a college would represent an ideal for training in health psychology, training in all other areas could be comparable to that now found in large divisions of large departments located in Arts and Sciences or other wholly academic colleges.

REFERENCES

Dickey, F. G. 1980. National Commission on Allied Health Education. *The Future of Allied Health Education*. San Francisco: Jossey-Bass.

VandenBos, G. R., and W. F. Batchelor. 1983. Health personnel requirements, service delivery, and national policy: A conversation with Thomas D. Hatch. *American Psychologist* 38:1363.

34

Training Health Psychologists in Schools of Public Health

Karen A. Matthews and Judith M. Siegel

Schools of public health train professionals to prevent disease and promote health. These goals are accomplished through organized community effort, education of individual citizens, development of health services, and basic and applied research in such diverse areas as risk factors for disease, basic pathogenic processes, intervention and prevention strategies, and health economics. Health psychologists clearly have training and knowledge applicable to these public health efforts, but the emphasis in psychology programs differs substantially from the emphasis in schools of public health. The present chapter focuses on the unique benefits that can be gained from exposure to the public health emphasis through training health psychologists in schools of public health. It begins by discussing what these unique benefits can be, followed by a practical consideration of how to obtain these benefits. The final section discusses some of the structural and organizational issues involved in training health psychologists in public health, including a comment on the potential benefits of their training on public health activities.

Advantages of Training Health Psychologists in Schools of Public Health

Although schools of public health were established relatively recently in the United States, they can provide the health psychologist with a longstanding history and tradition of research and intervention that can be traced back to the seventeenth and eighteenth centuries (Rosen 1979). In response to the devastating epidemics and illnesses of those times, systematic efforts, usually under the control of political and economic leaders, were made to identify the causes of poor health and to develop ways to improve working and living

This chapter was written during the tenure of an Established Investigatorship from the American Heart Association with funds contributed in part by the American Heart Association Pennsylvania Affiliate and awarded to Karen A. Matthews.

conditions believed to contribute to poor health. Public health research conducted during the eighteenth and nineteenth centuries had a strangely modern ring. For example, monographs were published on the relationship between social circumstances and differential morbidity and mortality; on the health problems of occupational groups such as sewer workers and match factory employees; on the reasons for noncompliance with requests for smallpox vaccinations by the working class and peasants; and on the health aspects of social disintegration (see Rosen 1979).

The above examples of public health monographs not only demonstrate the historical origins of the public health perspective but also its problem-oriented nature. Indeed the emphasis in schools of public health on problem-driven, as opposed to theory-driven, research and intervention persists today. Perhaps an illustration of this point will make it clearer. Between 1966 and 1969, seven cases of adenocarcinoma of the vagina were seen at a Massachusetts hospital. A particularly striking feature of the cases was the age of the women: all were younger than twenty-two years. Adenocarcinoma of the vagina previously had been observed only in women at least thirty years old and mostly in older women. It appeared that a new health problem was emerging in young women. Public health investigators then designed a study to document the incidence of cancer of the vagina in young women at other hospitals and to identify factors which might account for the increased incidence, if found, among this age group. Subsequent research showed that the mothers of these young women were more likely to have been prescribed diethylstilbestrol for threatened miscarriage during their pregnancy than mothers with similar demographic characteristics who delivered at the same hospital during the same time (Poskanzer and Herbst 1977). This case history demonstrates that public health efforts are typically triggered by the identification of the new health problem, not by the desire to elaborate theory. Training health psychologists in schools of public health would encourage this orientation and lead them to investigate and to intervene on the crucial health problems of the day.

At present, the problem-oriented public health approach has led to considerable research on chronic diseases because they constitute seven of the ten major causes of death (as of 1973). (In contrast, in 1900 only four of the ten major causes of death could be considered to be chronic diseases.) Furthermore, research has shown that behavioral factors are implicated in fifty percent of the deaths from the ten leading causes (Hamburg, Elliott, and Parron 1982). The examples of alcohol, cigarette smoking, and diet have been referred to throughout this volume. For example, alcohol consumption has been associated with accidental drownings and has been estimated to be related to more than one-third of adult male drownings. At least half of the deaths from motor vehicle accidents involve excessive alcohol intake (Sexton 1979). Such facts have led to a strong emphasis in the public health arena on prevention and early intervention with those behavioral risk factors that show promise of change. Training health psychologists in schools of public health allows them to have special input on prevention and intervention with behavioral risk factors and to become acquainted with the public health model of prevention and intervention.

In regard to the latter point, the public health model of prevention and intervention is based on a specific model of disease. In this model, disease is conceptualized as the outcome of host susceptibility, environmental factors, and the pathogenic agent(s). Intervention entails changing the relationship among the host, environment, and agent. An illustration of the public health model of disease comes from the work by Kasl, Evans, and Niederman (1979) on the epidemiology of infectious mononucleosis in a sample of 1,400 cadets at the West Point Military Academy. The causative agent is the Epstein-Barr virus. In this study, those host factors that predicted subsequent mononucleosis included the absence of the antibody to the Epstein-Barr virus as well as a high level of motivation combined with the relatively poor academic performance. Environmental factors included being in a competitive, demanding scholastic setting and having a father who was an "overachiever." Intervention on any of the three factors—preventing exposure to the Epstein-Barr virus, reducing student motivation or increasing performance, or withdrawing from an overly demanding scholastic setting—should reduce risk of the illness. Rather than psychology's emphasis on changing individual behavior in intervention, the public health approach to intervention focuses on changing the relationship among the three risk factors and therefore tends to be oriented more toward environmental change than psychology tends to be. This point leads to our next advantage for health psychologists in schools of public health.

Health psychologists can benefit from the population approach in schools of public health to health problems. In this approach, there is an emphasis on the community and how the health care system is used in order to understand health problems and their treatment. An illustration of the population perspective can be found in a series of studies by Bruhn, Philips, and Wolf (1982). They noted that individuals residing in Roseto, Pennsylvania, had a lower prevalence of coronary heart disease than did persons living in surrounding communities. Yet the risk factor levels did not seem to differ among the communities, although the Roseto diet contained more calories and fat than the average American diet. Rather than focus on individuals' attributes for an explanation of the low risk experienced in Roseto, Bruhn et al. investigated its social and cultural organization. They reported that many inhabitants were from Roseto, Valfortore, Italy. They had a tight social structure, knew each other well, and could call upon each other for aid and friendship in that they were related to one another. Bruhn et al. concluded that in spite of the heightened risk commonly associated with a diet like the Roseto diet, the social network of Roseto and the support it offered insulated its inhabitants from the heightened risk for coronary heart disease experienced by many persons living in surrounding communities.

Up to this point, we have cited five advantages of training health psychologists in schools of public health which, in fact, can be summarized succinctly into one: the benefit of exposure to the public health perspective with its long history and tradition, problem-oriented approach, emphasis on prevention, model of intervention focusing on environmental change, and unit of analysis being the population, community, or group (see also Runyan et al. 1982 and chapter 12 by Faden for a discussion of these points). The exposure to the public health perspective was also the most frequently mentioned advantage of employment in schools of public health volunteered in a survey completed by eighty percent of the psychologists in those schools (Matthews and Avis 1982). As one respondent stated, "I like the interdisciplinary, prevention-oriented approach that acknowledges that many of the problems are environmental, systemic, and a function of the delivery system rather than simply intrinsic to the client."

Two other advantages prominent in the psychologists' survey responses are relevant here: the interdisciplinary approach of a school of public health and the excellent opportunites for research. The respondents cited advantages like, "provides for a much broader outlook on health and disease" and "the intellectual challenge of trying to apply everything I know or can learn about the behavioral sciences to health problems." At a time when the major health problems are chronic illnesses with multiple causes, including behavioral ones, an interdisciplinary atmosphere should promote systematic, comprehensive research and intervention. Moreover, ongoing research in schools of public health on important health problems provides a challenging "laboratory" for elaboration of theory developed in other contexts and for testing new interventions. Training health psychologists in schools of public health increases the likelihood that they can take advantage of such opportunities.

Obtaining the Advantages of Training in Schools of Public Health

There are several ways that health psychologists can obtain the benefits of the public health perspective. One way is through didactic coursework. Although the organization of schools of public health varies across universities, most have either departments or divisions which focus on the following areas: (1) epidemiology; (2) biostatistics; (3) environmental and occupational health sciences; (4) nutritional sciences; (5) health services; (6) behavioral sciences and health education; and (7) population and family health. Below we elaborate on what these seven specific content areas have to offer the health psychologist.

The health psychologist who enrolls in epidemiology courses can benefit from instruction in epidemiology of specific diseases. Because epidemiologists study the distribution of diseases in population, they do not have the advantage of using random assignment in the true experimental sense. Thus, a major focus in epidemiology is on the methods of undertaking such research, including issues of sampling, selection of controls, computation of disease rates and relative risks, confounding, and drawing causal inferences. Instruction in biostatistics provides knowledge of the appropriate statistical tools for evaluating epidemiologic and other population-based studies. Although coursework in statistics is generally a part of the psychology curriculum, biostatistical training may be a useful complement in that it covers research designs with unequal cell sizes, multiple correlated predictor variables, nonlinear relationships between independent and dependent variables, and dichotomous dependent variables. Other epidemiology courses of potential use to health psychologists are those concerned with the epidemiology of specific diseases or disabilities, and may include: infectious and tropical diseases; neurologic disease; cardiovascular disease; cancer; and injuries. Of particular interest to the health psychologist are courses in social epidemiology which examine the social, cultural, and psychological determinants of disease.

Didactic training in the areas of environmental and occupational health sciences or nutritional sciences will be most useful to the health psychologist with a background in physiology. Areas of study include biological effects of air pollution, chemical behavior of aquatic systems, environmental toxicology, occupational safety and health, and both the biological and clinical aspects of nutrition.

Training in health services can serve a dual purpose for the health psychologist. First, health services cover a specific content area that may enhance the skills and research expertise of the health psychologist. Included within the rubric of health services is the study of the structure and function of health organizations, health planning, health administration, health policy and regulation, health financing, and health care. The second advantage of didactic training in health services is that health psychologists can operate more effectively in health care settings if they possess a working knowledge of the organization of the health care system.

Curriculum offered in behavioral sciences and health education represents the most direct application of the principles of psychology and sociology. Didactic training focuses on the psychosocial determinants of health status (physical and mental), the psychosocial determinants of health promotion, and evaluation of public health interventions. Determinants of health status studied by behavioral scientists and health educators include social variables (e.g., social class), psychological variables (e.g., stress), health beliefs, and health practices. Health promotion is studied both at the community level (e.g., community organization, community health education), and at the individual level (determinants of change in health-related behavior, health education in clinical settings). Furthermore, evaluation strategies appropriate for each setting are examined.

Didactic training in population and family health may be of the greatest interest to health psychologists who have a background in developmental or social psychology (particularly with an emphasis on sex roles). Population health courses emphasize population problems, human reproductive behavior, sexuality, and family planning programs and policy. Family health courses emphasize human growth and development, with a specific focus on the health problems of women, mothers, infants, and children in the context of both the family and the community.

A second major avenue through which health psychologists can benefit from training in schools of public health is through involvement in ongoing research projects. Public health research often involves a team of investigators representing a variety of disciplines including public health, medicine, the life sciences, and the social sciences. Although public health research shares a common perspective, there is considerable diversity in the range of problems that are studied. In order to provide concrete examples of the types of research in which health psychologists might become involved, two research projects are described below: a basic research project and an intervention research project.

The Pittsburgh Noise-Hypertension Project was undertaken to evaluate the impact of long-term noise exposure upon blood pressure. Previous research, in the United States and the Soviet Union, implicated long-term exposure to high levels of ambient noise as a risk factor for hypertension. To address the role of noise in hypertension, workers in two factories in the greater Pittsburgh area were selected for study participation. The factories and their work forces shared many recent characteristics in common but differed in their level of ambient noise at the work site. The research team consisted of two epidemiologists (one was also an M.D.), an M.D.-biostatistician, two psychologists (the authors of this chapter), an audiologist, and one epidemiology doctoral student, all of whom were interested in other aspects of the factory environment, as well as noise. In addition to blood pressure measurement, audiometric testing, and completion of a medical history, participants completed questionnaires concerning their perception of the work environment, their overall job satisfaction, the quality of their interaction with co-workers and supervisors, and their individual behavioral characteristics (e.g., Type A behavior pattern, anger, anxiety). Thus, the Pittsburgh Noise-Hypertension Project assessed the sources of job stress (including noise), the relationships of job stress to blood pressure, and the possible behavioral and physical mediators of the hypothesized relationship between job stress and blood pressure.

In contrast to the Pittsburgh Noise-Hypertension Project which examined possible etiological factors in disease, the Multiple Risk Factor Intervention Trial (MRFIT) attempted to change known risk factors for coronary heart disease (CHD) in men at high risk and to examine the presumed concomitant reduction in CHD morbidity and mortality (MRFIT 1982). A multi-center project, MRFIT solicited the participation of over 12,000 men who were in the upper ten percent of the risk factor distribution based on the Framingham Heart Study for the following risk factors: elevated blood pressure, smoking history, and levels of serum cholesterol. MRFIT was designed to lower blood pressure pharmacologically, to assist in smoking cessation efforts, and to reduce cholesterol levels via diet. Behavior change programs were implemented, compliance was assessed, and the program was evaluated at each site. In many MRFIT sites, psychologists were involved in designing, delivering, and evaluating the interventions.

Structural and Organizational Training Issues

There are a number of practical considerations involved in obtaining the benefits of the didactic material and research opportunities available in schools of public health. These include whether or not to seek exposure to the public health perspective at the predoctoral and postdoctoral level, to earn a graduate degree in the area, and to make efforts to establish health psychology training programs with a public health emphasis within a school of public health or within a psychology department. Discussion below addresses each of these issues.

Predoctoral versus Postdoctoral Training

Training of health psychologists in schools of public health can occur at the pre- or postdoctoral level. Training of the predoctoral health psychologist in a school of public health would probably be similar to the training of other public health graduate students. That is, the student would select an area of concentration (e.g., epidemiology or behavioral sciences and health education), but would also take courses from other divisions/departments within public health as well. This breadth is desirable at the predoctoral level because the student has not yet specialized in a particular aspect of health psychology. Thus, predoctoral coursework in a school of public health would serve the purpose of shaping research interests rather than supplementing them, as may be the case with postdoctoral coursework. Depending upon the program taken in psychology, predoctoral health psychologists might take some of their basic statistics and methods courses in a school of public health. While the postdoctoral health psychologist would already have a familiarity with statistical inference, for example, the predoctoral health psychologist may elect to take the elementary courses in biostatistics, particularly if the predoctoral trainee has a strong interest in the more advanced biostatistics courses. The same may hold true for courses on attitude and behavior change, for example.

The postdoctoral student in health psychology would most likely take public health courses that could enhance an already established area of research expertise. For example, the postdoctoral fellow interested in the Type A behavior pattern might take courses in cardiovascular disease epidemiology, social epidemiology, and biostatistics. A postdoctoral fellow interested in the physician-patient relationship might take courses in interpersonal dynamics in health services, patient education, and communication in health promotion and education. In other cases, the postdoctoral health psychologist may seek training in a school of public health not to supplement existing research interests, but to develop new ones. For these postdoctoral students, the appropriate coursework would be more familiar to that of the predoctoral student.

With regard to research involvement in schools of public health, the distinction in roles between predoctoral and postdoctoral health psychologists is similar to that which exists in traditional psychology programs. Predoctoral students may take a more active role in data collection and analysis while postdoctoral students would play a larger role in study design, supervision of data collection and/or analysis, and data interpretation. In a smoking cessation program, for example, postdoctoral students may utilize their knowledge of interpersonal communication to design a segment of the intervention; predoctoral students may gain research experience through actual delivery of the intervention.

The descriptions presented above are examples of the kind of training that might be appropriate for pre- and postdoctoral health psychologists in schools of public health. According to these descriptions, the predoctoral program would foster an integration of psychology and public health, whereas the postdoctoral program would provide a more in-depth study of a particular aspect of public health. Each program has its value, and thus we are not advocating predoctoral training at the expense of postdoctoral, or vice versa. We believe that the strongest health psychology program is one that can offer training in public health at both the pre- and postdoctoral levels.

DEGREE PROGRAMS IN PUBLIC HEALTH

Enrolling in a master's program in a school of public health at either the pre- or postdoctoral level has distinct advantages. (The discussion here centers on master's degrees rather than doctoral degrees as it is assumed that this would be the most practical option for a doctoral-level health psychologist.) First, a public health degree is a professional degree (as opposed to an academic degree) and will increase the employment opportunities for the health psychologist. This is true for employment in professional agencies or organizations, as well as for employment in academic positions within schools of public health. The training required to earn the degree will provide the health psychologist with a good grounding in public health, and the degree itself will enhance the credibility of the health psychologist within the health care profession. A second advantage of enrolling in a degree program is that it increases the sense of commitment to the endeavor and also provides a structure to the didactic experience with the school of public health. The health psychologist enrolled in a degree program may feel more connected with mainstream public health and, because of degree requirements, will have a clear picture of what is to be accomplished in the school of public health.

Naturally, there are also disadvantages to enrolling in degree programs. Because a degree program is more structured than simply choosing courses of interest, the health psychologist may feel constrained by requirements.

While the postdoctoral fellow may be able to waive certain master's courses, this is less likely for the predoctoral trainee. In addition, the predoctoral student may find it difficult to meet simultaneously the demands of the public health and psychology programs. Not only are there required courses, but there are also requirements of some combination of fieldwork, comprehensive exams, and a thesis. Not surprisingly, a degree program is considerably more rigorous than nondegree pursuits in schools of public health.

LOCATION OF HEALTH PSYCHOLOGY TRAINING

Health psychology training programs which include a public health emphasis could be located in either a department of psychology or a school of public health. If located in a department of psychology, advising and a major part of the didactic coursework would take place in psychology, with additional training in public health. Most faculty-student interaction would occur among psychologists, as psychology departments tend to be staffed exclusively by psychologists.

Health psychology programs located in schools of public health should also be staffed primarily by psychologists, but might include medical sociologists, medical anthropologists, or epidemiologists. Training could take place both in the school of public health and in the affiliated department of psychology, but the advising and physical location of the program would be in public health. While this model has the advantage of greater interdisciplinary exposure, it is currently less feasible than the psychology department model because most schools of public health do not have a critical mass of psychologists in tenure-ladder positions who could administer such a program. At this time, it appears that a practical approach would be for health psychology programs with a public health emphasis to be based in an academic psychology department. Core faculty members of the health psychology program, however, should be located and have their major appointment in a school of public health.

Summary and Concluding Comment

This chapter has focused on how health psychologists can benefit from training in the public health perspective in schools of public health, how to obtain the benefits of this perspective through didactic material and involvement in research projects, and what practical structural and organizational considerations are involved in selecting a program of study in public health in combination with a program in health psychology. To conclude our discussion, we wish to point out that health psychologists are not the only beneficiaries of their training in the public health perspective. Researchers in public health can also benefit from exposure to health psychologists (see also Singer and Krantz 1982). In contrast to the applied orientation of public health, psychologists can offer a theoretical perspective with regard to health, both in terms of individual and organizational behavior. Psychologists can offer their expertise in the measurement of host and environmental factors. Of particular importance are the skills for the psychologists in the conceptualization and measurement of stress. Similarly, psychologists' experience and sophistication in the areas of intervention and prevention are most useful. Finally, psychologists' knowledge of psychophysiological processes that may connect the brain, behavior, and disease are invaluable to the public health enterprise. Joined together, the psychological and public health perspectives can complement one another in the effort to understand the important health problems of our day.

REFERENCES

Bruhn, J. G.; B. U. Philips, Jr.; and S. Wolf. 1982. Lessons from Roseto twenty years later: A community study of heart disease. *Southern Medical Journal* 45:575–80.

Hamburg, D. A., G. R. Elliott, and D. L. Parron. 1982. *Health and behavior: Frontiers of research in the biobehavioral sciences.* Washington, D.C.: National Academy Press.

Kasl, S. V., A. S. Evans, and J. C. Niederman. 1979. Psychosocial risk factors in the development of infectious mononucleosis. *Psychosomatic Medicine* 41: 445–66.

Matthews, K. A., and N. E. Avis. 1982. Psychologists in schools of public health: Current status, future prospects, and implications for other health settings. *American Psychologist* 37:949–54.

Multiple Risk Factor Intervention Trial: Risk factor changes and mortality. 1982. *Journal of the American Medical Association* 248:1465–77.

Poskanzer, D. C., and A. L. Herbst. 1977. Epidemiology of vaginal adenosis and adenocarcinoma associated with exposure to stilbestrol in utero. *Cancer* 39: 1892–95.

Rosen, G. 1979. The evolution of science. In *Handbook of medical psychology,* edited by H. F. Freman, S. Levine, and L. G. Reeder. Englewood Cliffs, NJ: Prentice-Hall.

Runyan, C. W., R. F. DeVellis, B. M. DeVellis, and G. M. Hochbaum. 1982. Health psychology and the public health perspective: In search of the pump handle. *Health Psychology* 1:169–80.

Sexton, M. M. 1979. Behavioral epidemiology. In *Behavioral medicine: Theory and Practice,* edited by O. F. Pomerlau and J. P. Brady. Baltimore: Williams & Wilkins Co.

Singer, J. E., and D. S. Krantz. 1982. Perspectives on the interface between psychology and public health. *American Psychologist* 37:955–60.

35
Educating Health Psychologists: Lessons to Be Learned at School

Jean R. Eagleston and Carl E. Thoresen

Few would disagree today with the belief that our physical and emotional health and well-being are primarily determined by how we live—our particular patterns of eating, drinking, working, exercising, relaxing, and relating. These patterns of living result, in large part, from experiences, direct or vicarious, acquired over time in various contexts, including type of community, socioeconomic status, parental and family characteristics, subcultural factors, schools, and the mass media.

In a significant sense we *learn* to be healthy or to be sick. In effect our experiences teach us how to think, what to feel, when to take action and what to do. The ancient wisdoms of Hippocratic medicine concerning lifestyle are finally catching up to us in the aftermath of the modern medical model, a perspective that has viewed diseases as caused by a single identifiable microbe or germ.

We are beginning to realize that all causes have their prior causes (e.g., cigarette smoking as a "cause" of cardiovascular diseases or carcinoma having its own causes) and that causes produce effects that in turn become causes of other effects. Thus, instead of preventing or treating disease by pinpointing a particular microbial pathogen and eradicating it, we are faced with a host of "behavioral" (and environmental) pathogens that become intricately woven over time into complex patterns that markedly influence health and disease status (Matarazzo 1983).

Unfortunately, no substantiated theory of disease or of health exists; rather, a conglomerate of mostly descriptive or functional models offer hypotheses about what factors may influence various processes possibly linked to health or disease status (Hamburg, Elliott, and Parron 1982; Weiner 1981). Part of the problem is one of scope. Commonly, issues are studied from the narrow perspective of a specialty area within a particular discipline, without examining how the organism as a whole functions relative to the problem under study. Inquiry is clearly needed at many different levels, from the extremely microscopic study of intracellular activities to the highly macroscopic appraisal of cross-cultural influences on health and disease. Any comprehensive, let alone valid, theory of health or disease will need to incorporate concepts that span a broad range of factors.

Given the current complexities in understanding the many determinants of health and disease, how might the health psychologist be best trained? The answer seems straightforward: broadly. At least at initial or introductory levels, a health psychologist needs to understand physiological, behavioral, environmental, and cognitive processes. Further, most psychologists preparing to work with health and disease issues should have at the core of their scientific and professional training substantial knowledge and skills in the cognitive and behavioral areas—phenomena that are primary in the discipline of psychology. Consider a recent definition of health psychology:

> . . . specific educational, scientific and professional contributions of the discipline of psychology to the promotion and maintenance of health, the prevention and treatment of illness, and the identification of the etiologic and diagnostic correlates of health, illness, and related dysfunction.
>
> (Matarazzo 1980, 815)

Clearly, a prime focus in this definition is on how to help people stay healthy and how to prevent illness, disease, and sickness. (See Thoresen and Eagleston 1985 for a discussion of the distinction between illness, disease, and sickness.) Others have documented the crucial role played by routine habits and thinking patterns in health and disease (Hamburg, Elliott, and Parron 1982; Weiner 1981). What stands out in these thoughtful discussions of the interplay between brain, behavior, and environment is the need to understand and use effective methods to help people change—to modify their behaviors, to restructure their environments, and to alter their ways of perceiving and construing reality. These problems are decidedly educational, concerning how to arrange learning experiences that will effect the necessary changes. Hence the need is to bring the professional areas of education to bear on the problems of helping people change their behavior and their environments.

Professional training in schools of education in the United States today is not limited to producing teachers, principals, and school administrators. Instead the focus in many graduate programs is on producing educators in the broadest sense of the word—professionals who are able to help others learn effectively through a variety of methods in a variety of settings. Because of the compatibility between educational models and psychological theory, many counseling psychology programs are based in schools of education. In the remainder of this paper we will introduce briefly the field of counseling psychology and present a rationale for an educational model as we build the case for schools of education being an appropriate training site for health psychologists. Finally we will describe a Health Psychology specialty track within a Counseling Psychology Program based in the Stanford University School of Education.

Counseling Psychologists Trained in Educational Models

The field of counseling psychology has long recognized the need for an educational perspective in helping people solve problems. Counseling psychologists along with clinical psychologists contribute a perspective, knowledge, and skills that are focused on the application of interventions and treatments. The design, implementation, and evaluation of the efficacy of treatment programs are familiar activities for the counseling psychologist. While current training in counseling psychology may emphasize other topic areas, such as career decision making and interpersonal competence, the skills of the counseling psychologist also can be applied to: (1) the promotion and maintenance of health through the development of healthy habits and lifestyle (e.g., exercise, diet, relaxation), and (2) the prevention and treatment of disease through changing unhealthy behaviors, especially ones that may be associated with certain chronic diseases and health problems (e.g., cigarette smoking, excessive salt intake, sedentary habits).

Fortunately, there is considerable overlap between the potential contributions of counseling and clinical psychologists as well as with the other applied subfields such as school, industrial, and community. Counseling psychology, however, may offer some unique contributions in the health area because it is such a broadly based applied psychology specialty (Thoresen 1980). A three-part definition of counseling psychology was proposed by Ivey (1979): "(1) diversity and competence in many activities with an accompanying respect for the need of many, rather than one, approaches; (2) a firm commitment to the importance of the person's environmental considerations; and (3) an emphasis on positive mental health and development" (p. 3). Traditionally, the developmental, educational, prevention, and personal growth domains have been central in the field of counseling psychology (Fretz and Mills 1980). Educational models have prevailed with an emphasis on structuring learning experiences to facilitate change, particularly among normal populations, that is, people who lack severe pathology, who are instead experiencing difficulty in handling the developmental tasks of ordinary living (e.g., making education and career choices, maintaining close personal relationships, raising a family). This same perspective, emphasizing normal development and personal growth, coupled with an orientation toward prevention can clearly be applied to preventing illness and promoting health.

Counseling psychologists are "at home" in a wide variety of settings. The training of counseling psychologists usually equips them to work with clients on an individual basis or in small groups, as well as to provide consultation to public and private agencies and organizations. Private practice or mental hospitals may be a common employment setting for clinical psychologists and some counseling psychologists. Typically, however, schools, colleges, community agencies, and work organizations other than hospitals are the sites in which counseling psychologists provide services. This familiarity with a variety of settings and with providing consultation to individuals, small groups, and organizations can readily serve the needs of the specialty areas of health psychology and behavioral medicine.

Rationale for an Educational Model

In many ways the enhancement of optimal health along with the prevention and amelioration of diseases requires an educational strategy. An educational model emphasizes teaching people *how* to think, *how* to solve problems, and *how* to make decisions. One of the primary failures of traditional education was the belief that information sufficed, especially in the field of health education (Dwore and Matarazzo 1981). Besides receiving health information, whether it is dispersed by a physician, pamphlet, or pharmacist, people need to be taught how to use that information, particularly how to act upon knowledge in the face of competing personal and social-environmental factors, including complex issues of self-control (Thoresen 1984).

An educational model incorporates concepts and methods from several disciplines, not just physiology or psychology, in constructing curriculum to produce and maintain change. Conceptualizing health and disease problems as educational issues encourages a focus on the person in question as a student, someone who needs to learn how to do something, whether it be a different way to think about carcinoma, a new method to use in avoiding the temptation to smoke, or a strategy to restructure a highly stressful work environment. The task of the practicing health psychologist—at least one of the major tasks—is to function as an educator in the sense of arranging for effective learning experiences. Sometimes the health psychologist might function directly as a teacher with an individual or a group. Other times the health psychologist may orchestrate the learning by planning the nature and sequence of experiences to be utilized by others. The key point is that an educational paradigm has much to offer those concerned with the prevention of disease as well as treatment coupled with the promotion of good health.

Obviously educational settings themselves at all levels (preschool to adult education) are ideal settings for health promotion and disease prevention. Indeed, aside from the mass media, schools, colleges, and community centers are probably some of the best contexts for primary prevention—for keeping people healthy and for reducing premature disease states. The formative years of childhood and adolescence offer the opportunities to "imprint" a variety of attitudes and beliefs, as well as behaviors, concerning health.

Unfortunately, educational settings too often may offer dated and at times superficial knowledge about far too few health-related matters. Commonly the approach has been only to inform students but not to teach them how to act differently based on information. One exception may be driver education. For example, in some schools driver education in the form of information is combined with "behind the wheel" supervised driving practice. Typically, however, this comprehensive educational approach is not used to address health issues. A tremendous, as yet untapped, potential for health promotion exists in educational settings. We will briefly describe two research programs that are using an educational model in a school setting.

Smoking Prevention with Junior High School Students

A group of researchers within the Stanford Heart Disease Prevention Program have focused on developing smoking prevention programs for young adolescents (e.g., Perry et al. 1980; Telch et al. 1982). The junior high school setting was identified as crucial in modifying behavior and "inoculating" students against the environmental and cognitive demands to start smoking. In this intervention, high school students were trained to guide seventh-graders in the development of skills to resist personal and social pressures to smoke. During the academic year a total of seven sessions (45 minutes each) were conducted by high school students to teach 353 seventh-graders how to resist various factors believed to be related to the adoption of cigarette smoking (e.g., prolonged peer pressure and mass media advertising). Comparisons with 217 seventh-graders in another school, serving as control subjects, revealed differences between schools in the proportion of students who reported smoking at the nine-month follow-up that were significant (5.3% versus 10.3% p < .05). Over a two-year period, the relative increase in the percentage of control subjects smoking was significant (from 10.3% to 18.8%, p. < .02), while the increase of those receiving the smoking prevention treatment was modest (from 5.3% to 7.1%).

This program of research is exciting not only because it produced statistically and clinically significant results, but also because it vividly illustrates the use of an educational model for health promotion. Important features of the intervention include: (1) treatment taking place in the school, a setting where pressures to smoke typically are present, (2) use of slightly older peers (rather than highly trained, professional adults) as teachers and role models, and (3) attention to *how* to resist personal and peer pressures to begin or continue smoking. The intervention did not emphasize giving information on the negative health consequences of smoking, but rather used techniques such as modeling and role play to assist students to learn and practice the decision-making and interpersonal skills necessary to prevent smoking behavior.

ASSESSING CHRONIC STRESS IN CHILDREN AND ADOLESCENTS

In comparison to smoking prevention, in the area of chronic stress we are a bit less knowledgeable about personal and environmental factors that may cause prolonged stress for school-age children and adolescents (Garmezy and Rutter 1983). The Health in Youth Project at Stanford is investigating the physical health, social behavior, and academic performance correlates of chronic stress in fifth, seventh, and ninth grade students. In this project chronic stress is conceptualized as an undesirable state the person experiences over time, resulting from a perceived imbalance between demands and resources to meet the demands, coupled with maladaptive responses used in meeting the demands. The maladaptive responses can occur singly or in concert across four domains: physiological, behavioral, cognitive, and environmental. The assessment of responses in these four domains, as well as perceived demands and perceived resources, is the focus of our current research that has involved working with over 800 students in more than twenty schools.

Thorough assessment hopefully will lead to a better understanding of the phenomenon of chronic stress as it is experienced by younger people. Such an increased understanding of the relevant demands, resources, and responses could form the basis for designing an intervention program that could be incorporated into the school curriculum. We know that effective stress management with adults entails more than the advice to relax. With children and adolescents it also seems clear that an intervention program would need to provide more than just advice or information, for example, teaching about physiological (e.g., diet and exercise), cognitive (e.g., modifying self-talk and changing appraisals), and behavioral-environmental (e.g., social skills, support networks) resources (Thoresen and Eagleston 1983).

An Example of a Health Psychology Training Program Based in a School of Education

PREDOCTORAL TRAINING

A Health Psychology specialty track within the Counseling Psychology Program was approved by the School of Education at Stanford University in 1983. The curriculum for the Health Psychology specialty track currently is under development. Following the guidelines for predoctoral training recommended by the National Working Conference on Education and Training in Health Psychology (Stone 1983), table 35.1 presents an outline of sample coursework that could satisfy the requirements for mastery of knowledge and skills areas. The formalization of a health psychology program has demanded that a few new courses be developed, but the majority of the content areas can be addressed by courses offered by a variety of university and medical school departments—psychology, education, philosophy, sociology, human biology, medicine, and family, community, and preventive medicine. In fact, this outline of suggested coursework vividly illustrates the interdisciplinary cooperation that is essential for comprehensive training in health psychology.

PRACTICUM AND INTERNSHIP EXPERIENCES

In addition to the general psychology and health psychology training that may be obtained predominantly through coursework, the predoctoral training of health psychology students needs to involve *experience* in the career functions typically associated with a professional psychologist, namely: (1) research, (2) intervention (e.g., counseling/therapy with individuals, small groups, families), (3) consultation, (4) teaching, and (5) administration and management. Through practicum and internship placements in a wide range of agencies and settings, students are receiving "hands-on" experience in at least four of the above areas during their predoctoral training. Further, these training experiences address becoming a professional psychologist and include an opportunity to deal with issues such as ethics and

TABLE 35.1 Sample Coursework Requirements for Mastery of Required Knowledge and Skills Areas

Content Area		Representative Coursework*
	GENERAL PSYCHOLOGY TRAINING	
A. Scientific and Professional Ethics	Ed 432 Phil 78	Doctoral Seminar in Health Psychology Medical Ethics
B. Legal Issues	Ed 432 Psych 125 Psych 353	Doctoral Seminar in Health Psychology Psychology and Law Psychopathology and Mental Health Law
C. Professional Standards	Ed 432 Ed 238A–C	Doctoral Seminar in Health Psychology Counseling and Health Psychology: Supervised Applications
D. Research Design and Methodology	Ed 232/Psych 253 Ed 250D Med 201	Science and Research in Counseling & Health Psychology Statistical Analysis in Educational Research II: Exp. Design Epidemiology
E. Statistics	Ed 250A–C *or* Psych 60, 152, 153 Ed 321A, B	Statistical Analysis in Educational Research I and II Statistical Methods; Analysis of Data; Statistical Theory, Models, and Methodology Quantitative Methods in Qualitative Research
F. Psychological Measurement	Ed 252 Ed 255 Ed 236	Introduction to Test Theory Human Abilities Psychological Assessment

G. History and Systems of Psychology

Typically satisfied by previous coursework in
General, Abnormal, and Personality Psychology

H. Human Behavior
1. Biological bases

Psych 108	Neuropsychology
Psych 189	Endocrines and Behavior
Psych 189	Cellular Neurophysiological Approaches to Behavior
Soc 122	Introduction to Sociophysiology

2. Cognitive-affective bases

Psych 209	Perception
Psych 210	Cognitive Psychology
Psych 254	Principles of Personality Change

3. Social bases

Psych 212	Social Psychology
Psych 360	Family Influences on Cognitive Functioning and Educational Achievement
Psych 362	Research Seminar in Child Development and Early Education

4. Individual differences/
Psychological bases

Psych 211	Development Psychology
Psych 213	Personality
Psych 216	Abnormal Psychology

HEALTH PSYCHOLOGY TRAINING

A. Biological Basis of Health and
Disease

Hum Bio 111	Human Physiology
Hum Bio 166	Biosocial Aspects of Cardiovascular Disease

B. Social Basis of Health and Disease

Soc 111/FCPM 250	Social Issues in Health Care
FCPM 256	Economics of Health and Medical Care

(Continued on next page)

TABLE 35.1 (*continued*)

C. Psychological Basis of Health and Disease	Psych 335	Behavioral Medicine: Psychological Factors in Cure and Care
	Ed 235	Chronic Stress: Theory, Research and Clinical Practice
D. Health Policy and Organization	FCPM 222	Social Controversy and Policy Analysis in Medicine
	FCPM 279	Management of Hospitals and Other Health Care Institutions
	FCPM 391	Political Economy of Health Care
E. Health Assessment and Intervention	Ed 216	Cognitive Behavior Modification
	Ed 234	Individual Counseling Methods
	Ed 432	Doctoral Seminar in Health Psychology

PROFESSIONAL TRAINING

A. Assessment	Ed 214	Evaluation Research Methods
	Ed 236	Psychological Assessment
B. Intervention	Ed 238A–C	Counseling and Health Psychology: Supervised Applications
C. Consultation	Ed 338A–C	Internship in Counseling and Health Psychology
	Ed 208A, B	Introduction to Curriculum
D. Evaluation	Ed 214	Evaluation Research Methods
	Ed 278	Introduction to Issues in Evaluation

*These are *suggested* courses. Evidence of competence in a knowledge/skill area can be demonstrated through prior or alternative coursework or experiences.

professional standards, professional communication (i.e., writing, speaking), and personal development of a healthy life-style.

POSTDOCTORAL TRAINING

While predoctoral training in health psychology is becoming more available, we believe postdoctoral training will continue to be the more frequently used vehicle for obtaining the advanced skills training demanded in this subspecialty area. Postdoctoral training programs offer the opportunity to refine research, teaching, clinical and/or administrative skills. As we consider postdoctoral opportunities in our geographical area, it appears that specialized training can be obtained relative to:

Content area—for example, the two-year program offered by the Stanford Center for Research in Disease Prevention, where the focus is in part on cardiovascular disease and experiences, ranges from laboratory and field research to teaching and supervising predoctoral students to clinical intervention

Skills area—for example, programs in local HMOs in departments of pediatrics or obstetrics and gynecology where the emphasis is to refine direct service skills or a program in a nonprofit contract research organization where research skills and experiences could be expanded

Settings—for example, the health promotion programs in local companies or in the Stanford University Cowell Student Health Center

In brief summary, the training of health psychologists can benefit substantially from incorporating an educational approach. The perspective of counseling psychology with its emphasis on primary prevention and the amelioration of normal developmental problems and concerns in many contexts should facilitate the tasks of the health psychologist in promoting health, preventing disease, and aiding in the treatment of a broad range of health and disease problems.

REFERENCES

Dwore, R. B., and J. Matarazzo. 1981. The behavioral sciences and health education: Disciplines with a compatible interest? *Health Education* 12 (May/June): 4–7.

Fretz, B. R., and D. H. Mills. 1980. Professional certification in counseling psychology. *The Counseling Psychologist* 9(1): 2–17.

Garmezy, N., and M. Rutter, eds. 1983. *Stress, coping, and development in children.* New York: McGraw-Hill.

Hamburg, D. A., G. R. Elliott, and D. L. Parron, eds. 1982. *Health and behavior:*

Frontiers of research in the biobehavioral sciences. Washington, D.C.: National Academy Press.

Ivey, A. E. 1979. Counseling psychology—The most broadly based applied psychology specialty. *The Counseling Psychologist* 8(3): 3–6.

Knowles, J. H. 1977. *Doing better and feeling worse: Health in the United States.* New York: Norton.

Matarazzo, J. D. 1980. Behavioral health and behavioral medicine: Frontiers for a new health psychology. *American Psychologist* 35: 807–17.

———. 1983. Behavioral immunogens and pathogens: Psychology's newest challenge. *Professional Psychology: Research and Practice* 14: 414–16.

Perry, C., J. Killen, M. Telch, L. A. Slinkard, and B. C. Danaher. 1980. Modifying smoking behavior of teenagers: A school-based intervention. *American Journal of Public Health* 70: 722–25.

Stone, G., ed. 1983. Proceedings of the National Working Conference on Education and Training in Health Psychology. *Health Psychology* 2(5): 1–153, supplement section.

Telch, M. J., J. D. Killen, A. L. McAlister, C. L. Perry, and N. Maccoby. 1982. Long-term follow-up of a pilot project on smoking prevention with adolescents. *Journal of Behavioral Medicine* 5: 1–8.

Thoresen, C. E. 1980. Reflections on chronic health, self-control and human ethology. In *The present and future of counseling psychology,* edited by J. M. Whiteley and B. R. Fretz. Monterey, CA: Brooks-Cole.

———. 1984. Strategies for enhancing health. In *Behavioral health: Handbook of health and disease prevention,* edited by J. Matarazzo, S. Weiss, J. Herd, N. Miller, and S. Weiss. New York: Wiley.

Thoresen, C. E., and J. R. Eagleston. 1983. Chronic stress in children and adolescents. *Theory into Practice* 22: 48–56.

———. 1985. Counseling and health. *The Counseling Psychologist* 13: 15–87.

Weiner, H. 1977. *Psychobiology and human disease.* New York: Elsevier-North Holland.

———. 1981. Brain, behavior and bodily disease: A summary. In *Brain, behavior and bodily disease,* vol. 59, edited by H. Weiner, M. A. Hofer, and A. J. Stunkard. New York: Raven Press.

36

Schools of Professional Psychology as Sites for Training Health Psychologists

Nelson F. Jones

The National Working Conference on Training in Health Psychology at Arden House in 1983 explored in depth the full range of issues in educating health psychologists. In that regard it also looked to the likely places and patterns of employment to identify appropriate goals, content, style, and sites for training. Recommendations were forthcoming on many of these issues, although some of the recommendations, particularly in regard to training sites, ran counter to current educational trends in the field.

For instance, the recommendation that all health psychology service training be in the scientist-professional model was not accompanied by any explicit recommendation for dealing with the large number of psychologists now being trained in the professional practitioner model who are already moving into one or another aspect of health psychology. Assumptions were verbalized by the conferees, as they have been elsewhere (Snepp 1979), that health psychology training, or even basic doctoral training in psychology for that matter, is suitably gained only in a multidisciplinary university setting. Again, a large number of graduates from freestanding professional schools are already entering the practice of health psychology, and reversing the trend is unlikely at this point.

Attaching exact numbers to these trends is difficult, because as health psychology is practiced today it is very often integrated into clinical practice. Certainly not all clinicians practice in health psychology and, for those who do, widely varying proportions of their practices fall into the health psychology area. Full-time health psychology specialists exist, but they currently provide only a small part of the care being dispensed (Grzesiak 1983). The large number of clinical psychologists being graduated by professional schools will continue to have a foothold in this field, the extent of which it may not be possible to count or define. If health psychology is to emerge as an identifiable specialty with recognizable standards, and if we are to provide the most effective training for rendering services, it is essential that these issues be addressed. Defining the field in such a way as to ignore an existing and growing body of service providers will not necessarily make them go away, even if that, indeed, turns out to be desirable.

While the concerns voiced by the Arden House conferees were in terms negative to "professional schools" generally or to the Psy.D. as a professional degree, the actual issues of concern in training institutions are much more specific. They appear to be stability and adequacy of faculty, availability of needed academic and clinical teaching resources and numbers—the feared mass production of inadequately trained practitioners. Practitioners trained in professional programs, it is feared, would be incapable of pushing the field ahead because they may lack the training necessary to think critically and/or to conduct research. Whatever the merits of these concerns, there is a strong emotional component to them which will be slow to yield to logical argument, and there are few data with which to address an evaluation of the issues. Only the existence of large numbers of professional school graduates is clear.

Development of Professional Schools in Psychology

Discussion of the origin of professional schools in psychology, the arguments in favor of them, problems and complexities presented, and some mechanisms for quality control may be of help in understanding professional schools as sites for doctoral and/or postdoctoral training in health psychology.

As Schofield (1982) has pointed out, by 1965 psychology was caught in a situation in which the approved training sites, academic departments of psychology, could not and were not interested in training the sizeable numbers of practitioners needed if the profession was to reach its potential. "Within 20 years of its beginning, the profession of psychology seemed about to wither for lack of personnel" (p. 4).

Two training conferences and much discussion later, the concepts of a professional degree, the Doctor of Psychology, and a practitioner (as opposed to a scientist-practitioner) training pattern were officially accepted by the American Psychological Association. Several detailed accounts of this process exist (Korman 1974; McNamara et al. 1982). The first school to engage in large-scale training under the professional training mandate was the California School of Professional Psychology, a freestanding institution with four campuses now enrolling about 900 students or approximately twenty percent of all doctoral students in clinical psychology.

As it became apparent that such a freestanding institution could prosper, others were initiated. Concurrently, several university-based professional programs were established and, in 1976, the National Council of Schools of Professional Psychology was established at a meeting initiated by the APA Board of Professional Affairs. That group now has a membership, in its various categories, of twenty-nine schools. Full membership requires that a program be regionally accredited, be accredited by APA, that it consist of a separate administrative unit which is identified as a school of professional psychology or be an identifiable program in a department of psychology, that it be administered by a psychologist and have substantial control of its own faculty, student body and curriculum, that the primary programs be at the doctoral level and in an area of applied intervention such as clinical, counseling, industrial/organizational or school psychology.

There is a wide range of size, administrative structures, faculty staffing patterns, physical resources and educational philosophies represented within the NCSPP, as will be discussed subsequently in more detail. To date, no school of professional psychology has identified itself as entirely or even primarily dedicated to training health psychologists. Almost all, however, offer clinical psychology programs with training which bears on the area of health psychology, and almost all differ from each other in major ways.

A number of schools accredited by neither APA nor a regional accrediting body exist which advertise degrees in psychology but which have made no effort to become part of the NCSPP. These schools will presumably continue to operate outside any standard-setting organization, since state charters do not require accreditation. The single most effective factor controlling their proliferation is that their graduates usually are not eligible for licensing (Wellner 1978).

Any question about schools of professional psychology as sites for training of a specific nature must take account of the ways in which such schools differ and how an individual school meets the training requirements of the content area in question. A list of the dimensions along which schools of professional psychology differ may help in understanding how such schools do or do not meet those requirements. It is a complex picture.

The first of those dimensions is the nature of the degree offered and the second is the administrative structure of the school. Some professional programs within universities and some freestanding professional schools offer the Ph.D. and espouse the Boulder model of scientist-professional training, albeit with an emphasis on "professional." The Institute of Advanced Studies at Adelphi University and the four campuses of the California School of Professional Psychology are examples. Both university-affiliated and free-standing programs also offer the Psy.D. degree, assuming a practitioner training model but differing in the extent to which research training and productivity are emphasized. The School of Professional Psychology at Wright State University in Ohio and the freestanding Oregon School of Professional Psychology are representative of this group. An added branching of the issue of university affiliation has to do with the presence of two Psy.D. programs in medical school or hospital settings (Hahnemann Medical College in Philadelphia and the Forest Institute in the Chicago area) and Ph.D. programs in the same kinds of settings (Oregon Health Sciences University).

Within university programs there is still diversity in administrative arrangements which influences the style and content of training. Some programs, such as Baylor University's Psy.D. program, are housed within a department of psychology along with other traditional Ph.D. programs and the resources those programs make available to Psy.D. students. Some programs are separate departments within a graduate college (University of Denver) and some are colleges within the university but not part of an arts and sciences graduate school (Rutgers). Both of the latter arrangements provide access to university faculty in other areas of psychology, although not so readily as in those programs which are part of a department of psychology. Freestanding professional schools, on the other hand, must provide all needed faculty resources within the professional program. Thus, the focus on professional training, which is what brought these programs into existence, is often achieved at the expense of training in basic psychological science or adequate research supervision when instructional programs are isolated from other university resources.

Designation and Accreditation of Doctoral Programs in Psychology

All programs seeking designation as programs in psychology by the National Register of Health Service Providers in Psychology or seeking APA accreditation must offer a minimum of general psychology and research exposure. Those standards are reviewed in this volume in chapter 14. The various professional programs now designated or accredited meet or, in more cases, exceed these standards. Some require a dissertation (regardless of whether the degree offered is a Ph.D. or a Psy.D.) and others require a less formal scholarly production, but all require some final written product. Accreditation and its less stringent evaluation companion, designation as a program in psychology, become effective mechanisms of quality control and are especially important because of their strong appeal to students paying heavy tuition.

Practicum Settings

Another dimension of particular relevance to health psychology is access to health care settings for practicum experience at the predoctoral level. Again, there is a wide variability among professional programs regarding such access. Some graduate programs, of both service-delivery and research persuasions, are closely connected with health science centers and have easy, built-in mechanisms for making this training available. Others have informal but stable arrangements and some have none. Predictable and varied experience on this dimension was seen as essential by the 1983 Arden House conferees. Resources for meeting the requirement will simply have to be assessed for individual programs through the accreditation mechanism. Generic accreditation standards (APA 1983) already exist for laboratory and practicum training which will serve for evaluating health psychology training needs as well.

What becomes clear as a result of reviewing all this apparent confusion is that one cannot make specific assumptions about the nature of a professional program, as those programs exist today, without knowing a great deal more about it than its title. Movement in the direction of the Psy.D. degree and the professional school or professional program as a training site has been substantial and appears to be continuing. Of course to date most of these programs are clinical, but then most training for practice in health psychology is conducted in clinical programs.

The National Council of Schools of Professional Psychology has instituted a sweeping evaluation of the nature and quality of professional programs (Callan, Peterson, and Stricker 1986) and the Committee on Accreditation of APA has for several years wrestled with the complexities of adapting and applying accreditation standards to professional programs.[1] These quality control mechanisms should result, at the very least, in "truth in packaging" for those programs which have been evaluated. Prospective students and employers should be able to identify the kind of training conducted by the programs.

---

1. As a member of the Education and Training Board of APA, the Executive Committee of the Council for the National Register of Health Service Providers in Psychology, the Task Force on Review of Accreditation Criteria of APA, and as accreditation site visitor and *ad hoc* appeal panel member for the APA Committee on Accreditation, the author has been an active participant for several years in the process of translating APA accreditation standards, which were originally developed with university departments of psychology in mind, for evaluation of novel (and sometimes litigious) programs. New versions of the standards and of the *Accreditation Handbook* (APA 1983) reflect the subtleties of this process.

Judging Suitability for Training in Health Psychology

Whether professional programs are appropriate by nature and quality for the training of health psychologists will depend on the extent to which a given program meets the standards set out by Division 38 and incorporated into the accreditation procedures for evaluating programs. That is, of course, a statement applicable to any doctoral program. For standards to be maintained, there must be support for the accreditation process from universities, from postdoctoral training programs, from credentialing agencies, and from employers. Accreditation cannot and should not result in complete homogeneity among programs (APA 1983), but no assumptions about quality or lack of it are safe if they are based solely on the labeling of a program.

Respecialization

Only the Institute of Advanced Studies at Adelphi University offers a formal postdoctoral program at this time, although one or two others do have respecialization programs. For the most part, such programs have focused on clinical training for psychologists whose doctoral degrees have been granted in other areas. As health psychology becomes a recognized specialty and, hopefully, offers employment opportunities, professional schools will be asked to offer respecialization as well as basic doctoral training. Again, there is nothing inherent in the concept of the professional school to preclude doing so. The quality of health psychology education available will depend upon the resources available to the school, and settings dedicated to training for patient care may well have the best available resources for training in health care service delivery. Sufficient numbers of faculty of appropriate background and orientation, clinical resources, access to research populations and resources, and the very important element of socialization into the profession through association with peers and mentors with the same interests must be carefully and continually evaluated in any program, be it traditional or innovative, predoctoral or postdoctoral. The accreditation mechanisms needed to monitor these issues promise to be expensive, with little hope of any substantial support other than from the programs themselves. Responsible professional schools, as well as health psychology programs in other settings, will participate in and support this evaluative effort. The need to reinforce that responsibility is crucial, and it can only be met by cooperative efforts among educators in all settings, credentialing agencies, and professional organizations. They must maintain standards and publicize them widely to the public, to prospective students, and to employers. Cultivation of communication and coordination among elements of this net must be a top priority of the profession from the outset. That seems the best guarantee available of quality in educational efforts wherever they occur.

REFERENCES

American Psychological Association. 1983. *Accreditation Handbook.* Washington, D.C.

Callan, J. E., D. R. Peterson, and G. Stricker. 1986. *Quality in professional psychology training.* Washington, D.C.: American Psychological Association.

Grzesiak, R. C. 1983. Employment opportunities in health psychology: Three and one-half years of "Monitor" advertisements. In *Sourcebook in health psychology,* edited by C. D. Belar and C. Swencionis. Washington, D.C.: American Psychological Association.

Korman, M. 1974. National conference on levels and patterns of professional training in psychology. *American Psychologist* 29: 414–49.

McNamara, J. R., N. F. Jones, A. G. Barclay. 1982. Contemporary professional psychology. In *Critical issues, developments and trends in professional psychology,* edited by J. R. McNamara and A. G. Barclay. New York: Praeger.

Schofield, W. 1982. Clinical psychology in transition: The evolution of a profession. In *Critical issues, developments and trends in professional psychology,* edited by J. R. McNamara and A. G. Barclay. New York: Praeger.

Snepp, F. 1979. An interview with the Dean of the Graduate School of Applied and Professional Psychology. *Rutgers Professional Psychology Review* 1 (1): 2–3.

Wellner, A. M., ed. 1978. *Educating and credentialing in psychology.* Washington, D.C.: American Psychological Association.

37

Health Psychology in the Twenty-first Century

The Editors

An attempt to look into the future is, to the novice, at first intriguing and even exciting, but when the first idle thoughts have been jotted down and the realization dawns that one is going to have to produce many pages of plausible and even substantiated forecasts, the intrigue turns to anxiety, with terror lurking not far away. The feeling is compounded as one looks at the predictions made ten to twenty years ago and sees how wildly off the mark they often are. To bind anxiety, one sets about the task methodically, seeking a scheme of constraints that can make the task manageable.

This was the process by which we approached the writing of this chapter. We read a number of sources that discussed the world of tomorrow, the future of health care, and speculations on the next developments in psychology. Working from a systems perspective, we listed a dozen domains of society, the health system, and the science and discipline of psychology that will surely affect the future of health psychology (see table 37.1). The causal pathways linking these domains to each other and to health psychology are without doubt extraordinarily complex, and it is probably just as well to think of everything as being linked to everything else directly and reciprocally and thus implicitly through all possible indirect paths. Since we are unable to consider all of the possible paths in this system, we can choose more or less arbitrarily those that appear interesting to follow, and that is what we have done here.

Consider the list of domains presented in table 37.1. If in each domain there were only three issues of importance, and if the possible futures of each of those issues could be reduced to a binary alternative (e.g., nuclear war or no nuclear war), we would nevertheless be faced with the possibility of over 70 billion (2^{36}) futures from which to choose. In spite of the obvious impossibility of its being correct, a set of predictive assumptions was made concerning these twelve domains, and they were used to generate specific predictions about the future of health psychology. The results of this process were then circulated among the editors for their critique and emendation. Thus we arrived at a set of predictions that at least five of the eight of us think are more likely than not to characterize health psychology in the year 2010, a date only barely into the twenty-first century, but one beyond which even the foolhardy are loathe to venture with specific statements.

Basic Assumptions Regarding the World as a Whole

The one assumption that must be made if there are to be any sensible predictions about health psychology throughout the world is that there will be no large scale nuclear war. The editors are all agreed that the other alternative leads to a desolated, savage, and unpredictable world in which scholarly and professional work would be impossible. This no-war assumption appears to us to rest on another assumption which falls within the domain of political/ economic systems, that there will be a shift away from confrontational, militaristic, and terrorist efforts to secure advantages for small segments of the world's population and toward a global consciousness and commitment to sharing and preserving the resources of the earth. We don't expect this shift to be completed within the quarter century ahead but to be well underway and to represent the dominant viewpoint in most of the major world powers.

While the majority of the people in the most powerful nations will increasingly be approaching the world's problems from the perspective of what is good for the earth, its people, and its ecology, the problem of terrorism by individuals, factions, and even small and unstable nations may still be a serious threat and could in fact constitute a major health problem. The alienation and fanaticism that underlie terrorist activities will have to be addressed as are predispositions to disease, and our human propensity to "blame the victim" will need to be kept in mind as we do so.

World population growth rates will have declined, although the total population of the earth will still be increasing. In the technologically developed nations, growth rates will be near to zero, and there will even be shrinking populations in some areas. The older segments of the population will be growing markedly, while the number in the thirty to sixty age range will be small. By contrast, in areas where growth rates are still high, populations will have large excesses of children and young adults. The total population of the earth will be about 6.9 billion, of whom 5.6 billion (81 percent) will be residents of the poor and underdeveloped areas. Corresponding figures for 1984 are 4.8 billion and 3.6 billion (75 percent) (Statistical Abstract 1985).

TABLE 37.1 Domains of Variables that Will Influence the Future of Health Psychology

1. Demographic characteristics of populations
2. Availability of resources
3. State of technology
4. Political/economic systems in place
5. Public beliefs, attitudes, behaviors
6. Health problems to which resources are allocated
7. Financing of health care services
8. Health care delivery practices
9. Health values and beliefs of the public
10. Psychological theory
11. Psychological methods
12. Social context of psychology

The pressures of this greatly expanded population come up against critical limitations on the earth's resources. Energy from nuclear fusion will still not be available in commercial quantities, although its feasibility will have been demonstrated, and it will be reckoned as becoming a major source within another generation. Solar power, collected in desert areas and beamed to population centers will be a growing source, and pilot projects to study the cost effectiveness of collecting power in space will be underway. Thus, the world's energy problems will appear to be on the verge of solution. The major resource problems will be the availability of pure water, clean air, and waste disposal sites. The world will still be skirting the brink of ecological disaster, threatening the viability of fish in the lakes and oceans and of forests and orchards on the land. Critical depletion of the oxygenic capacities of the earth's plant cover will be recognized as a serious possibility, and re-forestation will be a major worldwide commitment. Changes in world climate due to particulate pollution, to increases in carbon dioxide content of the atmosphere, and to large-scale relocation of power and water will be a continuing concern with regard to its impact on agriculture.

Changes in technology will be dominated by four factors: continued reductions in the size and cost of electronic information processing and display equipment, the development and widespread adoption of robotics, great expansion of the capability to transmit power economically over long distances, and vast expansion and application of the potential of genetic engineering in agriculture and the chemical and pharmaceutical industries. The resulting high-technology culture, coupled with the sophisticated control processes that will be required to manage the threat to ecological systems, will require massive improvements in the effectiveness of our educational systems—changes which fortunately we will be able to accomplish with the aid of the electronic media and, particularly, computer-based instruction. Successful implementation of the possibilities in education, however, will depend on our success in improving the social morale of our cultures and our children by gaining widespread acceptance of the humanistic value—sharing and preserving the earth—mentioned above.

Current political and economic systems will be simply unable to accommodate the changes necessary to deal with the problems of the next twenty-five years. Systems based on commands coming from a centralized planning directorate will not be able to match the complexity of the systems that they seek to control, and their commands will prevent effective functioning of the system. Systems based on regulated self-interest will be the victims of various versions of the "tragedy of the commons" (Hardin 1968) and be unable to meet the problems of the global system. Systems that rely on constant growth of personal and military consumption of extracted and manufactured goods to provide full employment cannot succeed in the face of limited resources and automation and robotization. At this stage in its evolution, the global system can only function as a vast collection of hierarchical subsystems aligned and coordinated by a common global purpose. Both ancient and contemporary wisdom of survival provide such a purpose—the well-being of the planet and of all the people on it. We predict (or at least hope) that the world's leaders and the world's people will recognize in time that their primary purposes must be the satisfaction of the survival needs of every human and the provision of the opportunity for intellectual and spiritual growth within the constraints of ecological viability. A necessary implication of this realization will be the need for a massive worldwide shift from resource depleting values (cars, boats, elaborate houses, constant travel) to values that can be realized at greatly reduced costs of material resources (games, scholarship, art, electronic communication, personal services). Coercive control is inherently costly to resources, so that the overtly or covertly coercive systems prevalent in most societies today must evolve toward a basis in educated consensus. In the short run, it will probably be necessary to increase the use of individual incentives ("bottle laws"), tax incentives, and outright coercion (limits on the fuel consumption of engines), but these measures will be coupled with educational programs that will, over a period of years, lead to internalized control.

The various kinds of changes described in the preceding paragraphs are clearly reciprocally interdependent with the beliefs, attitudes, and behaviors of the world's people. Great changes in these human attributes are implied, and one may well question whether the necessary changes can occur within the span of the few years over which our forecasts are made. Our assertion that they can is based in part on evidence that massive changes in ideology do occur quickly under certain circumstances and on our belief that the circumstances of the next quarter century will be such as to foster great change. At the individual level, these dramatic changes go by the name of "conversion" or "transformation" (Snow and Machalek 1984).

Substantial shifts can also occur in large groups or segments of populations as well (Funkenstein 1978). There is some tendency, on the part of those who observe them but do not take part, to fear such changes. This fear is understandable for those who are vested in preserving conditions as they are, but the fear as well as the processes of change will be studied by those who recognize the need for radical change. These fears will lead to substantially exacerbated polarization between those who are narrowly focused on the benefits of technology, adherents of an antitechnological reaction, and an ultimately ascendant, synthesizing group that opts for technology in the service of the emerging ecological and human values.

These, then, are some of the major changes we anticipate in the world in general. They will affect health psychology in three ways: directly, through their effects on the lives of health psychologists, and indirectly, through their effects on the health system and through their effects on the development of psychological theory and methods. We turn next to a consideration of changes we anticipate in the health system.

Changes in the Health System

At the outset of this section, we want to make clear that we view the health system broadly and in particular that we see it as including but being much more than the health care system. We build on the broad definition of chapter 3, which includes, in addition to the various components of the health care system, the environmental hazards to our health, the resources used to combat these hazards and overcome their ill effects, and the institutions by which resources are allocated to these tasks and by which health behaviors (both positive and negative) are fostered as well as the various behaviors involved in participating in health care as a patient. We include also the opportunities that exist for developing a reserve of health—a potential to resist the impact of health hazards (Audy 1971; Schwartz 1984) and to move toward "salutogenesis" and "behavioral health" (Antonovsky 1979; Matarazzo 1980).

From this perspective, it appears that the greatest change to be expected in the years ahead is a shift in the allocation of resources from the present focus on extending the lives of older persons in affluent societies to providing the basis for healthy lives to poor but younger people in poor countries. This shift will not necessarily mean that renal dialysis and coronary bypass surgery will become unavailable to the affluent, since these health care services are not heavy users of material resources. At least 77 percent of the costs of a bypass operation go directly to pay for the services of health care personnel; 8 percent to pay for the labor used in manufacturing hospital supplies and constructing the health care facilities used, another 8 percent for interest and other direct expenses, and only about 7 percent to the tangible resources used (based on figures derived from California Health Facilities Commission 1983; and Cohen, Solnick, and Stephensen 1982). The resource shift does mean that there will be massive increases in world resources assigned to prenatal and infant care in the underdeveloped areas and to the elimination of the debilitating endemic diseases that afflict millions and rob them of much of their capacity to build sound life-styles—diseases such as malaria and schistosomiasis. In 1980, there were about 100,000 coronary bypass operations performed in the United States (Rapaport, 1982) at an average cost of about $20,000 (Cohen, et al, 1982). The cost of this surgery, for 100,000 Americans, is probably more than the combined expenditures for control of malaria, which caused more than a million infant deaths in tropical Africa each year in the 1970s, and schistosomiasis, which is believed to affect 200 million (World Health Organization 1981). In a world where the welfare of *all* humans is an overriding goal, there must be a proportionate shift in the resources allocated to these problems.

In the interest of gaining the resources for the shift described above, as well as to accommodate the widely held view that health care constitutes too large a share of our gross national product, there will be continuing emphasis on cost containment coupled with a growing focus on prevention rather than cure of illness. Cost containment in the United States will be approached both by altering the organization of health care delivery sites and by changing the methods of payment for health care services. There will be increased use of health care teams, with more and more procedures performed by subprofessionals with technological support (Maxmen 1976; Tarlov 1983). The sacred role of physicians, weakened already by increasing specialization and reliance on high technology, will be further undermined by computer-based diagnostic systems that can be operated by technicians to outperform the most highly skilled physician working without such support. Robotic support will make exquisitely sophisticated surgical procedures much more widely available. These factors together with overt economic pressures will shift physicians' incomes toward parity with those of other persons with postgraduate educations.

Expansion of cost containment mechanisms such as Diagnostic Related Groups (DRGs) will provide incentive for health care providers to move toward prepaid medical care as a means of controlling costs arising from a small percentage of all individuals (Anders et al. 1983). Then differential rates for persons who practice good health behaviors will permit sharing of health care costs in a way that emphasizes personal responsibility. Court challenges to this concept will lead to a codification by insurance companies and health maintenance organizations of risk factors that can and cannot be significantly influenced by personal actions.

Charges for health care or insurance will be only one of the factors associated with increasing participation in health-promoting and self-care activities. The general shift toward an appreciation of ecological systems will foster holistic health values, as will the increased valuation of nonmaterial aspects of well-being. Many health clubs, support groups, and guidance services will be formed to take advantage of this trend. Personal health focus is likely to link with the antitechnology attitude that will be prevalent in the early part of the period. As a part of the widespread synthesizing response, there will be a very marked increase in the emphasis on humanistic use of medical technology. Humanistic/technological health care will build on the basis of fostering autonomy and responsibility in patients. Providers will perform skillful and complex procedures and make increasingly subtle discriminations with the aid of computers and robotic extensions of their capacities for exquisitely precise manipulation. The technological support available to providers will enable them to spend more time with patients in education and values clarification.

Bioethics will become increasingly central as the capacity to diverge from "natural processes" continues to grow (Mankin 1983). It will be necessary to come to grips with the question regarding the minimum quality of life that warrants its prolongation. Criteria providing justification for genetic manipulations will be necessary. The rights of individuals to refuse treatment become more critical to specify as the results of those treatments increase in predictability and efficacy. In a closely similar vein, the rights of individuals to choose their treatment and to take responsibility for their own health care become more consequential as expert knowledge of probable outcomes of treatment choices become more precise.

Along with the trend toward life-style changes as a means of promoting health there will be much strengthening of the commitment by communities and governments to eliminate health hazards from our environment. The trends begun in the past decade with assaults on dioxin, PCBs, pesticides, and herbicides will be extended. Passive restraints in automobiles will become mandatory, smoking in public places will be banned, government subsidies to tobacco growers will be ended, discharge of polluted wastes into air and water will be strictly controlled, driving under the influence of intoxicants will be more severely punished than it is presently. By the year 2010, the idea that one person can deliberately endanger the health of others for profit or self-indulgence will be unthinkable. On the other hand, the concept of choice between alternative risks will be much more widely appreciated—the notion that to reduce some risks we must be willing to increase others.

What Lies Ahead in Psychology?

Large gains in psychological competence and theoretical grasp will rest on a modified paradigm that synthesizes several of the quasi-paradigms of the present. The debates over whether behavior is genetically programmed through evolutionary processes (e.g., Wilson 1975), or operantly conditioned by the contingencies that our social world presents us (Skinner 1953), or arises from meanings developed through cultural evolution (Mead 1953), or results from complex influences of social forces that *construct* the individual out of their interplay (Henriques et al. 1984) will give way to a synthesizing recognition that we are influenced at all of these levels of determination. The substitution of intentional self-control for programming by biological, environmental, cultural, political, or economic factors will be recognized as a principal aspect of human development, both historically and in the lives of individual humans. Increasing the scope of such intentional control by individuals will be recognized as the primary objective of parenting, education, and psychotherapy. This recognition will be accompanied by the recognition that the self-knowledge and self-consciousness of humans establish a boundary—a watershed—between the biological and the human sciences that requires different research approaches at the two levels. The science of unconscious, unreflective systems is inherently different from science that deals effectively with systems that are aware of their nature. It will be widely accepted that Gergen's (1982) critique of experimental method in psychology was basically sound, although applicable only to relatively well-informed and unconstrained humans. Given this recognition, the value of experimental studies for clarifying processes at the different levels of influence will be recognized by those who focus their work at "higher" levels. Within this multilevel paradigm for the study of human psychology we will thus be able to gain in our understanding of the processes at each level and of their complex and subtle interactions.

The Future of Health Psychology

In our view, health psychology is the application of the knowledge and competence of all of psychology to the problems of the health system. In this final section, therefore, we must restate briefly what we have predicted for the health system and for psychology. We predicted that the health system of the twenty-first century will be dominated by a philosophy, both in our own country and throughout the world, calling for good health for all of the world's people to be achieved through a combination of the removal of health hazards from the environment, strong support for and even mandating of health promoting behaviors, and health care supported by an extremely sophisticated technology that displaces, to a considerable degree, the highly skilled and knowledgeable practitioners of our day. Psychology will have developed an integrated view of humankind in which each individual is seen as seeking to develop the capacity to choose a life-style increasingly freed from the constraints of biology, conditioning, the irrational forces of the unconscious, and the coercion of social forces and institutions. The distinction between mental health and physical health will have largely disappeared, and health will be recognized as the personal capacity to pursue one's goals unhampered by malfunctions of mind or body. Rather than viewing rationality as the effective pursuit of the socially approved or as an illusory ideal or delusion of humankind, we will see it as a boundary condition descriptive of choices that can be made when values are clear, probabilities of contingencies accurately represented, and psychological constraints at a minimum.

Against this background, the primary activity of health psychologists will be the fostering of the engagement of individuals with the developmental process and assisting them in discovering how to overcome the obstacles to their individual development. Both research and practice will be called for in this endeavor. Both technological interventions, such as increasingly sophisticated biofeedback, and educational and counseling approaches will be significantly expanded. Health psychologists in the United States and in other developed countries will study the impacts of beliefs and values on the health of those who hold them. The capacity of beliefs, values, and subsequent behavior to mediate the impact of hazards will continue to be a major aspect of such work, and much more explicitly so than it now is. Since the possible variations in beliefs and values appear to have no limit, this activity would be one that could continue indefinitely, although it might eventually become quite routine.

The major changes in the health system that we have forecast may be largely complete in the "first world" countries by 2010. During the years when they are taking place there will be much need for psychological assistance to members of the professions whose roles are undergoing drastic change. Design and guidance of retraining programs will call for the participation of many psychologists.

The project of bringing health to all of the world's people will be in full swing in the early part of the twenty-first century. This enterprise will require a massive involvement of the world's psychologists working in conjunction with philosophers, anthropologists, and others in adapting the developmental ideal so that it makes a proper interface with the great variety of human cultures. Although in the early stages this project will often appear as no more than the continuation of the trend toward "Westernization of the underdeveloped," a much more sensitive approach will emerge that uncouples the concept of the development of human consciousness and freedom from the high technology and particularly from the consumerist values that have been dominant during the past century in Western countries. A significant aspect of this movement will follow from the widespread recognition that most of the world's cultures embody the development ideal in some form, so that what transpires will be a linking up of those strands in a context of mutual respect and the dissemination of the ideal much more widely within every culture. In this movement, the concept of health will play a key role, since it is a universally recognized value that varies little from one culture to another.

Within our own culture, there will be a great growth of entrepreneurial facilities—health clubs and the like—devoted to the fostering of the health ideal. Mutual support groups and growth groups will also flourish, and many of them may employ professionally trained guidance personnel to foster their work.

Psychologists trained in health will also be needed to study and treat the consequences of the intensified emphasis on self-regulation. For example, some have suggested that attributing greater control to people in their self-care may lead to their erroneously blaming themselves for causing their health problems, which would lead to guilt and distress (Millman 1980). Certainly, work will be needed to understand the parameters of effective self-management within the coming technocratic era.

Coda

As was said at the beginning of this chapter, specific predictions are very likely to be wrong and general trends almost as likely to be so. Professional futurists deal not in such predictions, but in scenarios—alternative pictures of what the world *might* be like. In our own modest venture into the future, we have really presented only a single scenario, and a very optimistic one. It is based upon a very fundamental assumption which gives it a good chance of being generally if not specifically accurate. This assumption is that, to the extent the future is predictable (that is, to the extent it isn't dominated by unpredictable natural catastrophes such as the earth's being struck by a massive meteor), it is shaped by human beliefs about what is possible and what is desirable. Starting from this assumption, we have taken the position that, technologically, much is possible but that recognition of the limits of the earth's resources will become a dominant constraint within the period of our forecast. Psychologically, we have assumed that people *can* change quickly when the need to do so is made clear. In the sphere of values, we believe that preservation of the species and of our earth are recognized as fundamental goals of virtually all of those who have conceptualized these goals as possible. Finally, we have assumed that a value, whether instrumental or ultimate, for the sharing of opportunity among all humans will become dominant within the next generation.

The forms of our optimism are apparent. The alternative assumption with regard to any of the six propositions would have grave implications for the future health of our earth and its people. Since human beliefs tend to be self-confirming, we invite our readers to join us in these healthy beliefs and in their dissemination.

REFERENCES

Anders, G. T., L. C. Beck, D. R. Sweeney, and J. T. Martin. 1983. Looking ahead: Medical practice in the future. *Pennsylvania Medicine* 86 (no. 9): 43–46.

Antonovsky, A. 1979. *Health, stress, and coping.* San Francisco: Jossey-Bass.

Audy, J. R. 1971. Measurement and diagnosis of health. In *Environ/Mental,* edited by P. Shepard and D. McKinley. Boston: Houghton Mifflin.

California Health Facilities Commission. 1983. *Aggregate hospital data for California: Report period ending June 30, 1981—June 29, 1982.* (CHFC Report II–83–9). Sacramento, CA: California Health Facilities Commission.

Cohen, H., M. Solnick, and A. Stephensen. 1982. The financing of coronary by-pass surgery. *Circulation* 66 (Suppl. 3): III-49–58.

Funkenstein, D. H. 1978. *Medical students, medical schools, and society during five eras: Factors affecting the career choices of physicians 1958–1976.* Cambridge, MA: Ballinger.

Gergen, K. 1982. *Toward transformation in social knowledge.* New York: Springer-Verlag.

Hardin, G. 1968. The tragedy of the commons. *Science* 162:1243–48.

Henriques, J., W. Hollway, C. Urwin, C. Venn, and V. Walkerdine. 1984. *Changing the subject: Psychology, social regulation, and subjectivity.* New York: Methuen.

Mankin, H. J. 1983. Orthopaedics in 2013: A prospection. *The Journal of Bone and Joint Surgery* 65-a (no. 8): 1190–94.

Matarazzo, J. D. 1980. Behavioral health and behavioral medicine: Frontiers for a new health psychology. *American Psychologist* 35:807–17.

Maxmen, J. S. 1976. *The post-physician era: Medicine in the twenty-first century.* New York: John Wiley & Sons.

Mead, M. 1953. National character. In *Anthropology today,* edited by A. L. Kroeber. Chicago: University of Chicago Press.

Millman, M. 1980. *Such a pretty face.* New York: Norton.

Rapaport, E. 1982. An overview of issues. *Circulation* 66 (Suppl. 3): III-3–5.

Schwartz, G. E. 1984. President's column. *The Health Psychologist* 6(2): 1–2.

Skinner, B. F. 1953. *Science and human behavior.* New York: Appleton, Century, Croft.

Snow, D. A., and R. Machalek. 1984. The sociology of conversion. *Annual Review of Sociology* 10:167–90.

Statistical Abstract. 1985. Washington, D.C.: U.S. Bureau of the Census.

Tarlov, A. 1983. Shattuck lecture—The increasing supply of physicians, the changing structure of the health services system, and the future practice of medicine. *The New England Journal of Medicine* 308:1235–44.

Wilson, E. 1975. *Sociobiology: The new synthesis.* Cambridge, MA: Harvard University Press, Belknap Press.

World Health Organization. 1981. *Global strategy for health for all by the year 2000.* Geneva: World Health Organization.

———. 1982. *Seventh general programme of work.* Geneva: World Health Organization.

Contributors

David B. Abrams
Assistant Professor of Psychiatry and Human Behavior
Brown University Program in Medicine
Providence, RI 02906

Nancy Adler
Professor of Medical Psychology
Health Psychology Program
Department of Psychiatry
School of Medicine
University of California, San Francisco
San Francisco, CA 94143

David G. Altman,
Associate Director
Health Promotion Resource Center
Stanford Center for Research in Disease Prevention
Stanford University
Stanford, CA 94305

Norman B. Anderson
Assistant Medical Research Professor
Department of Psychiatry
Duke University Medical Center
Durham Veterans' Administration Medical Center
Durham, NC 27710

Cynthia Belar
Chief Psychologist and Clinical Director of Behavioral Medicine
Kaiser Permanente Medical Care Programs
Los Angeles, CA 90027

Thomas Boll
Professor and Director of Medical Psychology Program
Department of Psychology
University of Alabama
Birmingham, AL 35294

Jerry Cahn
Chief Executive Officer
Brilliant Image
New York, NY

Patrick H. DeLeon
Executive Assistant to Hon. Daniel Inouye
U.S. Senate
Washington, D.C. 20510

Jean R. Eagleston
Research Associate
Health Behavior Research Program
Center for Educational Research (CERAS)
Stanford University
Stanford, CA 94305

Ruth R. Faden
Professor
Department of Health Policy and Management
School of Hygiene and Public Health
Johns Hopkins University
Baltimore, MD 21205

Michael J. Follick
Associate Professor of Psychiatry
Brown University Program in Medicine

Director, Clinical Psychology Internship
  Consortium
The Miriam Hospital
Providence, RI 02906

Wilbert E. Fordyce
Professor
Rehabilitation Medicine and Pain Service
University of Washington School of Medicine
Seattle, WA 98195

Joanne L. Fowler
Clinical Assistant Professor of Psychiatry
Brown University Program in Medicine
The Miriam Hospital
Providence, RI 02906

Johanna Freedman
Staff Member, Bush Center
Department of Psychology
Yale University
New Haven, CT 06520

Howard S. Friedman
Professor of Psychology
Department of Psychology
University of California, Riverside
Riverside, CA 92521

Robinsue Frohboese
Special Litigation Section
Civil Rights Division
United States Department of Justice
Washington, D.C. 20534

Margaret Gatz
Professor
Department of Psychology
University of Southern California
Los Angeles, CA 90089-1061

Judy E. Hall
Executive Secretary
State Board for Psychology
New York State Education Department
Cultural Education Center
Albany, NY 12230

Daniel A. Hatton
Department of Medical Psychology

School of Medicine
Oregon Health Sciences University
Portland, OR 97201

Joseph Istvan
Department of Medical Psychology
School of Medicine
Oregon Health Sciences University
Portland, OR 97201

James S. Jackson
Research Scientist and Professor of
  Psychology
Institute for Social Research
The University of Michigan
Ann Arbor, MI 48106

Mary A. Jansen
Dean for Professional Affairs
California School of Professional Psychology
Fresno, CA 93721

Nelson F. Jones
Professor and Director
School of Professional Psychology
University of Denver
Denver, CO 80208-0208

Ronald B. Kurz
Independent Practice
5401 Westbard Avenue
Bethesda, MD 20816

Gilbert Levin
Professor
Department of Epidemiology and Social
  Medicine
Department of Psychiatry
Albert Einstein College of Medicine
Bronx, NY 10461

Joseph D. Matarazzo
Department of Medical Psychology
School of Medicine
Oregon Health Sciences University
Portland, OR 97201

Karen A. Matthews
Associate Professor of Psychiatry,
  Epidemiology and Psychology

University of Pittsburgh School of Medicine
Department of Psychiatry
Western Psychiatric Institute and Clinic
Pittsburgh, PA 15213

Manfred J. Meier
Professor and Director of Health Psychology
Clinic and Neuropsychology Laboratory
University of Minnesota, School of Medicine
Minneapolis, MN 55455

Neal E. Miller
Department of Psychology
Yale University
and Emeritus Professor
The Rockefeller University
New Haven, CT 06520-7447

Paul D. Nelson
Accreditation Officer
American Psychological Association
Washington, D.C. 20036

Thomas D. Overcast
Partner in the firm of White, Overcast and
  Thomas
Edmonds, WA 98020

Cynthia G. Pearson
Lecturer
Department of Psychology
University of Southern California
Los Angeles, CA 90089-1061

Nathan Perry
Chair
Department of Clinical Psychology
University of Florida
Gainesville, FL 32610

Rodger P. Pinto
Director of Behavioral Medicine
Behavioral Counseling Associates
Ormond Beach, FL 32074

Judith Rodin
Professor
Department of Psychology
Yale University
New Haven, CT 06520

Neil Schneiderman
Professor of Psychology and Biomedical
  Engineering
University of Miami
Coral Gables, FL 33124

Lee Sechrest
Chair, Department of Psychology
University of Arizona
Tucson, AZ 85721

Judith M. Siegel
Associate Professor of Public Health
Division of Behavioral Sciences and Health
  Education
School of Public Health
University of California, Los Angeles
Los Angeles, CA 90024

Jerome E. Singer
Chair, Department of Medical Psychology
Uniformed Services University of the Health
  Sciences
Bethesda, MD 20814

George S. Stone
Professor of Medical Psychology
Health Psychology Program
Department of Psychiatry
School of Medicine
University of California, San Francisco
San Francisco, CA 94143-0844

Bonnie R. Strickland
Professor of Psychology
Department of Psychology
University of Massachusetts at Amherst
Amherst, MA 01003

Charles Swencionis
Assistant Professor of Epidemiology & Social
  Medicine, and Psychiatry
Albert Einstein College of Medicine
Bronx, NY 10461

Shelley E. Taylor
Professor of Psychology
Director, Health Psychology Program
University of California, Los Angeles
Los Angeles, CA 90024

Carl E. Thoresen
Professor of Education and Psychology
School of Education
Stanford University
Stanford, CA 94305

Edison Trickett
Professor of Psychology
Department of Psychology
University of Maryland
College Park, MD 20742

Steven Tulkin
Chief Psychologist
Kaiser Permanente Medical Center
Hayward, CA 94545

Gary R. VandenBos
Associate Executive Director
American Psychological Association
Washington, D.C. 20036

Wendy Weicker
Graduate Trainee
Department of Psychology
University of Southern California
Los Angeles, CA 90089-1061

Stephen M. Weiss
Chief, Behavioral Medicine Branch
National Heart Lung and Blood Institute
National Institutes of Health
Bethesda, MD 20205

Camille Wortman
Professor of Psychology
Institute for Social Research
University of Michigan
Ann Arbor, MI 48106

Index

Abboud, F. M., 271
Abdellah, F. G., 321
Abdominal pain, 212
Abortion counseling, 225
Abrahams, J. P., 363
Abrams, David B., 137, 139, 140, 143, 145, 146
Academy of Behavioral Medicine Research, 22–23, 61
Accidents, in children, 291, 297
Accreditation, 43, 113, 125, 322, 331, 413–23; in allied health professions, 473–74; defined, 52–53; and health psychology as specialty, 55, 56; of internships, 196–97, 200, 340, 346–47, 353; issues in, relating to health psychology, 420–23; philosophy and practices of, 414–15; of postdoctoral programs, 194–97, 200, 382–83, 386; of predoctoral programs, 197–98, 338–39, 346–48; of schools of professional psychology, 507–11; standards and criteria for, 417–20
Accreditation Handbook, of APA, 339–40, 345, 418, 509n
Achterberg-Lawlis, J., 124
Acute illness model, 287
Adams, D. F., 270
Adaptation principle, 153, 156–57, 160
Adelphi University Institute of Advanced Studies, 507–8, 510
Adenocarcinoma of the vagina, 482
Adiar, John, 266
Adler, N. E., 24, 95, 97, 99, 234, 340
Administration: employment opportunities in, 233, 234, 237–39; training for, 399–400

Adolescents, 497–99
Advisory councils, 94
Aged, health problems of, 247, 303–16
Age Discrimination Act, 221
Aid for Families with Dependent Children, 238
Albino, J. E., 155–56
Alcohol, Drug Abuse, and Mental Health Administration (ADAMHA), 80
Alcoholism, 3–4; programs for, 220, 222, 223, 482–83
Alderman, M., 138
Alexander, C. B., 123
Alexander, F. G., 272, 288
Alexander, H., 295
Alexion, N. G., 141
Allied Health Professional Personnel Training Act, 474
Allied health profession schools, 450, 473–80
Altemeier, W. A., 291
Altman, David G., 232
Alzheimer's disease, 306, 313, 314
American Association for the Advancement of Science, 182
American Association of State Psychology Boards (AASPB), 48–53, 194, 198, 382
American Board of Professional Psychology (ABPP), 54–57, 192–94, 198, 199, 372, 373, 382, 384, 385, 410
American Cancer Association, 367
American Cancer Society, 70
American College of Obstetricians and Gynecologists, 252
American Dental Association, 241
American Heart Association, 70, 80, 84, 367; Council on Epidemiology, 241

American Hospital Association, 138
American Medical Association, 473–74
American Medical Student Association, 180
American Orthopsychiatric Association, 241
American Psychological Association (APA),
125, 378, 474, 476; and abortion counseling, 225; *Accreditation Handbook,*
339–40, 345, 418, 509n; on aging,
312–13; Congressional Fellowship Program, 179; on continuing education,
199–200, 406–8, 410–12; on employment of psychologists, 233, 234; "Ethical
Principles of Psychologists," 203–25; and
health policy, 179, 181, 182, 389, 400–
401; on internships, 196–97, 329, 352–
53; on medicine and psychology, relationship between, 18; postdoctoral program
accreditation by, 197–98; predoctoral
training and curriculum standards of,
43–58, 192–98, 414–23, 445; and professional schools of psychology, 506–10;
on respecialization, 405, 411; on specialties in psychology, 43, 53–58, 338,
372, 383–86, 410; survey on training
backgrounds by, 325–26, 328, 329; Task
Force on Health Research, 20–21, 35, 61,
454; Task Force on Evaluation of Education, Training, and Practice, 400–401;
Task Force on Legal Issues, 217
——, Division of Health Psychology, 4–5,
122, 182, 203; establishment of, 4, 21–
22, 56, 58, 61; health psychology defined
by, 16, 27
American Psychologist, 20, 390
American Public Health Association, 241,
265, 266
American Society of Allied Health Profes-
sions (ASAHP), 474
American Telephone & Telegraph Company,
138
Anders, G. T., 519
Anderson, D. C., 330
Anderson, David E., 85
Anderson, J. E., 290
Anderson, K. O., 100
Anderson, Norman B., 271
Anderson, O., 266
Anderson, R., 266
Aneshensel, C. S., 251, 259, 260
Animal experimentation, 10–11; in applied

research, 111; in basic research, 78,
83–84; ethics of, 214; legal considerations
in, 223–24
Animal Welfare Act, 224
Annual Review of Public Health, 171
Anorexia nervosa, 294
Antonovsky, A., 260, 517
Anxiety, and asthma, 289
APA Monitor, 234
Apprenticeships, 46–47, 322, 341, 351–60;
and assessment centers, 408; development
of, 351–52, 372–73; and employment,
235, 240; in health policy, 396; recom-
mendations concerning, 354–58. *See
also* Internship programs
Arden House Conference. *See* National
Working Conference on Education and
Training in Health Psychology
Army Air Force Program, 11–12
Arnett, J., 69
Arons, S., 222
Arthritis, 123, 305
Ashmore, R. D., 235
Asian Americans, 265, 266
Asken, M. J., 329, 454
Assessment: in child health psychology,
291–94; ethics of, 213
Assessment centers. *See* Learning and assess-
ment center concept
Association for Fitness in Business, 241
Association of Psychology Internship Centers
(APIC), 329, 382
Association for the Advancement of Psychol-
ogy (AAP), 48–49, 400
Association of Academic Health Centers,
467
Association of Schools of Public Health
(ASPH), 166
Asthma, 123, 288–89, 296
Atchley, R. C., 305
Atkins, C. J., 95
Atkinson, Richard, 180
Attention deficit disorders, 292–93
Audy, J. R., 517
Avis, N. E., 72, 236, 484
Azrin, N. H., 296
Ajzen, I., 95

Babbitt, Irving, 458
Bandura, A., 83, 95

Baquet, C., 266, 268
Barcai, A., 296
Barry, P. Z., 168
Baruch, D. W., 288
Batchelor, W. F., 181, 475
Bauer, R. B., 139, 296
Baum, A., 122, 169, 265, 275
Baylor University, 327–28, 508
Beauchamp, D. E., 168
Beezley, P., 295
Behavioral assessment of children, 294
Behavioral cardiology research, doctoral program with emphasis in, 443–45
Behavioral medicine, 22–23, 77, 330; concept of, 61–63; doctoral programs with emphasis in, 431–33; employment in, 234
Behavioral sciences, training in, 485, 486
Behavior therapy, 221, 295–96
Belar, Cynthia D., 68, 326–30, 332, 335, 339, 340, 361, 363, 371, 375, 420, 421, 425, 426, 445 n, 448, 459, 462
Benjamin, L. T., Jr., 232
Benne, K. D., 397
Bennis, W. G., 397
Benson, D. F., 306
Benson, H., 142, 276
Bereavement, 93–94
Berger vs. Board of Psychologist Examiners, 48
Berkman, L. F., 171, 275, 303, 312, 313
Berman, A. J., 10
Berman, J., 222
Bernstein, A., 122–23, 251
Bernstein, B., 250
Berry, R. E., 4
Bersoff, D., 225
Besdine, R. W., 310
Beta blockers, 276
Bevan, W., 175, 178
Bibace, R., 69
Billington, R. J., 159
Binner, P. R., 144–45
Bioethics, 519
Biofeedback, 11, 93, 125, 142, 212, 276
Biostatistics, 71, 485
Birth control. *See* Contraception
Bjurstrom, L. A., 141
Blacks: culture and research involving, 154, 156, 157; hypertension in, 65, 85–86,

245–46, 266–78; in U.S. population, 265–66
Blackwell, B., 275
Blakelock, E. H., 273
Blaming the victim, 154, 167–68
Blanchard, Edward, 22, 69
Blazer, D., 304–6
Blendon, Robert, 471
Blitch, C. L., 223
Blumenthal, J. A., 305
Bok, D., 461, 462
Boll, Thomas J., 293–94, 339, 340, 445, 454, 462
Bonk, C., 289
Bordage, G., 36
Borreliz, M., 220
Borysenko, J., 363
Bosmajian, L. S., 123
Bott, E. A., 18
Botwinick, J., 305
Boulder Conference on Graduate Education and Clinical Psychology, 5, 192, 321–22; on internships, 252–53, 358–60; on postdoctoral training, 372–73, 376, 377, 383, 391; and psychology curriculum, 43–47, 57
Boulder model. *See* Scientist-practitioner model
Bowers, W. J., 223
Boyle, E., Jr., 277
Bradley, L. A., 122
Brady, J. V., 10
Bray, D. W., 408
Bricklin, P., 57, 383–85
Brod, J., 270
Brody, E. M., 305, 309
Brogan, D. R., 255
Broman, C. L., 273
Bronfenbrenner, U., 153
Brooks, R. H., 170
Brown, G. W., 260
Brown, R. A., 140
Brown, Roger, 165
Brownell, K. D., 140
Bruch, H., 295
Brucker, B. S., 11
Bruhn, J. G., 483–84
Brunner, H. R., 269
Bry, B. H., 453
Buck, R. L., 18

Bugen, L., 238
Buklad, W., 175
Bullough, B., 266
Bullough, V. L., 266
Bulman, R. J., 100, 103
Burns, W. J., 286
Bush, J. W., 170
Bush Foundation, 391
Bush Programs in Child Development and
  Social Policy, 391
Butler, R. N., 311, 313
Butterfield, E. C., 291

Cafferta, G. L., 251
Cahn, Jerry, 232
California Health Facilities Commission,
  518
California School of Professional Psychology,
  506–8
Callan, J. E., 509
Campbell, Donald T., 91, 114, 157–58, 401
Campbell Soup Company, 138
Cancer, 103, 124; breast, 257; childhood,
  290; in minority groups, 268; uterine,
  252; vaginal, 482
Caplan, G., 132
Caplan, N., 154, 390, 393
Cardiac catheterization, 210
Cardiovascular disease, 62, 92, 327–28,
  331; in aged, 305; ethical issues in treat-
  ment of, 209–10, 214; expenditures for,
  257, 518; in women, 254–55. *See also*
  Coronary heart disease (CHD);
  Hypertension
Cardiovascular reactivity studies, 84–87
Carmen, E., 249, 250
Carmody, T. P., 18, 236, 335, 458, 461
Carpenter, P. B., 175, 177, 178
Carpenter, P. J., 234, 240, 325–26
Carriger, B., 23
Carrington, E. R., 250, 254
Carroll, J. S., 235
Carter, Jimmy, 460
Cartwright, L. K., 36
Cassel, J., 270
Cathcart, L. M., 139
Cattell, J. McKeen, 351
Center for Disease Control, 3
Chadwick, J. H., 138, 140
Chambers, K. T., 224
Charvat, J., 270
Chein, I., 91

Chesney, A. P., 273, 275
Chesney, M. A., 138, 140, 141, 143, 378 n
Chicago Medical School, 438–40, 447
Child psychology, 44, 54, 55, 234, 285–86,
  330–31, 383
Children, 378; abuse and neglect of, 223,
  291, 296–97; health problems of, 246–
  47, 285–98, 498–99
Chin, R., 397
Chlorpromazine, 9, 10, 75
Christie, A. B., 306
Chronic illness, 3, 119, 211, 339; adaptation
  to, 123–24; in aged, 304–5, 313; public
  health research on, 482–84
Churchill, M. P., 290
Ciminero, A. R., 296
Cinciripini, P. M., 123
*City of Akron v. Akron Center for Re-
  productive Health, Inc.*, 225
Civilian Health and Medical Program of the
  Uniform Services (CHAMPUS), 176,
  225–26
Clark, A. H., 257
Clark, L. D., 10
Clark, L. F., 100
Clark, V. A., 251, 259, 260
Clarkson, T. B., 64, 78
Clayman, David A., 21, 22, 234, 240, 325–26
Cleary, P. D., 167, 251, 260
Clinical neuropsychology, 328, 329, 372,
  383, 384, 410
Clinical psychology, 19, 374, 495, 496; and
  allied health professions, 473–74; and
  child health psychology, 285, 290, 291;
  development of, as discipline, 44–45,
  54–57, 358–59, 371–72, 384, 415–19;
  internships in, 196, 352, 353; training in,
  as health psychology background, 125,
  131–32, 321–22, 325–29, 338–39, 365,
  420, 427–35, 438–40, 445, 505; treat-
  ment methods in health psychology and,
  205–7
Clinical services. *See* Health care services
Clinics: employment at, 233; training-
  research, 457
Cluss, P. A., 124
Coates, T. J., 71, 167
Cognitive-behavioral therapy, 125
Cognitive functioning, and aging, 305–6
Cohen, F., 24, 36, 101, 234, 340
Cohen, H., 518
Cohen, Louis, 476

Cohort, and aging, 307–8, 310
College of Health Related Professions, at
    University of Florida, 473–79
Collins, D. L., 169
Committee on Allied Health Education and
    Accreditation (CAHEA), 473–74
Committee on Standards of Providers of Psy-
    chological Services (COSPOPS), 383–84
Common law, 217
Communication, 235; between professionals,
    211, 462; patient-practitioner, 253–54; of
    research results, 99–100
Community, 70, 165, 483
Community psychology: ecological meta-
    phor in, 120, 151–62; systems approach
    in, 128
Competence, 204–7, 219
Competency-based training, 407–8, 412
Compliance, 66, 100–101, 124; in aged,
    313–14; in black hypertensives, 275–76;
    in children, 294; research in, 83
Computers, 79, 80, 519
Comroe, J. H., Jr., 75
Conant, J. B., 9, 75
Conference on Education and Credentialling
    in Psychology, 194–96, 336
Confidentiality, 101–2, 208–9, 222, 223
Congressional Fellowship Program, 179
Congressional Research Service, 238
Congressional Science Fellowship, 239
Consumer psychology, 54–55
Contagious diseases, 223
Continuing education, 113–14, 199–200,
    325–26, 403–12
Contraception, 251–52, 257–58
Control, sense of, 314–15
Control Data "Stay Well" program, 143
Converse Rubber Company, 142
Conway, T., 92
Cook, C. A., 276
Cook, T. D., 91
Cooper, C. L., 141
Cooperstock, R., 250
Coronary heart disease (CHD), 167; bypass
    surgery for, 518; public health studies of,
    483–84, 487; worksite programs and risk
    of, 137–46
Corso, A. P., 304
Costa, P., 305, 309
Council for the National Register of Health
    Service Providers in Psychology, 49, 193–
    97, 199

Council of Graduate Departments of Psy-
    chology (COGDOP), 48–52, 57, 382
Counseling psychology, 125, 196, 325–26,
    328–29, 338, 355, 372, 419–20; educa-
    tional model of training for, 495–503
Cousineau, D., 269
Cowen, E. L., 151
Cowley, W. H., 460
Crandall, R. C., 305
Crapo, L. M., 311–12
Crary, W. G., 20
Crawford, R., 168
Credentials, 189, 191–201; beyond entry-
    level, 198–99; continuing education,
    199–200; entry-level, 193–98; postdoc-
    toral research, 365–66. See also Ac-
    creditation; Apprenticeships; Education
    and training; Licensure
Crisis therapy, 125
Crouter, A., 291
Cultural pluralism, 154–56
Cummings, J. L., 306
Curricula. See Education and training
Cycling of resources, 153, 156–57, 160
Cyrs, T. E., 409

Dahl, L. K., 277
Danaher, B. G., 139
Daniel, R. S., 18
Darley, J. M., 237
Davidson, M. J., 141
Davis, C., 69
Dawber, T. R., 254
Deafferented limb experiments, 10
Deafness, in children, 292
Deasy-Spinetta, P., 290
DeBacker, G., 138
de Champlain, J., 269
Deckel, A. W., 169
Dekker, D. M., 289
DeKraai, M. B., 223
DeLeon, Patrick H., 67, 176, 178, 179, 181,
    182, 220, 225, 226, 390
Dell, P., 270
Deltredici, A., 122–23
Dembroski, Theodore, 86, 167
Dementia, in aged, 306
DeMuth, N., 71
Dennis, W., 18
Dentistry, 42, 45, 373, 374
Depression: in aged, 306; following myocar-

dial infarction, 205–6; and women, 249–51, 260

Derryberry, M., 23

DeSantamaria, C., 167

Designation, 56, 331; defined, 52–53; of postdoctoral programs, 382; of professional psychology programs, 507–11; of programs for health service providers, 194–98. *See also* Accreditation

Deuschle, K., 266

Developmental disabilities, 286–87

Developmental psychology, 44, 240, 285, 297

Devereux, R. B., 87

Diabetes, 123, 156, 211, 212, 288, 294

Diagnostic related groups (DRGs), 69, 519

Diamond, E. L., 85

Dickey, F. G., 474

DiMatteo, M. R., 33, 36, 62, 101, 362, 364

DiNicola, D. D., 33, 36, 101

Disease, public health model of, 483. *See also* Health, concept of

Dishman, R. K., 167

Doctor of Philosophy degree. *See* Ph.D. degree

Doctor of Psychology degree. *See* Psy.D. degree

Doleys, D. M., 296

Dörken, H., 69, 175–77, 225

Douglas, B. H., 277

Downing, M. P., 237

Dramaix, M., 138

Drazen, M., 140, 141, 144

Dressel, P. L., 460

Dripps, R. D., 75

Driver education, 497

Drotar, D., 286–87, 295

Drugs and medications: for aged, 313–14; alternatives to, 122–23; programs for abuse of, 222, 223; women's use of, 249–51

Durbeck, D. C., 141

Dwore, R. B., 67, 70, 378 n, 380, 440, 462, 496

Dynes, R. R., 169

Eagleston, Jean R., 494, 499

Ebert-Flatteau, P., 454

Eckstein, J. W., 271

Ecological metaphor, 151–62

Education, schools of, 450–51, 494–503

Education and Credentialling in Psychology, 194–96

Education and training, 3–12, 321–23; in child health psychology, 286–87; and competence, 204–7; continuing, 113–14, 199–200, 325–26, 403–12; current status of, 325–33; in health care services, 116, 117, 124–27, 193–94, 204, 336–41, 356, 358, 371–87, 454–55, 468–70; in health-related disciplines, 62, 71–72; in research, 5–6, 78–80, 107–18, 193–94, 354, 357–58, 361–68, 395–96; for respecialization, 403–5, 411; of women in health care system, 255–56, 260–61. *See also* Accreditation; Apprenticeships; Credentials; Designation; Internship programs; Practica

——, postdoctoral, 204, 322–23, 343; accreditation of, 197–98, 200, 382–83, 386; in allied health setting, 476–78; assessment centers in, 408–9; descriptions of, 330–31; and employment, 236–37; in health policy studies, 389–402; for research, 361–68; in schools of education, 503; in schools of professional psychology, 510; in schools of public health, 488–89; for service providers, 371–87; women in, 260

——, predoctoral, 204, 322–23, 335–48, 373; accreditation of, 194–97, 338–39, 346–48; in allied health setting, 476–77; breadth and depth in, 324–25; curriculum standards for, 41–59, 195–96; descriptions of, 326–29, 425–48; funding of, 329, 400; in schools of education, 499; in schools of professional psychology, 508–9; in schools of public health, 488–89; for service and nonservice providers, 193–94, 336–42

——, sites for, 449–51; academic medical centers, 450, 467–72; allied health professions schools, 450, 473–80; quality of, 374–76; schools of education, 450–51, 494–503; schools of professional psychology, 451, 505–11; schools of public health, 450, 481–91; university departments of psychology, 449–51, 453–62, 446

Edwards, J. D., 235

Ehrenreich, B., 250, 251, 254, 258

Einstein/Ferkauf program, 468
Eland, J. M., 290
Elliott, G. R., 181, 242, 265, 266, 275, 482, 493, 494
Ellsworth, P. C., 95
Elstein, A. S., 36
Emergency care centers, 231, 237
Employment, 190, 231–42, 447; and public health training, 489; training during, 344
Encopresis, 288, 296
Engel, B., 69
Engel, G. E., 121
English, D., 254
Enuresis, 288, 296
Environmental health sciences, 485
Environmental Protection Agency, 80, 238
Epidemiology, 109; psychosocial, 458; training in, 66, 71, 124, 485
Epstein, L. H., 123, 124, 312
Epstein-Barr virus, 483
Erfurt, J., 138
Eron, L., 159
Esler, M., 274
Ethical issues, 6, 189, 519; APA on, 203–15; in health care services, 126; in health policy, 399; in research, 101–3
Ethnic groups. *See* Minority groups
Evaluation Research Society, 241
Evans, A. S., 483
Evans, G. W., 169
Evans, R. W., 220
Evans, Richard I., 22, 167, 204, 327
Ewart, C. K., 95, 167
Experimental psychology, 44, 48, 325–26, 351, 371–72, 443–45
Experimenting society, 401–2
Expert witness, 226
Eyberg, S. M., 294

Faden, A. I., 168
Faden, Ruth R., 168, 170, 484
Fairweather, G. W., 97, 98
Family: and aged, 306, 307, 311, 313; and child health, 291, 292, 294, 295
Family health, training in, 485, 486
Family therapy, 296
Faricy, W. H., 460
Farina, A., 250
Farquar, J. W., 167
Federation of Behavioral, Psychological, and Cognitive Sciences, 182

Feedback groups, 94
Fein, G. G., 168
Feinleib, S. G., 254
Feldman, Robert H. L., 443
Felix, Robert H., 352
Fellowships, 179, 239, 366–67. *See also* Funding
Fenderson, Douglas, 180
Ferguson, J. M., 122
Fertility, 257, 266
Feuerstein, M., 141, 143, 328, 378 n
Filskov, S., 340
Fischoff, B., 168
Fishbein, M., 95
Fisher, T. D., 250
Fishman, D. B., 175, 241
Fleming, R., 169
Flexner, Abraham, 191, 415, 468
Flynn, B. S., 138
Focus groups, 94
Folkow, B., 270
Follick, Michael J., 137, 140, 144–46
Food and Drug Administration, 224
Foot, A., 138
Ford, Gerald, 460
Ford Motor Company, 138, 139
Fordyce, W. E., 123
Forensic psychology, 372, 383, 384, 410
Forest Institute, 508
Foreyt, J. P., 139
Forman, S. G., 179
Fort, Charles, 112–13
Fowler, Joanne L., 140
Fox, R. E., 422
Foxx, R. M., 296
Fozard, J. L., 304
Francis, V., 255
Frank, G. W., 132
Fredericks, A., 84
Fredrikson, M., 270–71
Freedom of Information Acts, 222
French, T. N., 288
Frerichs, R. R., 251, 259, 260
Fretz, B. R., 495
Freud, Sigmund, 352
Friedman, Howard S., 62, 362, 364
Friedman, S., 296
Fries, J. F., 129, 305, 311–12
Frohboese, Robinsue, 127, 179, 226
Fulcher, R., 232, 233
Fuller, J. L., 10

Funding: of academic medical centers, 468, 471; of allied health programs, 474–75; for basic research, 80–82; legal considerations of, 225; of postdoctoral programs, 331, 374, 380–81; of predoctoral programs, 329, 400; of university-based psychology programs, 457–58, 460–61, 462
Funkenstein, D. H., 517

Gable, K., 220
Gaide, M. S., 84
Gaines, R., 291
Galante, N. A., 221
Galanter, R. B., 168
Garbarino, J., 291
Gardner, John, 180
Garmezy, N., 498
Gary, H. E., 273, 275
Gatchel, R. J., 169
Gatz, Margaret, 314
Gellman, M., 84
General Accounting Office, 238
General Foods, 139
Gentry, W. Doyle, 18, 22, 236, 273, 275, 329, 335, 354, 454, 462
Gergen, K., 520
German, M. L., 296
Giamatti, A. B., 461
Gillum, R. T., 267, 269, 277
Gimpl, M. P., 84
Ginsberg, M. R., 175, 183
Givelber, D. J., 223
Glass, D. C., 109, 307
Glass, G. V., 92
Glicksman, A. S., 103
Glidden, R., 414, 418
Gold, J. R., 329–30
Goldberg, R., 124
Golden, C., 328, 329
Goldstein, D. S., 269
Goodstein, L. D., 417
Gove, W., 259
Government employment, 238–39. *See also* Funding
Grabert, J., 285, 330
Gray, V. K., 311
Green, C., 24, 122, 337, 338, 340
Green, L. W., 138, 171
Greenhill, J. P., 250
Gregory, T. G., 185
Griffin, A., 224
Grignolo, A., 83–84

Grim, C. E., 271–72, 277
Groen, J., 289
Grotto, A. M., 139
Group therapy, 125
Grunberg, N. E., 265
Gruppenhoff, J. T., 178
Grzesiak, R. C., 234, 236, 505
Guillion, M. E., 296
Gutman, M., 83
Guyton, A., 269

Hahnemann Medical College, 508
Hall, G. Stanley, 17, 351
Hall, J., 57, 383–85
Hall, Judy E., 126, 203, 215
Hall, R. C. W., 124
Hall, R. P., 273, 275
Hamburg, David A., 23, 70, 181, 242, 265, 266, 275, 482, 493, 494
Hames, C. G., 277
Hamilton, C. A., 269
Hansen, B. A., 132
Harburg, E., 273–76
Hardin, G., 516
Harrel, George, 476
Harris, T., 260
Harrup, T., 132
Hartman, K. A., 36
Hartnett, S. A., 273
Harvard University, 351
Harwood, A., 265
Hastrup, J., 270
Hatch, Thomas D., 475
Hatton, Daniel C., 326
Haug, M. R., 309, 311
Haynes, R. B., 140–41, 145
Haynes, S. G., 254
Hazards, 167–69, 223
Headache, 212; migraine, 122–23
Health, concept of, 17, 28, 30–31, 493–94, 521
Health and Human Service Fellowship, 239
Health behavior, doctoral program with specialization in, 440–43
Health Belief Model, 23
Health care costs, 76, 231–32, 237, 518
Health Care Financing Administration, 238
Health care services, 62, 67–71, 121–34; for aged, 309–10; eligible providers of, 131–32; employment opportunities in, 233, 234, 237–38; institutional barriers to practice of, 128–31; legal restrictions

on, 220–21; public health school training in, 485–86; research versus, 109–11; scope of, 122–24; training and credentials in, 116, 117, 124–27, 193–94, 204, 336–41, 356, 358, 371–87, 454–55, 468–70

Health care system, 6, 32–33, 36; women in, 250–56

Health counseling, 128

Health education, 138–39, 485, 486

Health insurance, 48, 49, 225–26, 239, 519

Health in Youth Project, 498–99

Health maintenance organizations (HMOs), 67, 69–71, 128–29, 225, 231, 237, 367, 503

Health policy, 62, 120, 175–85; and aged, 311–12; apprenticeships in, 355–56; development of, 175–78; postdoctoral training in, 389–402; roles for health psychologists in, 178–83; sample activities in, 183–85; women's issues in, 256–58

Health promotion, 69–71

Health psychology: defined, 15–16, 27–28, 58, 77, 494; development of, 3–5, 16–24; education and training in (*see* Education and training); future of, 513–23; knowledge base of, 75–76; and other health professions, 61–73; and other segments of psychology, 41–59; professional issues in, 189–90; research in (*see* Research); scope of, 27–39; and segments of the population, 245–47

Health Psychology (journal), 4, 5, 22, 35–36, 56, 447

Health system, 28; future of, 517–18, 521–22; overview of, 30–34; as research site, 38–39; salient psychological problems of, 34–37

Heart disease. *See* Cardiovascular disease

Hebb, D. O., 312–13

Heber, F. R., 296

Hedlund v. Superior Court, 223

Helmer, O. M., 272

Henderson, J. B., 139

Henriques, J., 520

Henry, J. P., 270

Heppner, P. P., 237

Herbsleb, J., 219

Herbst, A. L., 482

Herd, J. A., 65

Herr, S. S., 222

Hertz, P., 168

Hetherington, H., 460

Heyden, A., 277

Hibbard, M., 183

Himmelfarb, S., 309

Hines, C., 224

Hinton, J. M., 103

Hirai, H., 11

Hiskey-Nebraska Test of Learning Aptitude, 292

Hispanics, 265, 266

Hochbaum, G. M., 23

Hogan, D. B., 366, 453

Hoiberg, A., 65, 71

Hollenberg, N. K., 270

Holmgren, R. L., 235

Hospitalization: of aged, 308; of children, 290–91

Hospitals, 67, 115; employment of psychologists in, 233, 236, 447; and health care costs, 237; internships in, 353; pediatric, 286–87, 353. *See also* Health care system

Hosticka, C. J., 183

Hostility, suppressed, and hypertension, 272–74

Houseworth, S. A., 271

Houston, B. K., 270

Houston Project, 167

Howell, M., 250, 255

Hoyer, W. J., 363

Huber, B. J., 241

Hughes, H., 326, 328, 329, 371, 420, 421, 425, 426, 445 n, 448, 459, 462

Hughes, M., 259

Hunsinger, S., 297

Hunter, E. J., 103

Hurst, J. L., 421

Hyperactivity, 292–93

Hypertension, 69, 122–23, 156; in aged, 305; basic research in, 83–86, 92; in blacks, 65, 85–86, 245–46, 266–78; and noise, 486–87; relaxation therapy for, 212; worksite programs for, 137, 140–41

Hypertension Detection and Follow-Up Program, 274

Hypnotherapy, 208

Hysterectomy, 251–52, 258

Ince, L. D., 11

Income, of psychologists, 233, 236

Industrial health psychology, 44, 48, 54, 55, 331–32, 372

Informed consent, 221–22

Injury, during malpractice, 220–21
Institute of Medicine (IOM), 23, 181
Instruments and devices, legal control of, 224
Intelligence quotient (IQ), 296–97
Interdependence principle, 153, 156–57, 160
International Association of Applied Psychology, 56
Internship programs, 46–47, 205, 322; in academic medical centers, 469; accreditation of, 196–97, 200, 340, 346–47, 353; in allied health center, 476–77; descriptions of, 329–30; development of, 352–54; and employment, 235; in health policy, 396–97; in schools of education, 499–503
Intervention: community research as, 161; public health model of, 483
Irwin, C. E., 31
Iscoe, I., 151
Istvan, Joseph, 326
Ivey, A. E., 495

Jackson, J. J., 265, 275
Jaffe, J. H., 139
James, S. A., 273–75
James, William, 16–17, 42, 351
Janis, I. L., 36
Jansen, M., 261
Jarnfelt, A., 251
Jarvik, L. F., 305
John Henryism, 273–74
Johns Hopkins University, 335, 351
Johnson, E. H., 273
Johnson, J. E., 93, 100
Johnson, Lyndon, 460
Johnson, M. E., 200
Johnson, M. R., 295, 296
Johnson (Robert Woods) Fellowship, 179, 239
Johnson & Johnson "Live for Life" program, 143
Joint Commission on Accreditation of Hospitals (JCAH), 176
Jones, D. H., 269
Jones, K. R., 310
Jones, Nelson F., 200
Jordan, S. C., 138, 140
Jorgensen, R. S., 270
Journal of Behavioral Medicine, 22, 447

Journals, communicating research results in, 99–100
Judicial Fellowship, 239
Jung, C. G., 352

Kaiser-Permanente Medical Center, 130, 132–34
Kalnins, I. V., 290
Kalsbeek, W. D., 273
Kane, R., 250
Kannel, W. B., 277
Kanzler, M., 139
Kaplan, J. R., 64, 78
Kaplan, R. M., 95, 170
Kaple, James, 390
Karoly, P., 297
Kasl, S. V., 171, 274, 303, 312, 313, 483
Kasper, A. S., 251
Kasper, J., 251
Kassirer, L. B., 221
Katz, R. M., 289
Kaufman, A., 293
Kaufman, N., 293
Kaufman Assessment Battery for Children (K-ABC), 293
Kellogg Foundation, 474
Kelly, G. S., 398–99
Kelly, J. G., 151–53, 159–60
Kelman, H. C., 91
Kenney, R. A., 304
Kerr, C., 460
Kesler, J. A., 222
Kessler, R. C., 99
Khan, A. U., 289
Kilburg, R. R., 175, 176, 183
Kimberly Clark, 139
Kimble, G., 184
Kirscht, J. P., 36, 255
Klaber, M. M., 291
Kleban, M. H., 305, 309
Klerman, G., 250, 260
Klose, K. J., 84
Knapp, H. D., 10
Knapp, S., 213, 225
Knowles, J. H., 3, 166
Koepke, J. P., 83–84, 272
Koocher, G. P., 453
Korman, M., 506
Kornitzer, M., 138
Korsch, B. M., 253, 255
Kovar, M. G., 303, 309, 311

Krantz, D. S., 65, 70–72, 122, 167, 265, 307, 491
Kraut, A. G., 181, 182, 225, 226
Kravitis, J., 266
Krupka, L., 314
Kubie, L. S., 396
Kubler-Ross, E., 295
Kucharski, L. T., 310
Kuperman, S. K., 328, 329
Kurz, Ronald B., 285, 286, 291, 353
Kutner, N. G., 255

Lake, B. W., 85
LaLonde, M., 3, 166
Lamy, P. P., 313
Lane, J. D., 271
Langer, E. J., 158
Langford, H. G., 277
Lansky, S. B., 290
Lapointe, L., 269
Laporte, W., 141
Laragh, J. H., 269
Larned, D., 252, 258
Lau, R. R., 36
Lavigne, J. V., 286
Law: issues of, and health psychology, 6, 126–27, 189–90, 217–26; as profession, 41, 42, 45, 47, 373, 374, 414
Lazarus, L. W., 314
Lazarus, R. S., 36, 101
Learned helplessness theory, 91–92
Learning and assessment center concept, 408–12
Learning disabilities, 293
Lehmann, J. W., 276
Lehr, E., 292, 293
Leichner, P., 69
Leserman, J., 255
Leventhal, H., 36, 83, 100, 167
Levin, P. J., 232
Levine, Murray, 128–31, 134, 303
Levy, C. L., 221
Levy, L. H., 421
Levy, S. M., 92
Lewis, C. E., 255
Lewis, Irving J., 467, 471
Lewis, M. A., 255
Lewis, M. I., 311, 313
Li, V. C., 167
Licensure, 113, 125, 219, 359; and continu-

ing education, 410; and credentialling system, 192–94, 198–99; and curriculum development in psychology, 47–49; and postdoctoral training, 373; for research, 365–66; and schools of professional psychology, 507; and specialization, 56, 131, 385
Lichtenstein, E., 139
Lichtman, R. R., 101
Life-style: and age, 312; and culture, 207; and health behavior, 166–67
Light, K. C., 84, 270, 272
Linden, V., 141, 144
Linscheid, T. R., 296
Lipid biochemistry, 64
Lipowski, Z. J., 288
Lofholm, P., 313
Long, Earl K., Memorial Hospital, 429
Long, R. T., 288
Louisiana State University, 427–29
Lubin, B., 18
Luft, F. C., 271–72

McAlister, A., 167
MacArthur Foundation, 23, 31, 80
McBride, A. B., 252
McBride, W. L., 252
McCall, R. B., 185
MacCanon, D., 80
McCaul, K. D., 167
McClelland, D. C., 409
McCrae, R. R., 307
McCubbin, H. I., 103
McDonald, R. H., 274
McDougall, A. K., 139
Machalek, R., 517
McHenry, D. E., 459
McKinlay, J. B., 253
MacKinnon, D. W., 409
McMillan, J. J., 20
McNamara, J. R., 24, 454, 455, 506
McNeil, B. J., 171
Macroexpertise, 398–99
Magrab, P. R., 292, 293
Maher, Brendan, 80, 127
Maisto, A. A., 296
Malaria, 518
Malpractice, 211–13, 220–21
Managerial prevention, 36
Mankin, H. J., 519
Mann, L., 36

Mann, P. A., 151
Manning, M. M., 95
Manton, K. G., 312
Manual for the Identification and Continued Recognition of Proficiencies and New Specialties in Psychology, 383–84
Manuck, S. B., 64, 78, 270
Manuso, J., 142
Marieskind, H. I., 249, 251, 257, 258
Marmot, M. G., 142
Marshall, John, 390
Martin, H. P., 295
Martin, R., 221
Mase, Darrel, 476
Masek, B. H., 312
Master of Business Administration (MBA) degree, 400
Master of Public Health (MPH) degree, 166, 400, 489–90
Masters, J. G., 391, 393, 394, 397, 400
Masur, F. T., III, 100, 329, 454
Matarazzo, Joseph D., 4, 18, 22, 24, 27, 43, 44, 49, 55, 58, 67, 70, 71, 79, 198, 236, 265, 321, 326–28, 331, 335, 338, 342–43, 363, 365, 371, 372, 375, 378 n, 380, 381, 383, 385, 387, 396, 417, 421, 422, 425, 426, 440, 448, 454–56, 458, 460–62, 493, 494, 496, 517
Matthews, K. A., 72, 92, 167, 236, 484
Mattson, A., 290
Matulef, N. J., 461
Maxmen, J. S., 518
Mead, L. M., 399
Mead, M., 520
Meagher, R., 24, 122, 337, 338, 340
Measurement: noninvasive, 65; understanding bases of, 127
Mechanic, D., 251, 260
Media, and health policy, 184–85
Medicaid, 225–26, 231, 237, 258
Medical centers: academic, training at, 450, 467–72; employment at, 237
Medical crises, 123
Medical Psychologist's Network, 21
Medical psychology, 327, 329, 331, 354, 427–29, 435–36
Medical schools, 115, 476; of academic medical centers, 468; employment of psychologists at, 236, 447–48; psychology teaching in, 18; university, 457–59
Medical sociology, 458

Medicare, 225–26, 231, 237, 238, 258, 311, 364
Medications. *See* Drugs and medications
Medicine, 336; and allied health, 474; practicing without license, 211–13, 224–25; as profession, 41, 42, 45, 47, 373, 374, 414; specialization in, 113–14. *See also* Behavioral medicine; Medical schools
Meltzer, R. H., 329–30
Mensch, I. N., 18
Mental illness, in aged, 306, 310
Mentors, 373–76, 381
Merrikin, K. J., 220, 221, 226
Mesibov, G. B., 296
Metres, P. J., 103
Meyer, A. J., 139
Meyers, G. C., 312
Meyers, J. C., 179, 226
Miami Beach Conference, 55, 57
Michael, J. M., 137
Michaels, D., 274
Mickel, C., 72
Microexpertise, 398–99
Migraine headache, 122–23
Military psychology, 54–55
Millard, R. M., 414–15
Miller, H., 288
Miller, J. B., 249, 250
Miller, Neal E., 5, 9, 11, 15, 22, 64, 75, 83, 127, 209, 265, 307, 338, 342, 343, 363, 454, 455, 457
Millman, M., 523
Millon, T., 24, 122, 125, 337, 338, 340
Mills, D. H., 495
Minority groups: cancer in, 268; social support in, 275; in U.S. population, 265–66; women of, 259. *See also* Blacks
Minors, and research, 221, 222
Minuchin, S., 296
Mitchell, G. W., 103
Money, J., 289, 290
Mononucleosis, infectious, 483
Moore, E. C., 250, 254
Moore, W. E., 191
Moos, R. H., 123, 144, 146, 155
Moral standards, 207
Morbidity, 3, 266, 311–12
Morrill, W. H., 421
Morris, M., 255
Morris, R., 222
Morrison, A., 390, 393

Morrow, G. R., 234, 240, 325–26
Mortality, 3, 259, 266
Moses, L. E., 114
Mosteller, E., 114
Mott, F. W., 10
Multidisciplinary practices, 225
Multiple Risk Factor Intervention Trial
(MRFIT), 487
Multiple sclerosis, 123
Mumford, E., 92
Munoz, R. F., 151
Muranaku, M., 271
Murphy, A. F., 138
Murray, J. P., 185
Myers, H. F., 274
Myocardial infarction. *See* Cardiovascular
disease

Nathan, R. G., 18
National Academy of Sciences Institute of
Medicine, 23
National Cancer Institute (NCI), 81; Office
of Cancer Communications Internship, 239
National Cancer Society, 80, 252
National Center for Health Statistics, 254,
257, 265–67
National Commission on Allied Health Edu-
cation, 474
National Council of Schools of Professional
Psychology (NCSPP), 507, 509
National Eye Institute (NEI), 81
National Heart, Lung, and Blood Institute
(NHLBI), 80–86, 331
National Institute of Allergy and Infectious
Diseases (NIAID), 81
National Institute of Arthritis, Diabetes, and
Digestive and Kidney Diseases (NIADDK),
81
National Institute of Child Health and Hu-
man Development (NICHD), 81, 82
National Institute of Dental Research
(NIDR), 81
National Institute of Environmental Health
Sciences (NIEHS), 81
National Institute of General Medical Sci-
ences (NIGMS), 81
National Institute of Health Research
(NIHR), 380–81, 386
National Institute of Mental Health
(NIMH), 43, 238, 331, 332, 352, 380–
81, 386, 430, 436, 443–44

National Institute of Neurological and
Communicative Disorders and Stroke
(NINCDS), 81, 82
National Institute on Aging (NIA), 81–82
National Institutes of Health (NIH), 56, 238,
332, 366–67, 380–81, 386, 443–44; *Ex-
tramural Programs*, 82; research funding
by, 79–82; Rotating Intern, 239
National Parkinson Foundation, 80
National Register of Health Service Providers
in Psychology, 48–53, 57, 122, 125,
198–99, 383, 385, 410, 508; Council for
the, 49, 193–97, 199
National Research Council, 233
National Research Service Awards (NRSA),
79–80
National Science Foundation (NSF), 80, 84,
232, 366
National Task Force on Education and Credentialing, 49
National Working Conference on Education
and Training in Health Psychology, 24,
191, 236, 331, 333, 421, 425, 462; on apprenticeships, 353–58; on basic skills of
psychologist, 235; on community psychology, 151, 162; on competence, 204; on
continuing education, 406–7; health psychology defined by, 77; on health-related
venues for health psychology, 62, 71–72;
on health services provision, 131, 376–
83; highlights of, 5–7; on legal issues,
217; on postdoctoral training, 196, 199,
344, 362–64, 376–83; on predoctoral
training, 193, 326, 336, 339–40, 454,
455, 499; on professional schools of psychology, 505–9; on research training, 78,
79; on specialties in psychology, 55, 57,
410
Native Americans, 265, 266
Nausea during pregnancy, 250–51
Negligence. *See* Malpractice
Negrete, V. F., 253
Neigher, W. D., 175, 241
Nelson, Paul D., 338
Nelson, S. D., 154
Nerenz, F., 36
Nethercut, G., 97
Neuropsychological assessment of children,
293–94
Neuropsychology, 55, 56, 234; clinical, 328,
329, 372, 383, 384, 410

Nevid, J. S., 140, 141, 144
New York Continuing Medical Education statute, 200
Niederehe, G., 363
Niederman, J. C., 483
Nixon, Richard, 460
Norepinephrine (NE), and hypertension, 269
North Karelia Project, 167
Novak, E. R., 250
Nowlin, J. B., 305
Nursing, 47, 68, 374, 474
Nursing homes, 237, 305, 312, 314
Nutritional sciences, 485

Obesity. *See* Weight reduction programs
O'Brien, R. M., 140
Obrist, P. A., 83–84, 267, 270, 272
Occupational health sciences, 485
Office of Strategic Services (OSS), 408
Office of Technology Assessment, 238
O'Keefe, A. M., 182
Olbrisch, Mary Ellen, 19, 204, 362, 371, 454, 456, 457
O'Malley, J. E., 290
O'Malley, P. L., 179
O'Neill, P., 152
On Vital Reserves: The Energies of Men; The Gospel of Relaxation (James), 16–17
Oregon Health Sciences University, 331, 443–45, 447, 508
Oregon School of Professional Psychology, 508
Orleans, C. S., 137, 139
Overcast, Thomas D., 127, 219, 220, 221, 222, 225, 226
Owen, F. W., 289

Pace, N., 140, 141, 144
Page, I. H., 268
Pain, chronic benign intractible, 123
Palinkas, L., 65, 71
Pallak, M. S., 176, 184
Parent training, 296
Parkinson, R. S., 138, 143
Parloff, M. B., 177
Parron, D. L., 181, 242, 265, 266, 275, 482, 493, 494
Partnerships, 225
Patel, C., 69, 142
Patterson, G. R., 296
Pauker, S. G., 171
Pavlov, Ivan, 30

Pavur, E. J., Jr., 310
Payton, Carolyn, 180
Pearlin, L. I., 307
Pediatric psychology. *See* Child psychology
Pennebaker, I. W., 36
Perceived control hypothesis, 158–59
Perl, M., 305
Perry, C., 497
Perry, N., 125, 131
Peters, J. M., 142
Peters, R., 142
Peterson, D. R., 191, 420, 422, 453, 454, 509
Petrillo, M., 295
Petrushevskii, I., 141, 144
Petty, N. E., 329
Pew Memorial Trust, 390
Ph.D. degree, 192, 193, 236, 325, 335. *See also* Education and training, predoctoral
Philips, B. U., Jr., 483–84
Physical fitness programs, worksite, 137, 141
Physiological psychology, 44, 54, 325, 443–45
Piccione, A., 330
Pierce, W. D., 155
Pittsburgh Noise-Hypertension Project, 486–87
Play therapy, 295
Pollack, E. S., 268
Pollard, M., 219, 225
Pollution, 515, 520
Population: growth of, 265–66, 514–15; training in, 485, 486
Population approach, 483–84
Porter, D., 142
Poskanzer, D. C., 482
Practica, 352; accreditation guidelines for, 345–48; in schools of education, 499–503; in schools of professional psychology, 509
Practice management, legal issues relating to, 225
Preferred provider organizations (PPOs), 69, 71, 128–29, 231, 237
Pregnancy, nausea during, 250–51
Prevention, 69–71, 119, 122; and aging, 483; and child health behavior, 296–97; managerial, 36; public health model of, 483
Price, D. K., 460
Price, R. H., 151
Professional conduct, legal standards of, 219–24

Professional corporations, 225
Professional psychology schools, 451,
　505–11
Professional relationships, 210–11, 220–22
Proficiencies, in psychology, 384–86
Proietti, J. M., 270
Prokop, C. R., 122
Psy.D. degree, 193–94, 325, 506, 508, 509.
　See also Education and training,
　predoctoral
Psychiatry, 3, 68–69
Psychoanalysis, 352, 383, 393, 396
Psychological Abstracts, 19–20, 35
Psychological Index, 17–18
Psychological tests, 213, 291–94
Psychology: accreditation in, 413–20; appli-
　cations of, versus applied research, 109;
　apprenticeships in, 351–52; curriculum
　development in, 41–53; definition and
　scope of, 15, 29, 191; employment in,
　232–33; future of, 520–21; graduate
　training beginnings in, 325; health psy-
　chology contributions to core of, 37–39;
　specialties within, 43, 53–59, 338, 371–
　72, 385–86, 418–20
Psychology and National Health Care, 20
Psychophysiology, 328
Psychosocial epidemiology, 458
Psychosomatic illness, in children, 286–90,
　296
Psychosomatic medicine, 61, 121
Psychotherapy, 19, 393, 396; with children,
　295–96; training in, 125
Public health, 23, 32–33, 120, 165–71;
　schools of, 450, 468, 481–91
Public Health Act, 475
Public statements, by health psychologists,
　208

Quarantelli, E. L., 169

Racial groups. *See* Minority groups
Raimy, V. C., 5, 45, 50, 191, 192, 352, 353,
　373
Rakowsky, G. W., 329
Rand Corporation, 390
Rand-UCLA Center for Health Policy Study,
　390, 392
Ransen, D. L., 158–60
Rapaport, E., 518
Raskind, C. L., 363
Raven, B., 364

Reagan, Ronald, 460
Records, legal obligations regarding, 222
Regan, Peter, 476
Rehabilitation Act, 221
Rehabilitation psychology, 36–37, 234
Reid, J. L., 269
Reimbursement, legal issues relating to,
　225–26
Reinsch, S., 95
Relaxation therapy, 212, 276
Renin, and hypertension, 269–70, 272, 274
Research, 19–20, 204, 499; on aging, 316;
　in allied health professions setting, 478;
　areas of, in health psychology, 34–37; be-
　havioral cardiology, doctoral program
　with emphasis in, 443–45; in community
　settings, 154–62; employment in, 233,
　234, 236, 239; on essential hypertension
　in blacks, 272, 277–78; ethics of, 213–
　14; and health care services, 109–11,
　127; judging quality of, 9–10; legal re-
　strictions on, 219–24; in medical centers,
　468–70; in psychology departments of
　universities, 454, 459–62; in schools of
　public health, 486–89; training and cre-
　dentials for, 5–6, 78–80, 107–18, 193–
　94, 354, 357–58, 361–68, 395–96; and
　women's issues, 257–60. *See also* Animal
　experimentation
———, applied, 62, 64–67, 75–76; basic re-
　search versus, 77, 91, 107–18; laboratory,
　107–8, 111; training for, 107–18, 357–58
———, basic, 62–64, 75–76; applied research
　versus, 77, 91, 107–18; apprenticeships
　in, 357; field, 78, 91–103, 107, 111;
　laboratory, 77–87, 91, 107–8
Respecialization, 322–23, 403–5, 411,
　510–11
Respiratory illness, 257
Responsibility, 203–4
Riecken, H. W., 99
Ries, L. G., 268
Riley, M. W., 310
Rittenhouse, J., 93
Robach, A. A., 351
Roberts, J., 267
Roberts, M., 367
Robinson, E. A., 294
Rodin, Judith, 22, 23, 158, 307, 314, 315
Roe, A., 45
Roeper, P. J., 273
Rogers, David E., 467, 471

Rogers, J., 139
Rosen, G., 481, 482
Rosen, G. M., 139
Rosenfield, S., 254
Rosenman, R. H., 141
Rosenstock, I. M., 23, 255
Rosenthal, R., 96
Rosnow, R. L., 96
Ross, S., 417
Rossi, P. H., 418
Rothenberg, P. G., 461
Routh, D. K., 290, 296
Rowland, M., 267
Rowlands, D. B., 269
Runyan, C. W., 23, 455, 484
Russo, D. C., 312
Russo, N. F., 249, 250
Rutgers University, 508
Rutter, M., 498
Ryan, W., 168

Sackett, D. L., 83, 140–41
Sales, B. D., 57, 219, 222, 223, 225, 226, 383–85
Sanford, F. H., 420
Sanger, S., 295
Sarason, S. B., 154
Saunders, A., 267
Scarr-Salapatek, S., 296–97
Schaefer, A. B., 288–89
Schistosomiasis, 518
Schlesinger, H. J., 92
Schneider, S. F., 156, 236, 338
Schneiderman, Neil, 22, 84
Schneiderman, T., 454
Schoenberger, J. A., 138
Schofield, William, 20, 21, 34–35, 61, 67, 506
School psychology, 328–29, 338, 372, 419–20
Schools, health psychology at, 67, 70
Schratz, M., 310
Schulz, J. H., 307
Schulz, R., 158
Schwab, J., 103
Schwalm, N. D., 167
Schwartz, Gary E., 22, 61, 77, 154–55, 328, 455–58, 517
Schwitzgebel, R. K., 224
Science: designation of core curricula in, 42–43; understanding of, 9

Scientist-practitioner model, 5–6, 327, 330, 478; and applied research, 110–11, 127; and apprenticeships, 354, 359; entry-level credentials for, 193–94; and postdoctoral training, 381; and professional schools of psychology, 451, 504–8; and university-based doctoral programs, 454, 455
Scott, C. R., 250
Scott, L., 139
Screening procedures, worksite, 138
Sealey, J. E., 269
Seaman, B., 251
Seaman, G., 251
Sears, R. R., 415
Sechrest, Lee, 125, 131, 362, 371, 454, 456, 457
Sechzer, J. A., 224
Selavan, I., 266
Self-care programs, 129
Self-efficacy theory, 95
Self-regulation theory, 297
Seligman, R., 295
Senate Appropriations Subcommittee on Labor, Health and Human Services, 182
Sever, P. S., 269
Sexton, M. M., 483
Shakow, D., 321–22, 415, 417, 422
Shanas, E., 307
Shapiro, A. P., 122–23
Shapiro, D., 267
Shartle, Carroll, 419
Shaw, E. G., 290
Sheps, Cecil G., 467
Sheridan, E. P., 375
Sherr, R. L., 329–30
Sherrington, C. S., 10
Shiloh, A., 266
Shipley, R. H., 137, 139
Short-term therapy, 125
Siegel, J. C., 307
Siegel, J. M., 171
Siegel, L. J., 326, 330, 361, 363, 375
Siegel, M., 222
Siegler, I. C., 304, 305, 309
Silver, R. L., 92
Singer, Jerome E., 22, 65, 70, 71, 72, 78, 109, 122, 167, 169, 275, 491
Skinner, B. F., 312–13, 520
Slovic, P., 167
Smetana, J., 95
Smith, A. F., 458

Smith, J. M., 289
Smith, P. C., 310
Smoking, 3–4; cessation programs for, 130, 132–34, 137, 139, 166–68, 206, 208, 222; by junior high school students, prevention of, 497–98; by women, 251, 259
Smyer, M. A., 307, 311
Snepp, F., 505
Snow, D. A., 517
Snowden, L. S., 151
Sobel, R., 291
Social context of health psychology, 154–56
Social ecology program, 436–38, 445
Social psychology, 325–28, 331, 429–30, 445
Society for Pediatric Psychology, 22
Society of Behavioral Medicine, 61, 241, 332
Socioeconomic status (SES), 153, 266, 274–75
Sodium retention, and hypertension, 271–72, 277
Soghikian, K., 132
Solanch, L. S., 123
Solnick, M., 518
Solomons, G., 288–89
Sorenson, J. E., 144–45
Specialization: need for, 113–14; in psychology departments, 459; within psychology, 43, 53–59, 338, 371–72, 385–86, 410, 418–20. *See also* Respecialization
Spinetta, J. J., 290
Spouse abuse, 223
Staerk, M., 289
Stambaugh, R. J., 390, 393
Stamler, J., 137
Stamps, P. L., 168
Stanford Three and Five Community Studies, 167
Stanford University, 43, 503; School of Education, 450–51
Stanley, D. T., 114
Stanley, J. C., 157–58
Stapp, J., 232, 233
Starr, P., 252
Stason, W. B., 170
State University of New York at Buffalo, 433
Statistical Abstract, 1985, 514
Statistics, 78–79; bio-, 71, 485
Steele, D. J., 36
Steger, H. G., 20
Steger, J., 123

Stein, M., 289
Stephensen, A., 518
Stern, S., 453
Stoeckle, J., 249, 253
Stone, George C., 18, 22, 24, 28, 30–35, 61, 62, 72, 170, 193, 204, 234, 235, 266, 326, 328, 340, 342, 367, 421, 440, 454, 455, 462, 499
Stoup, C. M., 232
Strain, J., 132
Street, W. J., 329, 454
Stress, 214; in aged, 307; in children and adolescents, 286, 290–91, 294–95, 498–99; and hypertension in blacks, 270–75; programs for managing, 108–9, 125, 137, 141–43, 156; public health studies of, 486–87, 491; research on, 167; in women, 255, 259–60
Stricker, G., 509
Strickland, B. R., 260
Strupp, H. H., 422
Stunkard, A. J., 137, 140, 144
Succession principle, 154, 156–57, 160
Sulzer-Azaroff, B., 167
Sundberg, N. D., 183
Supreme Court, U.S., 218, 225
Surgeon General, 3–4, 380
Surgery, 295; studies of patients of, 92, 93; for women, 251–52
Surwit, R. S., 267
Svarstad, B., 255
Swan, G. E., 330
Swazey, J. P., 9, 75
Sweeney, J., 81
Swencionis, Charles, 126, 203, 215
Syle, C. B., 259
Sympathetic nervous system (SNS), 268–72, 275, 276

Takanishi, R., 392, 396
Takooshian, H., 240, 242
Tanabe, G., 71
Tanney, F., 176
Tarasoff case, 223
Tarlov, A., 518
Taub, Edward, 10, 223–24
Tavel, E., 462
Taylor, C. B., 122
Taylor, S. E., 66, 91–92, 100, 101, 122, 123, 275, 364

Teaching: credentials for, 193–94; efficient, 8–9; employment in, 233, 234
Technology, 515–16, 519, 521
Telch, M. J., 497
Terminal illness in children, 295
Terrorism, 514
Terry, G. E., 290
Terry, P. J., 142
Thilly, C., 138
Thompson, E., 138
Thompson, R. J., 365
Thoresen, Carl E., 494–96, 499
Todd, A. D., 253
Todd, D. M., 152, 153
Tornatzky, L. G., 97, 98
Tourette's syndrome, 296
Trickett, Edison J., 152, 153, 155, 159–60
Tsuda, A., 11
Tulkin, Stephen R., 132
Tull, R., 124
Tuma, J. M., 285, 286, 288, 330, 367
Turnbull, H. R., 222
Type A behavior, 17, 84–86, 92, 141, 167, 209–10
Tyroler, H. A., 277

Ulcerative colitis, 289
Uniformed Services University of the Health Sciences, 435–36, 447
Universities, 115, 353, 447; employment of psychologists at, 233, 234, 236–37, 240; professional psychology programs of, 507, 508; training in psychology departments of, 449–50, 453–62, 476, 490. *See also* Education and training
University of Alabama in Birmingham, 427
University of California, 367; at Irvine, 436–38; at Los Angeles (UCLA), 390, 391, 429–30; at San Francisco, 328, 331, 440, 447
University of Denver, 508
University of Florida, 327, 330–31, 473–79; at Gainesville, 330–31
University of Georgia, 431–33
University of Houston, 331
University of Maryland, 440–43
University of Michigan, 391; Institute of Public Policy Studies, 394–95
University of North Carolina, 391
University of Pennsylvania, 351
University of Pittsburgh, 18

University of Southern California Medical Center, 252
U.S. Department of Agriculture, 224
U.S. Department of Defense, 80, 176
U.S. Department of Education, 80
U.S. Department of Health and Human Services, 80, 181, 224, 252, 257, 265, 266, 277
U.S. General Accounting Office, 310
U.S. Public Health Service, 23, 415, 450; Center for Disease Control, 3; Commissioned Officer Student Training and Extern Program, 239

Vail, Colorado, Conference, 43, 46
VandeCreek, L., 213, 225
VandenBos, Gary R., 176, 178, 181, 182, 225, 226, 475
Vasectomy, 252
Vener, A. M., 314
Verbrugge, L. M., 251, 260
Vernon, D. T., 290
Veterans Administration (VA), 43, 80, 225–26, 338–39, 353, 380–81, 386, 415
Veterans Cooperative Study, 276
Veysey, L. R., 458
Vick, R., 269, 271
Vickery, D. M., 129
Vincent, T. A., 152, 153, 155, 159–60
Vischi, T. R., 310

Waitzkin, H., 249, 253
Walder, L., 159
Walker, C. E., 296
Wallace, R. E., 222
Wallen, J., 249, 253
Wallston, B. S., 167
Walsh, M. E., 69
Walsh, M. R., 250
Washington, L. A., 159
Watson, R. L., 277
Weaver, T., 266
Webb, Wilse, 476
Webster, T. G., 18
Weight reduction programs, 137, 139–40, 206, 222, 276–77
Weinberger, M., 271–72
Weiner, H., 493, 494
Weinstein, M. C., 170
Weisberg, I., 290
Weisenberg, M., 20

Weiss, B., 168
Weiss, J. M., 10–11
Weiss, Stephen M., 5, 22, 61, 77, 457, 458
Weissman, M., 250, 260
Welfare of the consumer, 209–10
Wellner, A. M., 194–96, 507
Wellness programs, 33
Wellons, R., 261
Werner, C. M., 235
West, Andrew F., 458
West Point Military Academy, 483
Wexler, D. B., 221
White, R. M., 310
Whitehead, W. E., 123
White House Fellowship, 179, 239
Wiggens, J., 69
Williams, A. F., 23, 168
Williams, G. H., 270
Williams, M. L., 296–97
Williams, R. A., 267
Williams, R. B., Jr., 267, 271
Williamson, D. A., 123
Willis, P. W., 272
Wilson, E., 326, 328, 329, 371, 420, 421, 425, 426, 445 n, 448, 459, 462, 520
Wilson, J. R., 250, 254
Wingard, D. L., 171
Wisenbaugh, P. E., 269
Witmer, Lightner, 351
Wolcott, I., 250
Wolf, S., 483–84
Wolfson, J., 232

Wolinsky, F. D., 266
Women: health issues pertaining to, 245, 246, 249–61; life expectancy of, 307; minority group, 267, 271, 277
Women and Health Roundtable, 257
Women's Bureau, 261
Wood, J. V., 101
Woodward, C. V., 460
Woolander, S., 266
Worksites, health psychology at, 67, 70, 120, 137–46
World Health Organization, 518
Wortman, C. B., 92, 100, 103
Wright, L., 69, 285, 288–89, 296, 367
Wright, T. L., 95
Wright State University, 508
Wundt, Wilhelm, 16, 351

Yale University, 61, 391
Yarvote, P. M., 141
Young, J. L., 268
Young, K. E., 413, 414

Zanna, M. P., 237
Zarit, J. M., 313
Zarit, S. H., 306, 313
Zaro, J. S., 176
Zeidenberg, P., 139
Zigler, Edward, 180, 297
Zimmerman, R., 83
Zumeta, W., 236–37